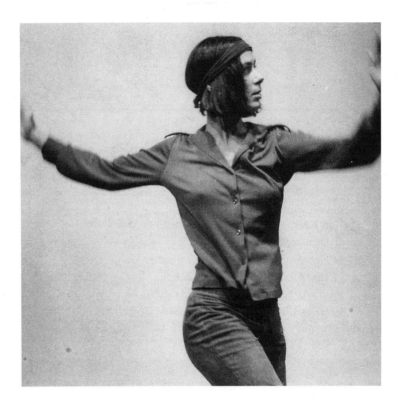

PAJ Books
Bonnie Marranca and Gautam Dasgupta
Series Editors

Art + Performance

A Woman Who . . .

Essays, Interviews, Scripts

Yvonne Rainer

A PAJ Book

The Johns Hopkins University Press   Baltimore + London

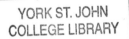

© 1999 Yvonne Rainer
All rights reserved. Published 1999
Printed in the United States of America on acid-free paper

9 8 7 6 5 4 3 2 1

The Johns Hopkins University Press
2715 North Charles Street
Baltimore, Maryland 21218-4363
www.press.jhu.edu

Library of Congress Cataloging-in-Publication Data will be
found at the end of this book.
A catalog record for this book is available from the British Library.

ISBN 0-8018-6078-4
ISBN 0-8018-6079-2 (pbk.)

Frontispiece: Yvonne Rainer performing *Trio A* at the Nova Scotia
College of Art and Design, July 1973.

Permissions credits may be found on page 439.

For Belle
who might have reached 101

Contents

IV   The Horse's Mouth

Photograph gallery follows page 134.

Acknowledgments

What I'd really like to do here is thank everyone with whom I've ever had a good conversation, beginning with my much beloved older brother Ivan and ending (? hopefully not!) with last week's conversation with my lover, partner, companion Martha Gever (who also, when editor of *The Independent,* commissioned two of these essays). I would necessarily include Nancy Meehan, Al Held, George Sugarman, and the late Ronald Bladen, conversations with all of whom were important to me in the fifties and early sixties. And then there were those wonderful discussions with Steve Paxton throughout the sixties that would become regretfully more intermittent in the following thirty years, and those with John Erdman, Mark Rappaport, Amy Taubin, Cynthia Beatt, and Annette Michelson in the seventies and early eighties. From the early eighties to the present it would be B. Ruby Rich, Joan Braderman, Ronald Clark, Peter Wollen, Laura Mulvey, Bérénice Reynaud, Martha Rosler, Ernie Larsen, Ilona Halberstadt, Sherry Millner, Su Friedrich, Lynne Tillman, Sheila McLaughlin, Thyrza Goodeve, and Gregg Bordowitz with whom I would have some great confabs. Whether or not I am now in communication with any of the above, the resonances of those interchanges linger on, especially the ones from my younger days when I was so much more impressionable and excitable. I've saved Trisha Brown for near-to-last, because my conversations with her started early and continue on with remarkable consistency. And of course many thanks to my editor Bonnie Marranca, without whom this volume would not have materialized.

Now that I've started this process of recollection and recognition, I must necessarily press on: gratitude to Judith Mayne, Peggy Phelan, and Mary Kelly for their ongoing support; to the Whitney Museum of American Art for providing me with a job at the Independent Study

Program since 1974; to the editors and conference organizers who commissioned/solicited these articles and interviews over the years, including the late Lyn Blumenthal, Ann Snitow, Rachel Blau DuPlessis, Simon Field, Constance Penley, Sandy Flitterman, Patricia Mellencamp, Janet Bergstrom, Elisabeth Hart Lyon, Noel Carroll, Steve Anker, Scott MacDonald. Now it's time to relinquish a mounting compulsion to be exhaustive and simply extend my thanks to those whom I have involuntarily omitted.

I Introductory Essays

Peggy Phelan

Yvonne Rainer: From Dance to Film

Encompassing material composed between 1966 and 1997, this collection offers a remarkable opportunity to reconsider some of the major transformations and impasses in art practice in the United States over the past forty years. Yvonne Rainer's long relationship to theater, dance, and film has inspired a great deal of critical commentary, but the vast majority of that discourse has been framed by the particular artistic or theoretical specialization of the writer. This volume illustrates the cross-disciplinary intellectual and artistic journey Rainer has been pursuing and the persistence of a set of central questions as they return across several media. Taken as a whole, Rainer's work represents both a disciplined and liberatory practice of writing—a practice of *graph*ing that encompasses choreo*graphy*, filmo*graphy*, and autobiog*raphy*. From the breathless clarion call of her 1965 NO manifesto,[1] to the close-up of newspaper text pasted across her own face in *Film About A Woman Who . . . ,* to the scrolling statistics that march across the bottom of the frames of *MURDER and murder,* Rainer has consistently insisted that there is no seeing that is not always the result of a specific form of literacy, a mode of reading that both reveals and conceals. Rainer is interested in making her reader conscious not only of what she reads, but of the way in which she reads. For Rainer, reading is a practice, a discipline, a way of approaching an idea, a person, an emotion, as complex as an artistic practice. Rainer's aspirations are immense, even at times stupefying. But for almost forty years she has consistently demonstrated that what is off-screen, not quite manifest, thoroughly frames what we can see, apprehend, be. The muscularity of Rainer's imagination has allowed us to glimpse—however fleetingly—a moving body, a narrative structure, a political ethics—in the act of becoming. Central to all of Rainer's work is a profound psychological ambivalence and intellectual skepticism that make the idea of a final conclusion, a fixed point of view, or even a sure architecture, extremely elusive. While in other artists, such an insistence on doubt often leads to a kind of wishy-washy relativism, the rigor and grace of Rainer's inquiry enact a habit of mind that insists that clear thinking is imperative, that beauty is possible, and that love, if always late, messy, and imperfect, must nonetheless compel our surrender and our conviction. For love is linked to art in its capacity to inspire us to remake ourselves, over and over again.

This volume makes clear that Rainer's work in dance and performance thoroughly infuses all of her work. Like the remarkable collage on the wall of *The Man Who Envied Women* (1985), or the long set of objects on the mantelpiece of *Journeys from Berlin/1971* (1980) to which her camera continually returns in the manner of a visual chorus, Rainer's writings meander across and return to the central questions of performance—what constitutes an act? what is required for the observation of action? What motivates an ethical act? a violent act? an erotic act? Can there even be an act that is not already framed by the space—material, political, psychic—in which it takes place? How does one act in a world in which it is impossible to know the results of one's actions in advance of their undertaking? Comprised of letters, interviews, theoretical speculations, and film scripts, Rainer's rhetorical performances are themselves well-crafted inquiries into the act of writing itself. Rainer makes us aware of the particular writerly pose each genre requires. Her refusal to employ only one form of address allows us to see each genre as a partial gesture, a specific language game useful (or not) for the enunciation of specific points of view. These rhetorical performances reveal a woman for whom truth and meaning always remain a little off stage, off frame, off page. These pages might be read, then, as a score for a performance whose enactment requires something more strenuous than the customary assumptions about reading as a quiet, passive experience. Sometimes stubborn, sometimes lyrical, sometimes literal, sometimes cast in the speech of a child, sometimes poetic, Rainer's writing expands the borders of both performance and writing.

i

"I want everything I make to reflect my whole life."
(Rainer: *Camera Obscura* Interview).

Rainer often claims that her decision to move from dance to film was motivated by her desire to work more directly with what she called "shared emotion." This claim seems to suggest that her minimalist dances lacked emotion, which is not true. But film seemed to promise a way out of a certain trap she had felt was endemic to modern dance. In a letter to Nan Piene written in January 1973, Rainer observed:

> Dance is ipso facto about *me* (the so called kinesthetic response of the spectator notwithstanding, it only rarely transcends that narcissistic-voyeuristic duality of doer and looker); whereas the area of the emotions must necessarily concern both of us. That is what allowed me permission to start manipulating what at first seemed like blatantly personal and private material. But the more I get into it, the more I see how such things as rage, terror, desire, conflict, et al., are not unique to my experience the way my body and its functioning are. I now—as a consequence—feel much more connected to my audience and that gives me great comfort (*Work*: 238).

Rainer wrote this shortly after she had completed her first feature-length film, *Lives of Performers* (1972). Her interest in abandoning the "narcissistic-voyeuristic duality of doer and looker" had been a consistent ambition of her dance choreography throughout the sixties.[2]

The particular challenge that the new dance taking place in the Judson Church in the early sixties made to its tradition had two aims: one involved a radical broadening of the kinds and qualities of movement that constitute dance, and by extension, the kinds of bodies capable of dancing, and the second addressed itself to the structure of the relationship between the spectator and the performer. Following the lead of Merce Cunningham, with whom she studied off and on for seven years, Rainer and other members of the Judson Dance Theater were interested in employing ordinary movement as an integral part of their dance vocabulary. By making dance less dependent upon the traditional notion of spectacle, the new dancers hoped to initiate and promote a much wider conception of the possibilities of dance. Thoroughly in keeping with the larger ideological project of democratizing power in the sixties, the new dance was also a movement against the elitism of classical dance's aestheticism. But what made some of the more progressive, even revolutionary aspirations of this choreography take a stutter step, was the persistent conservatism of the structure of the relationship between the dancer and the spectator.

In *Trio A*, her most celebrated piece of choreography, Rainer designed a series of movements which rejected formally delineated phrases and dissolved the rhythms between climax and rest characteristic of *ballet mecanique*. Designed to be performed by virtually anybody, *Trio A* does not require extraordinary physical prowess (although it does require a great deal of mental concentration and a good sense of balance). In it, Rainer seemed to solve some of the problems attendant upon "the dancer's dance" and successfully illustrated the art in task-oriented and ordinary movement. But even as this movement theory became increasingly clear and pragmatic, Rainer found herself continually duped by the psychological positioning of performing itself. Believing that dance left her only one stance, the narcissistic one, and the spectator another, the voyeuristic posture, she tried in *Trio A* to foreground these attitudes and the cognitive assumptions they left unmarked. "[T]he 'problem' of performance," Rainer maintained, "was dealt with by never permitting the performers to confront the audience. Either the gaze was averted or the head was engaged in movement" ("The Mind is a Muscle"). Although this feature of the dance in many ways anticipated her filmic concerns as we shall see in a moment, when I saw Rainer perform *Trio A* in 1987, I was immediately struck by the intense musicality of the movement. Although it has been performed to Wilson Pickett's "In the Midnight Hour," when I saw it, there was no score. The "melody" of the movement came from the intimate humming of breath and blood; as the movement phrases flow into one another without any pause to mark the end of one and the beginning of another, the movement of the body becomes absorbed in the sounds that accompany moving utterances. The continuous cacophony of these utterances contribute to an undisguised celebration of dance as thought. *Trio A* is scored to the sentient physicality of thought itself.

Choreographing *Trio A*, Rainer hoped to undermine what were to her at the time the polarized operations of narcissism and voyeurism integral to dance spectacle, and to challenge their apparent inevitability by disallowing the customary exchange of gaze between dancer and spectator. Although this four and a half minute dance enabled Rainer to isolate one possible solution to the problem of the performer-spectator relationship, it raised others. Rather than eliminating voyeurism, *Trio A* displaced it. Rainer had, perhaps unwittingly, initiated a kind of filmic voyeurism into live performance. Since voyeurism is contingent upon looking while remaining unseen oneself, *Trio A* encouraged a less inhibited voyeurism than the one usually operative in live performance where the spectator must confront the possibility of being seen by the performer. While this possibility is still present in *Trio A*, it is far more restricted because the performer's gaze "was averted or the head was engaged in movement." Thus, in short, *Trio A* produced a proto-cinematic relationship between spectator and performer.

Between 1966, when *Trio A* had its debut (as part of a larger piece appropriately entitled *The Mind is a Muscle, Part I*) and 1971, Rainer's "ongoing argument with, love of, and contempt for dancing" led her to develop an already apparent propensity to choreograph dances in which "things" were as important as "people" ("Statement"). Vacuum cleaners, red balls, staircases, mattresses, and eventually slides and films became much more than props for the performer: they functioned as sort of mute characters. Moreover, the physicality of these objects underlined the "objectness" of the physicality of dancing and, Rainer rather idealistically hoped, left the "subjectivity" of the dancer herself outside the performance—and thus not subject to the spectator's objectification.

> . . . [A]ction or what one does [on stage], is more important than the exhibition of character and attitude, and that action can best be focused on through the submerging of the personality; so ideally one is not even oneself; one is a neutral "doer" ("The Mind is a Muscle").

The idea of a "neutral doer" had made frequent appearances throughout dance history. Yeats' famous question, "How can we know the dancer from the dance?" is itself a consolidation of the notion that dance's beauty comes from the inseparability of the mover and the movement. By 1975, Rainer had distanced herself from the idealism implied in this position. "The problem is that in the attempt to justify and launch a movement as vital and audacious as that early 60's dance explosion, enthusiasm can easily become rhetoric. [. . .] For instance, the flaw in the ideal of the 'neutral doer.' I wrote that one can't 'do' a *grand jeté*, one has to 'dance' it. Well, neither can one 'do' a walk without investing it with character. From the beginning one of the reasons Steve Paxton's [a dancer and choreographer in Judson Dance Theater and a member of Grand Union] walking people were so effective was that the walk was so simply and astonishingly 'expressive of self'" (*CO* interview). But at the time, Rainer could not see this. Committed to the ideal of the neutral doer, in the early seventies Rainer had come to feel that her art gave her little room to explore the emotional and psychic questions that were pressing very urgently on both her work and her life. Dance, defined as an arena for the "submerging of personality," was an inadequate form for the expressions she most wanted to explore.

Rainer had been working with film since the mid-sixties. By 1970, she had made four films which were conceived as parts of dances: *Volleyball* (1967, 16 mm, b&w, silent, 10 min.); *Hand Movie* (1968, 8 mm, b&w, silent, 5 min.); *Rhode Island Red* (1968, 16 mm, b&w, silent, 10 min.); *Trio Film* (1968, 16 mm, b&w, silent, 13 min.); and *Line* (1969, 16 mm, b&w, silent, 10 min.). Rainer believed that these films were "an extension of [her] concern with the body and the body in motion" (*Work*: 209). In 1971, however, after her return from India, she decided to concentrate more fully on film. She did, however, keep the experiences of performing as her subject matter: *Lives of Performers* (1972) was Rainer's first full-length independent film.

While Rainer's film work has been repeatedly discussed in relation to feminist film theory, it is important to understand that her films are also revisions of the concerns she first articulated in dance. Dance is at once a presentation and representation of the body: it is a form in which artist and art work, "the dancer and the dance" seem inseparable. Feminist theory's attention to the representation of women's bodies and to the affective and psychic consequences of embodiment resonate deeply with many of the new dance's deepest concerns. *Trio A* in particular anticipates feminist film theory's attention to the structure of the gaze in terms that are resonant with Laura Mulvey's celebrated 1975 essay "Visual Pleasure and Narrative Cinema." The averted gaze of the dancer in *Trio A* anticipates Rainer's more radical experiment with short-circuiting the exchange of gazes between spectators and performers in her 1985 film, *The Man Who Envied Women*. Here, Rainer does not image the protagonist; the narrator/artist (Trisha Brown) is given a voice but no image in the film.[3] Rainer's manipulation of the visual exchange which provides the currency for representational economies such as film and dance has been a significant aspect of her work. While the legacy of Mulvey's essay has been a kind of wholesale examination of "the cinematic apparatus," Rainer saw very early on that the performer plays an integral part in representational economies which capitalize on "the narcissistic-voyeuristic duality of doer and looker." The evolution of Rainer's thinking through feminist film theory reveals the degree to which her background as a performer defines and shapes her filmic practice. As both a critique of the limitations of Mulvey's thesis (and the subsequent legacy it has had for feminist film theory) and a powerful illustration of the consequences of it, Rainer's post-1975 films and essays advance feminist film theory by challenging the visual/literal consequences of it—primarily from the perspective of performance.

Interestingly, however, Rainer had some important initial hesitations about feminism and was not eager to link her first two films, *Lives of Performers* (1972) and *Film About A Woman Who . . .* (1974), to an explicitly feminist project. In the fascinating *Camera Obscura* interview, Rainer questioned the editors' attempt to link her film practice with their film theory. The *Camera Obscura* editors, Constance Penley, Janet Bergstrom, Sandy Flitterman-Lewis, and Elisabeth Hart Lyon, suggested that Rainer's "radical formalism" was the expression of "radical political concerns." Rainer said this was "emphatically" wrong. The *CO* editors, although continually forced to qualify and reword their questions, could never shake their thesis about this connection and proposed that in *Film About A Woman Who . . .* Rainer was drawn to "situations which have their primary layer of meaning embedded in sexual politics" and that the film as a whole is a thorough critique of patriarchy. Their argument failed to convince Rainer who was pointing to Eustache's *The Mother and the Whore* as an example of a film whose *conventional form* contained a critique of patriarchy, i.e., "radical political concerns."

Rainer's hesitation about the equation "radical form equals radical politics" was not only a rejection of political/feminist readings of her films but also an expression of a useful hesitation about the evidence the *CO* editors had assembled to make their case. In 1980 she discussed the argument again with Noel Carroll:

> The fact that most of the situations in *Film About A Woman Who . . .* concern a woman's rage at a man, or men, doesn't in itself make a political statement about patriarchy, but maybe the disjunctive text-image relations and the demand these make on the audience and their implicit critique of dominant cinema—maybe all this constitutes a political position. It sounds good until you try to make particular correlations—like disjunction equals alert viewer equals critique of patriarchy and narrative coherence equals passive viewer equals status quo—without also making a convincing ideological analysis of narrative in cinema. This they didn't do.

Although Rainer's retrospective account of the interview is accurate enough, it obscures another thornier issue involved in the 1976 discussion. The *Camera Obscura* editors failed to recognize the degree to which Rainer sees her film work as an extension of her dance work. "But don't you see," Rainer asked them, "that I am, or was, a dancer? I'm very involved with space and motion, so it is going to come out in a lot of different forms. The space of the frame, metaphors for relationships, the physical space of intimacy, of avoidance, of attraction, flirtation or hostility" (*CO*). Following the lead of Maya Deren, another dancer turned filmmaker, Rainer understood her films to be an extension of the questions she had been working on as a movement performer. Like dance, films move across space and unfold in time. Moreover, because the movement of film so closely parallels the movement of dreams, Rainer hoped that they might achieve an emotional intimacy with their spectators that she feared her dances lacked.

Mulvey's essay, unlike the language of the *CO* editors, does speak very directly to the issues with which Rainer had been concerned. Mulvey's analysis of voyeurism and the structure of the gaze, enabled Rainer to see, more perhaps than she had been able to previously, her work as part of a wider revision of representational conventions. Mulvey's essay perhaps also coincided with Rainer's own need for a non-dance vocabulary. After over a decade ensconced in an artistic community as small as the avant garde dance world many people might feel a little claustrophobic, restless, hungry for new languages. Mulvey's attention to narrative film also provided the "ideological analysis of narrative in cinema" that Rainer complained the *CO* editors failed to bring to their discussion of her work.

ii

Rainer's interest in narrative was sparked by her trip to India in the winter of 1971. While there she spent about five weeks watching traditional Indian dance (Kathakali and Bharata Natyam mainly), in which performers reenact the epic stories of Indian mythology taken from the *Ramayana* and the *Mahabharata*. Watching these dances Rainer began to see narrative itself as an important tool in the expression of shared emotion. "Maybe we in the Western avant-garde are really fooling ourselves in our contempt for that question, 'What does it mean?'" Rainer wrote in her journal after seeing a Bharata Natyam dance (*Work*: 176). Rainer's recognition that a Kathakali dancer is able to project emotion is a bit like Hamlet's "Hecuba" speech:

> . . . this guy [Kunjan Nayar—the old dancer playing King Nala] actually projects *emotion*. His cheeks vibrate, he seems about to cry, he looks startled, he looks afraid, he looks puzzled, he looks proud. But all through extremely small changes in particular parts of his face. [. . .] I don't watch most people's faces that closely but it must all be there. His hands I couldn't read. I simply responded kinetically. I haven't experienced kinetic empathy for years (*Work* 180).

It was the projection of this kind of subtle emotion that Rainer wanted to have access to in her own work. Surprised as much by her emotional response as her physical one, Rainer began to recognize how much she wanted to connect her artistic and emotional lives. Inspired by the epic scale and compassionate empathy evoked in Indian dance forms, Rainer decided to work more directly with narrative, character, and mythology—not the *Mahabharata,* but contemporary United States' myths of nationhood, gender, and emotion.

In *Grand Union Dreams* (1971), the first dance she choreographed after returning to New York, dancers were divided into three groups—the Gods, the Heroes, and the Mortals. Although not quite "characters," they were close to that. As Rainer indicated in the program notes, this dance was the first version of her solution to the problem she found herself confronted with upon her return from India. She knew she was in an almost impossible situation. As one of the pioneering practitioners of the new dance, and as one of its most infamous theoreticians, she came back from India and essentially wanted to revive melodrama. It would seem that the momentum of Rainer's 1965 NO manifesto, an army of "no's" that lack the conventional period as end point, had led her to the ultimate renunciation—no more dance. "I'm at the point now of reevaluating and suffering and trying to figure out what I'm going to do next and how I'm going to do it," she remarked shortly after her return. "I've even thought of giving up art. That's how bad it's gotten. But that's what I know how to do best. So I'm going to go on. I have some kind of faith that what I saw in India will affect me, and it will produce, maybe in ways I can't predict now, a different way for me to work" (*TDR*: interview: 142).

The most immediate legacy of the trip to India in Rainer's early films is her revelry in her newly found license to project emotion. Rainer's attraction to emotional narrative also led her to conceive of her own life as a sort of "mythic" source. This, in turn, produced a kind of double consciousness about the ways in which art imitates life and life mimics art. Moreover, her double consciousness tends to make Rainer's films exceptionally, albeit darkly, comic and to allow her to take time to consider the personal consequences of ideological and aesthetic positions. Concerned both with creating scenes in which empathy is possible, while avoiding some of the violence of psychic "identification" common to narrative cinema, Rainer became interested in the politics of narrative. After completing *Kristina Talking Pictures* (1976), she wrote:

... my own involvement with narrative forms has not always been happy or whole hearted, rather more often a dalliance than a commitment. The reason lies partly in the nature of the predominating form of the narrative film. The tyranny of a form that creates the expectation of a continuous answer to "what will happen next?" fanatically pursuing an inexorable resolution in which all things find their just or correct placement in space or time—such a tyranny having already attained its epiphany in the movies [. . .], such a form has inevitably seemed more ripe for resistance, or at least evasion, than for emulation. ("A Likely Story")

Rainer's resistance to and evasion of narrative has led her to an increasingly overt examination of both the desire for "a just and correct placement in time and space" and of those "things" that make such a precise judgment and ethically clean placement impossible, or at least difficult. While she maintains that her later work has "demand[ed] a more solid anchoring in narrative conventions" ("More Kicking and Screaming from the Narrative Front/Backwater"), the conventions themselves are subjected to an increasingly overt critique. The most dramatic instance of this can be seen in the hallway scene in *The Man Who Envied Women*. There, while busily constructing a new narrative of seduction, she continually inserts film clips of Max Ophuls' *Caught*, thus revising (through literally re-editing) the convention of filmic seduction she is so self-consciously employing.

The common assumption about Rainer is that her aesthetic must be derived from a radical political and intellectual position. Well, yes and no. And this is what is, for me, the most interesting thing about Rainer as an artist. She is a fan of melodrama; she believes in an almost Aristotelian notion of empathy; she is completely and absolutely literal. Her objection to the tyranny of narrative comes mainly from her objection that the "Narrativizing Authority" creates coherence and unity where there isn't any in life; her experiments with narrative come from a deeply felt faith in mimesis—just not a mimesis that has ever been "represented" before.

Can the presentation of sexual conflict in film, or the experience of love and jealousy, be revitalized through a studied placement or dislocation of clichés borrowed from soap opera and melodrama? Can specific states of mind and emotion, or subtleties of social interaction, be conveyed in film without being attached, or being only provisionally attached, to particularities of place, time, person, and relationship? And can such subject matter be presented without being "acted out"—in both the theatrical and psychoanalytic senses —via simulated dialogue and action? Are faces such as belong to Katharine

Hepburn and Liv Ullman the only vehicles for grief and passion? ("A Likely Story")

Rainer's "banditry" of narrative forms then is motivated by her belief in the possibility of representing "grief and passion" that is more than skin-deep. Just as the Judson Dance Theater sought to democratize dance and the kinds of bodies and movements that constituted dance, so too does Rainer want to expand both the kinds of faces and the modes by which those faces inspire the spectator's identification and empathy. Her experiments with narrative in *Journeys from Berlin/1971* and *The Man Who Envied Women* have two distinct purposes therefore. On the one hand, she wants to point to the failures of traditional narrative structures to represent the full complexity of "reality," and she wants to create a new narrative which will, more accurately, reflect that complexity. *Journeys* and *The Man* are in this sense book end projects: in *Journeys* she critiques and rewrites the narrative dimension of filmic point-of-view through a temporal complexity, and in *The Man* she critiques and revises narrative point of view through an examination of filmic space.

In *Privilege*, Rainer juxtaposes documentary, cinema's most literal "realism," with a fictional representation of a white woman's memory of a rape—a traumatic memory that is, therefore, full of distortions, displacements, and what sometimes seem to be stray narrative threads. The documentary material includes footage from medical films and interviews with women who are experiencing menopause. The relationships between racism, sexism, and bodily traumas (both rape and menopause) are explored across different filmic surfaces (computer monitors, video, film, television). Again, Rainer's literal exploration of the disconnections between form and content help expose the ways in which cinematic "realism" and "visual pleasure" are themselves symptomatic responses to the violence of injustice, misrepresentation, and medical imperialism. Some of the more nagging problems of racial privilege are examined, if not successfully resolved, in the interview reprinted here, "Declaring Stakes."

In her most recent film, *MURDER and murder*, Rainer returns to the themes of *Lives of Performers* and to what is perhaps the most difficult and therefore most ubiquitous narrative genre of all, the love story. Her protagonists are a performance artist and mother named Doris who falls in love with a lesbian film theorist and professor named Mildred. Doris gets breast cancer in the film, and Rainer, in a beautifully erotic tuxedo that reveals her own mastectomy scar, performs the role of narrator and statistician, citing connections between chemical corporations and the health care industry that are as horrific as they are persuasive. The faces and bodies Rainer finds for her latest meditation on "grief and passion" are not the faces of Hepburn and Ullman. And yet, as she points out in her conversation with Thyrza Goodeve, these characters are both personally and professionally concerned with masquerade and performance. Rainer's work returns to the inescapable theatricality of the erotic and political relationship and demands that her spectator read and reread that performance before surrendering to the easy comforts of visual pleasure. As she confesses in "Skirting," while making *MURDER and murder*, her early sexual fantasies peopled with women who looked like Marilyn Monroe and Jayne Mansfield were invited "back into my living room from the back porch to which they had been banished for so many years." But when Marilyn and Jayne lie on Rainer's couch, they look a lot different than when they lounged across Hollywood's tighter screens.

iii

One of the most appealing things about Rainer is her willingness to return to her past and to allow her past to return to her. (Perhaps this is a carry-over from what she terms her "annoyingly persistent involvement with psychology" ["More Kicking"].) This volume is also a history of a self-portrait of the artist as indefatigable performer. In her expository essays with their impossibly long titles, Rainer continually charts her intellectual and artistic history. Therefore, when trying to construct a thesis about Rainer's art one must necessarily confront two distinct sets of texts: the performances and films she's made and the essays she's written about the performances and films she's made.

Although one might tend to think that the essays are more direct statements about what she attempts in her art, this is not the case at all. Rainer's essays are rhetorical performances as complex as *Trio A*. A short analysis of *Journeys* for example is entitled "Beginning With Some Advertisements For Criticisms of Myself, Or Drawing The Dog You May Want To Use To Bite Me With, And Then Going On To Other Matters," and begins by offering a series of objections (phrased as questions) that a spectator may have to her film. Her self-analysis of *The Man Who Envied Women* is entitled "Some Ruminations Around Cinematic Antidotes to the Oedipal Net(les) While Playing With de Lauraedipus Mulvey, or, He May Be Off-Screen, but . . . ," and it too begins with a rehearsal of The Audience's objections: "The Audience is once more perplexed after viewing my last film." Rainer's point in these essays is to acknowledge the difficulties her films create for her viewers and to assure them that she has thought through their objections. But the surplus of her rhetorical performance renders "the audience" a character in a script that extends well beyond the frame of her film. If autobiography is the explicit source for filmic narrative, then projection is likely to become more than a professional skill, indeed it might become a habit of mind. Rainer's intense explicitness about this habit, however, also allows the comic aspects of it to be seen. In *MURDER and murder*, Mildred and Doris stage a boxing match which allows them to become the spectacle that erotic conflict often leads us to long to find. But as the two spar and jab, it becomes increasingly difficult to know what they are fighting about: the mat is covered with statistics about breast cancer, the fight is set within old footage of other filmed fights, and the performers speak their lines and try to maintain their positions while being literally floored by the force of eroticism itself.

Just as Rainer complicates our understanding of the causes of breast cancer, the late onset of lesbianism, the nature of romance, so too does she complicate and extend the boundaries of genres: her art work and her writing perform different voices in a continuing conversation, pursued across different media and involving different fictional and real interlocutors, but intent on challenging our understanding of the nature of the act and the spectator's response to that act. Rainer herself explained the connection between her art practice and her writing when she told the *CO* editors: "Just as I make art to justify my existence, so I must sooner or later make words to justify my art."

It is characteristic of Rainer to seek justification and justice. Her ethical and intellectual approach to the complexity of emotion and politics is the hallmark of her work. The writing here records Rainer's journeys from choreography to film, from heterosexual to lesbian, from aspiring artist to acclaimed *auteur*. While most critics contend that Rainer's film work is in a complex and direct dialogue with feminist film theory, this truism can sometimes obscure the fact that Rainer's actual theoretical interests are extremely broad and continually pass through the paradigm of performance. Post-structuralist, feminist, Marxist, and now also queer theory illuminate the intellectual and psychic terrain traversed by Rainer's films. They continually circle around the claims of the past, the ethics of an act that one undertook when one could not possibly know its outcome. This inability to know has seemed to Rainer at times to be a source of rage, of grief, of compassion, of comedy. But it also has led her to a conviction that repetition and return might be a way to yield more compassion, consolation, empathy. Rainer's tango with the *CO* editors, for example, lead her, some ten years later, to return to the argument in her film *The Man Who Envied Women*. Trisha calls her brother and sister-in-law and returns us to Eustache's *The Mother and the Whore*. But this time, Trisha deconstructs the apparent superficiality of the film's title and cites Dorothy Dinnerstein's and Nancy Chodorow's investigations of the interests in keeping the mother and the whore psychological opposites. Trisha's voice-over is comic and accommodates the picking up of extensions and the need to make other plans. The return, in other words, is a conversation that includes multiple voices and gathers different textual and psychic conditions together. The argument is in every way opened up and extended. This is the kind of generative repetition that Rainer also wanted her early dances to discover in movement itself.

Yvonne Rainer's life and work over the course of almost forty years seem to me exemplary instances of an art practice that is vital and revitalizing. While the means through which thought and passion find expression change often in Rainer's work, she reminds us again how persistent and central our need for empathy is. In our inability to know in advance the results of our acts, Rainer reminds us that emotional intelligence is a hungry muscle much in need of exercise. In her journey from dance to film, Rainer has found a way to make her initial renunciatory "no" into a richly achieved "yes." In 1965, Rainer yelled "no to moving or being moved" but the rest of her effort has been geared toward finding the generative intelligence produced by, and necessary for, kinesthetic, political, and psychic empathy. A well-toned empathy increases our capacity to respond to the compelling possibilities of moving and being moved and remains our best hope for remaking ourselves and our worlds.

Notes

1. The NO manifesto was originally published in *Tulane Drama Review* 10, 2 (Winter 1965) as a postscript to Rainer's "Some Retrospective Notes . . ." It reads: "NO to spectacle no to virtuosity no to transformations and magic and make believe no to the glamour and transcendency of the star image no to the heroic no to the anti-heroic no to trash imagery no to involvement of performer or spectator no to style no to camp no to seduction of spectator by the wiles of the performer no to eccentricity no to moving or being moved" (Reprinted in *Work*: 51).

2. Jill Johnston's pieces for *The Village Voice* remain the best contemporary accounts of the impact of Rainer's distinctive movement style. Some of the best of these are reprinted in Johnston's collection, *Marmalade Me* (New York: E. P. Dutton, 1971). Two essays place Rainer's work in its broader context: "The New American Modern Dance" and "Judson 1964: The End of An Era." Sally Banes' study of Judson, *Democracy's Body: Judson Dance Theatre, 1962–1964* (Ann Arbor, Michigan: UMI Research Press, 1983) and Banes' *Greenwich Village, 1963* are the best historical and scholarly accounts of the context for this work. Annette Michelson was one of the first to realize the important theoretical aspects of Rainer's dance. See her prescient piece "The Dancer and the Dance: Part One" *Artforum* (January 1974): 57–64. Rainer's own interpretation of what she was doing can be found in *Work, 1961–73* (New York: New York University Press, 1974) and in an interesting interview with Trisha Brown conducted by Lizzie Borden, published in *Artforum* (June 1973): 79–81.

3. For a fuller discussion of the role of "aversion" in feminist film and performance see my essay, "Post-Structuralism, Feminism and Performance" (TDR: 1987) and my essay, "Spatial Envy: Yvonne Rainer's *The Man Who Envied Women*," in *Unmarked: The Politics of Performance* (New York: Routledge, 1993): 71–92.

Judith Mayne

Theory Speak(s)

This collection of interviews, essays, and recent filmscripts by Yvonne Rainer offers a wonderful opportunity to witness how this remarkable artist has changed, grown, and developed over the years. Those familiar with Rainer's work might be surprised that I use terms like "changed, grown and developed," since they are fully saturated with exactly the kinds of narrative assumptions that Rainer has always challenged in her work—assumptions about seamless identities, linear cohesion, and the achievement of insight. But while Rainer has always challenged narrative, she has never shied away from it. Rather she explodes the limits of narrative and visual possibility. Thus the changes, growths and developments traced in this volume are never predictable. We see how a dancer becomes a filmmaker, how an artist inspired by new theories of representation pushes the limits of those theories in her work, how a filmmaker comes out in many senses of the word, and especially how a woman who has been central to so many different forms of avant-garde and independent art sees herself in the midst of change. The very notion of change is understood dynamically in Rainer's work, having to do with changes in one's individual body, whether from aging or cancer; changes in the world, whether in terms of movements or global politics, and the connections between those old standbys of feminism, the personal and the political.

Rainer's latest film, *MURDER and murder*, has been heralded as her most accessible work to date (the term was also applied to her previous film, *Privilege*). Depending upon your point of view, this accessibility factor could mean that Rainer has sold out or has wised up; that she has been won over by identity politics and turned her back on theory, or that she has finally given up all that endless theory-speak that is either performed or implied in her earlier work; that she has lost it or found it. Once you start reading this collection, you become very suspicious of any such either/or propositions. Yet like narrative, which has consistently had a kind of push-me pull-you force in Rainer's work, either/or propositions have their own seductive quality, particularly insofar as the lure of theory is concerned. For at its most basic, theory offers a way of mapping complex terrains into easily negotiated territories. In Rainer's work, theory does plenty of mapping, but negotiating the territories is never easy.

I am particularly interested in how these collected pieces offer an opportunity to reflect upon theory—what it means to speak of works of art that are informed by theory, and how Rainer's various musings on the varieties of theoretical experience might be taken as suggesting some interesting ways of rethinking the theoretical enterprise. By "theory," I am referring primarily to the work associated with the politics of representation that in film studies just happens to be coincidental with Rainer's own film career. Her first film, *Lives of Performers*, came out in 1972, and the next two films, *Film About a Woman Who . . .* (1974) and *Kristina Talking Pictures* (1976) echo many of the concerns that preoccupied film theorists of the 1970s concerning the gaze and identification, the nature of cinematic desire, and the controlling effects of the cinematic apparatus. Yet unlike many so-called "theory films" of the era (a term coined by E. Ann Kaplan to describe films that were so directly influenced by film theory that they functioned as theoretical texts in their own right), Rainer's work could never be described as subscribing to a particular theoretical point-of-view. Rather, Rainer's films have taken theory as a point of departure, most obviously in questioning who speaks, who sees, and who tells. The famous *Psycho* scene in *Film About a Woman Who . . .* addresses simultaneously the segmentation of film (and its commodification) and the gender politics of female victimization. *Kristina Talking Pictures* explores the various ramifications of identity through image and language. Rainer's films also cite theory quite explicitly and at times quite humorously. In *MURDER and murder* a hair stylist cites Gayatri Spivak on the politics of home ownership; in *The Man Who Envied Women* the character of Jack Deller and filmmaker Jackie Raynal engage in an extremely dense theoretical discussion that parodies both the theory and the scene of heterosexual seduction. Theory is removed from its proper context, in other words, and subjected to narrative and visual manipulation as are a host of other discourses.

Rainer's films have been known as "difficult," in part because they are very wordy and full of various citations and investigations of contemporary theoretical discourse on representation, and also in part because Rainer rarely concedes any truth value to a single theoretical point. I am particularly struck in this collection by Rainer's insistence that theory be flexible, open to query, and a point of departure. Rainer's films can only be described as "theoretical" if one is willing to concede that theory has no purchase on truth, only on narrative. The same holds true for her essays and her interviews; theory is a mode of inquiry, never an end in itself. In "Thoughts on Women's Cinema: Eating Words, Voicing Struggles," Rainer proposes a hilarious list of what she calls "useless oppositions," including documentary versus fiction, experimental versus traditional narrative, and direct storytelling versus parody. Rainer's send-up may well have readers agreeing that these are "divide-and-conquer oppositions," but they also correspond to a very strong and influential tradition of what theory is, what film theory is, and in particular what feminist film theory is. Now Rainer has usually been put on the side of the theorists, that is, on the side of those who argue against any use of transparent cinematic form, classical narrative techniques, or character identification. At various moments throughout this collection, Rainer explains that her choice of cinematic styles has less to do with a theoretical principle and more to do with what seems right and appropriate to her at the time. I once attended a feminist film conference where Rainer and other filmmakers, representing different types of filmmaking—documentary, feature, and experimental—participated in a panel that seemed ripe for a kind of staging of useless oppositions. But instead of arguing from a lofty theoretical position concerning the bourgeois and patriarchal stakes of traditional representation, Rainer said quite simply that she couldn't conceive of making a film that was Hollywood in tone or inspiration—not that she was opposed to such a film but rather that it just wasn't something she thought she could do. I suspect that much of Rainer's appeal as a filmmaker might be this very refusal to speak in theoretical clichés or generalities.

Consider, for example, a memory of the movies that Rainer shares with her viewers (in *Film About a Woman Who . . .*) and her readers ("Some Ruminations around Cinematic Anecdotes . . . "). In the film the memory appears as follows: She was 9 or 10, and was taken with a scene in a Hollywood movie in which one woman rips another woman's dress off. "She had stayed in the movie theater long after her friends had left until that scene came around again. And she must have felt guilty about it, because she never told anybody, not her mother, not anybody." Theorizing about that memory and its appearance in the film, Rainer describes (in the essay, written more than a decade after the memory found its way into the film) a scenario of male sadistic identification, and an attendant sense of wonder as to where, in feminist psychoanalytic theories of spectatorship, that moment fits. For according to such theories, women are asked to identify doubly, to identify simultaneously with their own objectification and with the male position of objectifier. Conceding her own willingness, if not always eagerness, to align herself with the position of desired object, to be a good female viewer, Rainer cannot so easily read the memory of the thrill and pleasure of watching two women fight as a simple reflection of learned female spectatorship. I don't doubt Rainer's own reading of the scene and her response to it as having to do with the repression of anger. But more important, Rainer remembers watching the movies and sees not only how feminist film theory renders the moment ("male sadistic identification") but also sees what feminist film theory doesn't quite account for—the thrill, the rush, the excess. At the same time, Rainer's film work provides a sense of "something else" that theoretical discourse is so often at a loss to describe. It became common in feminist film theory, particularly in the 1980s, to bemoan the absence of anything that could properly be called feminist alternative cinema. Part of the problem was that virtually every version of an alternative could be found wanting in one way or another—one of the risks of the seduction of theory is that nothing seems to offer pleasure, nothing seems to be satisfying. Rainer imagines something else—in the conclusion of her essay, she imagines one woman asking the other about her dress. Over and over again in her films, Rainer imagines other, sometimes utopian possibilities, whether by removing the woman from the realm of the visual altogether (as in *The Man Who Envied Women*) or by showing us scenes of female drama that have not been shown quite in this way before (rape and menopause in *Privilege*; lesbian love and breast cancer in *MURDER and murder*).

Rainer is very suspicious of the claims of theory to account for desire and passion in their entirety, or to account for anything in an all-inclusive way. In 1976, *Camera Obscura*, the first journal devoted to feminist film theory, published its first issue, including the interview with Rainer included in this volume. I have a vague recollection that at the time of the publication of the *Camera Obscura* issue, I found Rainer somewhat "difficult" in the interview. But of course at that time I was very much convinced—as were the editors of *Camera Obscura*—that self-critical practice was the only way to go, that all art was ideologically shaped in fairly predictable ways, and that theory really did provide concrete and reliable means to divide the world into what was reactionary and/or patriarchal and what was not. I cringed when I read the interview again 20 years later; what I took at the time to be self-evident truths on the part of the editors seem remarkably pat and simplistic in hindsight. Rainer is a real nag in that interview, refusing to make any pronouncements about the political efficacy of her art, and in particular refusing to abstract the "audience" into a convenient grab-bag of projections. While Rainer agrees with her interviewers about the importance of the active process demanded of viewers in alternative film, she immediately qualifies any generalizations one might make about the audience: "When you talk about people who might be affected by a different kind of film, you're talking about yourselves, still a very tiny segment of the population." At the time, few theorists thought they were talking about themselves, or if they did speak of themselves it was in coded terms, hidden beneath the imperatives of the subject, desiring or speaking or otherwise. Now I would be succumbing to yet another useless opposition if I were to oppose feminist film theory to the kind of embodied, complex and contradictory practice that Rainer has developed in her films and in her writings. Let me suggest instead that throughout this collection, Rainer refuses to let theory rest on its laurels, as it were, and insists that theory must be tested, probed, and let loose in a frenzy of narrative possibilities. Rainer presents theory as a part of a number of different and sometimes competing narratives, and she consistently resists the tendency to abstract theoretical truths from those narrative contexts.

In an era when memoir seems to have replaced theory as the dominant intellectual discourse, it is tempting to see Rainer as a convenient bridge between the two domains, autobiography and critical theory. Of course it is much more complicated than that. Rainer is very explicit in her uses of autobiography and in its limitations. She is a constant literal presence in her films, and she draws on her own life, her own experiences as both source material and as a way of exploring connections and contradictions. She doesn't reduce theory to autobiography, but she unapologetically states the need, for her, to ground theoretical reflection in her life. It has become quite common in recent years to try to bridge the perceived gap between theory, understood either as abstract truth-telling or a master-narrative of how the world is, and the body, understood as lived experience or resistance to abstraction or performance. Yet all too often such attempts to create bridges propose yet another set of commodified abstractions. One of the features I admire most in Rainer's films, and particularly in *Privilege* and *MURDER and murder*, is the way she appears as a narrator, usually external to the central thread of the film, functioning somewhat like the lecturer in early cinema who accompanied film screenings to assist viewers in constructing their relationship to the film. Of course there is a huge difference between Rainer's dizzying displays of cinematic virtuosity, her complex layers of narrative, and the early cinema, but I think the comparison is worthwhile in the sense that Rainer stands alongside her audience, pokes and prods, but never acquires the authoritative and all-knowing presence of the omniscient narrator of classical film narrative. Rainer's achievement in *MURDER and murder* in this respect is particularly noteworthy. Her tuxedo-clad commentator/lecturer/narrator manages to be funny and provocative, moving and troubling at the same time.

Sometimes Rainer can be provocative to a fault. When I saw *Privilege* for the first time, I found myself challenged, as always, by Rainer's encounters between fiction and memory, and intrigued by her explorations into the realms of menopause and aging that seemed far away from the preoccupations of feminist film theory with the cinematic gaze (not so far as all that, as it turns out—one of the dominant tropes of the film is the desire to be looked at, and the attendant coming to terms with the real and traumatic implications of not being the object of the look, even when you thought you were past all that). But in this film, Rainer's analogies between racism and sexism, and in particular the creation of a lesbian character who seemed to function primarily as a screen for all of the sexual confusion of the main character, Jenny, really bothered me. Rainer's letter to me, included in this volume, was a result of discussions we had over the two days that she spent in Columbus showing the film and discussing her work. Recently I saw *Privilege* again and it occurred to me that what had bothered me most about the film's approach to lesbianism was that it seemed so confused, down to the last words spoken in the fiction of the film, between the two characters Jenny and the fictitious African American filmmaker Yvonne Washington, about whether or not Jenny had ever slept with Brenda, the lesbian. In other words, lesbianism seemed there and not there, much like Terry Castle's characterization of the ghosting effect so typical of classical representations of lesbians (in *The Apparitional Lesbian*).

And of course my reaction to the film was also a product of my own stake in theoretical discourse and my own stake as a viewer, i.e., my own desire to see lesbianism as something other than a shadow, a projection. Rainer's previous film, *The Man Who Envied Women*, was detached from the heterosexual world it portrayed with such irony, and it provided enormous pleasures of recognition, theoretical and otherwise. Ever clinging to the very linear narrative I had been taught to distrust, I expected *Privilege* to move further in the same direction. It did and it didn't. In retrospect—and as is made clear in Rainer's two letters to me—what I saw as confusion in the film vis-a-vis lesbianism was precisely an "issue" with genuine, complex, personal stakes for her.

It would be far too simple to see the changes evident in her most recent film, *MURDER and murder*, as some kind of direct result of the changes in Rainer's own life. The film combines a wide array of genres; it layers narrative upon narrative and it asks questions about how women represent themselves. The big difference between this film and Rainer's previous work is that Doris and Mildred are characters you can love, and they share a love story—but this is still a far cry from what most viewers would identify as a narrative in any classic sense of the word. And theory is there, throughout the film, in the longing gazes exchanged between the two lovers, and in the figures from their pasts that carry on a conversation with themselves and with the audience, and in the devastating effects of breast cancer.

Yvonne Rainer is an unrelenting theorist, in the sense that the terms of reflection may change, but the act of reflection is always there. Her films and her words offer theoretical reflection as always in flux, always changing. Theory never has a unified voice; sometimes it seems to be mocked, sometimes it seems to be cited with great reverence. Theory never has a sure footing, and as a result you often find theory in unexpected places in Rainer's work.

II First Person Political

The Mind is a Muscle

The following essay was written in 1966 and first published in Gregory Battcock's *Minimal Art: A Critical Anthology* (New York: E.P. Dutton, 1968), later appearing in *Work 1961–73* (Halifax: Nova Scotia College of Art and Design and New York: New York University Press, 1974), *Esthetics Contemporary,* edited by Richard Kostelanetz (Buffalo: Prometheus Books, 1989), and in *The Twentieth-Century Performance Reader* edited by Michael Huxley and Noel Witts (New York: Routledge, 1996).

In rereading it I am impressed, i.e., slightly embarrassed, by my historical myopia as evinced in such expressions as "ideas about man and his environment." Not to beat up on myself, I can't help but speculate on how I—or should I say "we"—could have been so obtuse. For starters, our unconscious sexism dictated an overdetermined identification with members of the more respected and rewarded gender. The piece also contains an overview of modern dance history the carelessness of which I can attribute simply to not having seen the work. Just as young dancers of the '90s can only follow '60s dance from so many removes—a book, some photos, a scrap of film—so my generation was hampered by a comparable lack of access to the work of thirty years earlier. How many of us had a sense of the dances of Jane Dudley, Sophie Maslow, the early work of Humphrey/Weidman, and of Graham herself? At that time I felt privileged to have had an older friend, the sculptor George Sugarman, who supplied me with ample descriptions of Graham in her heyday ("She was amazing; she drove people out of the theater"). I myself had been bowled over by seeing her dance Medea in *Cave of the Heart* in her late fifties. (She was amazing; she had me glued to my seat.) A more recent revelation was the Graham Company's 1995 revival of the 1936 *Steps in the Street* which, quite apart from its putative antiwar theme, stands on its own as a phenomenal and electrifying movement event. Seeing it in 1966 would surely have changed the way I thought of Graham as tied only to "dramatic and psychological necessity."

But here lies yet another mantra of the minimalist aesthetic that was so widely influential in the '60s: art must eschew topicality, metaphor, reference, organizational hierarchies. This is evidenced in my description of *Trio A,* with its aversion to "high points [and] focal climaxes." What becomes apparent in thinking about this area of '60s art-making is its formulation and enactment of lexicons and taxonomies limited by such excesses of curtailment as to call into question the intricacies of any previous method of ordering or invention. Certainly this is one way—albeit ambivalent on my part—of characterizing the avant-garde. John Cage's metaphor—banging his head against the wall of Schoenberg and harmony—is a simpler way of putting it: each successive age defines and tries to demolish or break through the wall that its predecessor has devised. Thus, Schoenberg's twelve-tone row becomes Cage's silence; De Kooning's gesture becomes Rauschenberg's erasure; Cunningham's arabesque becomes Steve Paxton's walk. It's not for me to describe my own strategies for the benefit of younger artists' challenges. In fact it is unclear to me whether the present generation is knocking its head against the walls of their predecessors, or just writing on them.

The material following "A Quasi Survey . . ." also appeared in *Work 1961–73.* Since its 1966 debut (by Steve Paxton, David Gordon, and myself at Judson Church), *Trio A* has lived on in many incarnations. In an interim version of *The Mind is a Muscle* (Judson Church, May 22, 1966), it was performed by William Davis, David Gordon, and Steve Paxton. At the end Peter Saul executed a balletic solo version, with pirouettes and jumps. In 1967 I performed it solo as *Convalescent Dance* (Angry Arts Week, Hunter Playhouse); in April 1968 I performed it in tap shoes at the end of the final version of *The Mind is a Muscle* at the Anderson Theater on Second Avenue. In 1968 Frances Brooks, the first of many untrained dancers who have learned it, performed it during a lecture-demonstration at the New York City Library of Performing Arts; in 1969 it was performed by a half-dozen dancers to the Chambers Brothers' "In the Midnight Hour" on the stage of the Billy Rose Theater in New York City. At the Connecticut College American Dance Festival of 1969, fifty students who had been taught *Trio A* by members of the group with whom I was in residence there, performed it for over an hour in a large studio for an audience that was free to roam to other events in the same building. In 1970 during the opening of the *People's Flag Show*, I and some members of the dance collective Grand Union—Lincoln Scott, Steve Paxton, David Gordon, Nancy Green, and Barbara Dilley—performed it in the nude at Judson Church with five-foot American flags tied around our necks. (The *People's Flag Show* was organized by Jon Hendricks, Faith Ringgold, and Jean Toche as a protest against the arrest of various people accused of "desecrating" the American flag, including gallery owner Stephen Radich, who had shown the "flag-defiling" work of sculptor Mark Morrel in 1967 and whose case traveled all the way to the Supreme Court, where it was thrown out on a technicality.) Around 1970 Michael Fajans, who had learned *Trio A* from Barbara Dilley, taught it to fifty students, at Antioch College who performed it on a large stage to "In the Midnight Hour"; in 1971 those members of the fledgling Grand Union who knew *Trio A* performed the nude/flag version at New York University's Loeb Student Center during the last throes of my *Continuous Project-Altered Daily* (the dance which, begun in 1969, gradually "atomized" into improvisatory programs by the Grand Union). It was here that Pat Catterson, who had learned *Trio A* from Becky Arnold and Barbara Dilley, joined us, performing it in reverse; shortly thereafter she again performed it in reverse (now fully clothed) during her own evening of work at Merce Cunningham's studio; later that year she and a group of her students performed it on the sidewalk outside my hospital window. In 1973 I incorporated it into the narrative of my multimedia *This is the story of a woman who . . .* ("She shows him her dance."); in 1978, five years after I had stopped performing, I performed it in Merce Cunningham's studio for a 16 mm film shoot (produced by Sally Banes, the film and video are distributed by the Dance Film Archive, University of Rochester). In 1979 the PBS TV series *Dance in America* produced a version with Sarah Rudner of the Twyla Tharp Company, Bart Cook of the New York City Ballet, and untrained dancer Frank Conversano; in 1980 I taught it to a group of French ballet and modern dancers in a workshop in the south of France (Les Fêtes Musicales de la Sainte-Baume). In 1981 during a Judson Dance Theater revival at St. Mark's Church produced by Wendy Perron, I performed it in a state of almost crippling adrenaline poisoning (otherwise known as extreme stage fright). The life of *Trio A* for the next eleven years eludes me. In 1992 I taught it to Clarinda MacLow, who performed it in the Serious Fun Festival at Lincoln Center; she in turn taught it to Jean Guizerix, formerly of the Paris Opera Ballet, who danced it during the 1996 Montpelier Dance Festival and later in Paris on a program organized by the French group Quatuor Albrecht Knust. More recently, in August 1997, Clarinda, I, and several students to whom she had taught it, danced *Trio A* at the Talking Dancing Conference in Stockholm (I introduced *my* interpretation as the "geriatric version"). I have lately been fantasizing about an hour-long *Trio A* performed by ten women over sixty (or maybe women and men—why not?) to "In the Midnight Hour," of course.

A Quasi Survey of Some "Minimalist" Tendencies in the Quantitatively Minimal Dance Activity Midst the Plethora, or an Analysis of *Trio A.*

OBJECTS	DANCES
eliminate or minimize	
1. role of artist's hand	1. phrasing
2. hierarchical relationships of parts	2. development and climax
3. texture	3. variation: rhythm, shape, dynamics
4. figure reference	4. character
5. illusionism	5. performance
6. complexity and detail	6. variety: phrases and the spatial field
7. monumentality	7. the virtuosic feat and the fully extended body
substitute	
1. factory fabrication	1. energy equality and "found" movement
2. unitary forms, modules	2. equality of parts, repetition
3. uninterrupted surface	3. repetition or discrete events
4. nonreferential forms	4. neutral performance
5. literalness	5. task or tasklike activity
6. simplicity	6. singular action, event, or tone
7. human scale	7. human scale

Although the benefit to be derived from making a one-to-one relationship between aspects of so-called minimal sculpture and recent dancing is questionable, I have drawn up a chart that does exactly that. Those who need alternatives to subtle distinction-making will be elated, but nevertheless such a device may serve as a shortcut to ploughing through some of the things that have been happening in a specialized area of dancing and once stated can be ignored or culled from at will.

It should not be thought that the two groups of elements ("eliminate" and "substitute") are mutually exclusive. Much work being done today—both in theater and art—has concerns in both categories. Neither should it be thought that the type of dance I shall discuss has been influenced exclusively by art. The changes in theater and dance reflect changes in ideas about man and his environment that have affected all the arts. That dance should reflect these changes at all is of interest, since for obvious reasons, it has always been the most isolated and in-bred of the arts. What is perhaps unprecedented in the short history of the modern dance is the close correspondence between concurrent developments in dance and the plastic arts.

Isadora Duncan went back to the Greeks; Humphrey and Graham[1] used primitive ritual and/or music for structuring, and although the people who came out of the Humphrey-Graham companies and were active during the thirties and forties shared sociopolitical concerns and activity in common with artists of the period, their work did not reflect any direct influence from or dialogue with the art so much as a reaction to the time. (Those who took off in their own directions in the forties and fifties—Cunningham, Shearer, Litz, Marsicano et al.—must be appraised individually. Such a task is beyond the scope this article.) The one previous area of correspondence might be German Expressionism and Mary Wigman and her followers, but photographs and descriptions of the work show little connection.

Within the realm of movement invention—and I am talking for the time being about movement generated by means other than accomplishment of a task or dealing with an object—the most impressive change has been in the attitude to phrasing, which can be defined as the way in which energy is distributed in the execution of a movement or series of movements. What makes one kind of movement different from another is not so much variations in arrangements of parts of the body as differences in energy investment.

It is important to distinguish between real energy and what I shall call "apparent" energy. The former refers to actual output in terms of physical expenditure on the part of the performer. It is common to hear a dance teacher tell a student that he is using "too much energy" or that a particular movement does not require "so much energy." This view of energy is related to a notion of economy and ideal movement technique. Unless otherwise indicated, what I shall be talking about here is "apparent" energy, or what is seen in terms of motion and stillness rather than of actual work, regardless of the physiological or kinesthetic experience of the dancer. The two observations—that of the performer and that of the spectator—do not always correspond. A vivid illustration of this is my *Trio A*: Upon completion two of us are always dripping with sweat while the third is dry. The correct conclusion to draw is not that the dry one is expending less energy, but that the dry one is a "nonsweater."

Much of the western dancing we are familiar with can be characterized by a particular distribution of energy: maximal output or "attack" at the beginning of a phrase,[2] recovery at the end, with energy often arrested somewhere in the middle. This means that one part of the phrase—usually the part that is the most still—becomes the focus of attention, registering like a photograph or suspended moment of climax. In the Graham-oriented modern dance these climaxes can come one on the heels of the other. In types of dancing that depend on less impulsive controls, the climaxes are farther apart and are not so dramatically "framed." Where extremes in tempi are imposed, this ebb and flow of effort is also pronounced: in the instance of speed the contrast between movement and rest is sharp, and in the adagio, or supposedly continuous kind of phrasing, the execution of transitions demonstrates more subtly the mechanics of getting from one point of still "registration" to another.

The term *phrase* can also serve as a metaphor for a longer or total duration containing beginning, middle, and end. Whatever the implications of a continuity that contains high points or focal climaxes, such an approach now seems to be excessively dramatic and more simply, unnecessary.

Energy has also been used to implement heroic more-than-human technical feats and to maintain a more-than-human look of physical extension, which is familiar as the dancer's muscular "set." In the early days of the Judson Dance Theater someone wrote an article and asked "Why are they so intent on just being themselves?" It is not accurate to say that everyone at that time had this in mind. (I certainly didn't; I was more involved in experiencing a lion's share of ecstacy and madness than in "being myself" or doing a job.) But where the question applies, it might be answered on two levels: (1) The artifice of performance has been reevaluated in that action, or what one does, is more interesting and important than the exhibition of character and attitude, and that action can best be focused on through the submerging of the personality; so ideally one is not even oneself, one is a neutral "doer." (2) The display of technical virtuosity and the display of the dancer's specialized body no longer make any sense. Dancers have been driven to search for an alternative context that allows for a more matter-of-fact, more concrete, more banal quality of physical being in performance, a context wherein people are engaged in actions and movements making a less spectacular demand on the body and in which skill is hard to locate.

It is easy to see why the *grand jeté* (along with its ilk) had to be abandoned. One cannot "do" a *grand jeté;* one must "dance" it to get it done at all, i.e., invest it with all the necessary nuances of energy distribution that will produce the look of climax together with a still, suspended extension in the middle of the movement. Like a romantic, overblown plot this particular kind of display—with its emphasis on nuance and skilled accomplishment, its accessibility to comparison and interpretation, its involvement with connoisseurship, its introversion, narcissism, and self-congratulatoriness—has finally in this decade exhausted itself, closed back on itself, and perpetuates itself solely by consuming its own tail.

The alternatives that were explored now are obvious: stand, walk, run, eat, carry bricks, show movies, or move or be moved by some *thing* rather than oneself. Some of the early activity in the area of self-movement utilized games, "found" movement (walking, running, etc.), and people with no previous training. (One of the most notable of these early efforts was Steve Paxton's solo, *Transit,* in which he performed movement by "marking" it. "Marking" is what dancers do in rehearsal when they do not want to expend the full amount of energy required for the execution of a given movement. It has a very special look, tending to blur boundaries between consecutive movements.) These descriptions are not complete. Different people have sought different solutions.

Since I am primarily a dancer, I am interested in finding solutions primarily in the area of moving oneself, however many excursions I have made into pure and not-so-pure thing-moving. In 1964 I began to play around with simple one- and two-motion phrases that required no skill and little energy and contained few accents. The way in which they were put together was indeterminate, or decided upon in the act of performing, because at that time the idea of a different kind of continuity as embodied in transitions or connections between phrases did not seem to be as important as the material itself. The result was that the movements or phrases appeared as isolated bits framed by stoppages. Underscored by their smallness and separateness, they projected as perverse *tours-de-force*. Everytime "elbow-wiggle" came up one felt like applauding. It was obvious that the idea of an unmodulated energy output as demonstrated in the movement was not being applied to the continuity. A continuum of energy was required. Duration and transition had to be considered.

Which brings me to *The Mind is a Muscle, Trio A.* Without giving an account of the drawn-out process through which this four-and-a-half-minute movement series (performed simultaneously by three people) was made, let me talk about its implications in the direction of movement-as-task or movement-as-object.

One of the most singular elements in it is that there are no pauses between phrases. The phrases themselves often consist of separate parts, such as consecutive limb articulations—"right leg, left leg, arms, jump," etc.—but the end of each phrase merges immediately into the beginning of the next with no observable accent. The limbs are never in a fixed, still relationship. and they are stretched to their fullest extension only in transit, creating the impression that the body is constantly engaged in transitions.

flattened phrase

Another factor contributing to the smoothness of the continuity is that no one part of the series is made any more important than any other. For four and a half minutes a great variety of movement shapes occur, but they are of equal weight and are equally emphasized. This is probably attributable both to the sameness of physical "tone" that colors all the movements and to the attention to the pacing. I can't talk about one without talking about the other.

The execution of each movement conveys a sense of unhurried control. The body is weighty without being completely relaxed. What is seen is a control that seems geared to the *actual* time it takes the *actual* weight of the body to go through the prescribed motions, rather than an adherence to an imposed ordering of time. In other words, the demands made on the body's (actual) energy resources appear to be commensurate with the task—be it getting up from the floor, raising an arm, tilting the pelvis, etc.—much as one would get out of a chair, reach for a high shelf, or walk down stairs when one is not in a hurry.[3] The movements are not mimetic, so they do not remind one of such actions, but I like to think that in their manner of execution they have the factual quality of such actions.

Of course, I have been talking about the "look" of the movements. In order to achieve this look in a continuity of separate phrases that does not allow for pauses, accents, or stillness, one must bring to bear many different degrees of effort just in getting from one thing to another. Endurance comes into play very much with its necessity for conserving (actual) energy (like the long-distance runner). The irony here is in the reversal of a kind of illusionism: I have exposed a type of effort where it has been traditionally concealed and have (concealed phrasing) where it has been traditionally displayed.

So much for phrasing. My *Trio A* contained other elements mentioned in the chart that have been touched on in passing, not being central to my concerns of the moment. For example, the "problem" of performance was dealt with by never permitting the performers to confront the audience. Either the gaze was averted or the head was engaged in movement. The desired effect was a worklike rather than exhibition-like presentation. *reference*

I shall deal briefly with the remaining categories on the chart as they relate to *Trio A*. Variation was not a method of development. No one of the individual movements in the series was made by varying a quality of any other one. Each is intact and separate with respect to its nature. In a strict sense neither is there any repetition (with the exception of occasional consecutive traveling steps). The series progresses by the fact of one discrete thing following another. This procedure was consciously pursued as a change from my previous work, which often had one identical thing following another—either consecutively or recurrently. Naturally the question arises as to what constitutes repetition. In *Trio A,* where there is no consistent consecutive repetition, can the simultaneity of three identical sequences be called repetition? Or can the consistency of energy tone be called repetition? Or does repetition apply only to successive specific actions?

All of these considerations have supplanted the desire for dance structures wherein elements are connected thematically (through variation) and for a diversity in the use of phrases and space. I think two assumptions are implicit here: (1) A movement is a complete and self-contained event; elaboration in the sense of varying some aspect of it can only blur its distinctness; and (2) Dance is hard to see. It must either be made less fancy, or the fact of that intrinsic difficulty must be emphasized to the point that it becomes almost impossible to see.

Repetition can serve to enforce the discreteness of a movement, objectify it, make it more objectlike. It also offers an alternative way of ordering material, literally making the material easier to see. That most theater audiences are irritated by it is not yet a disqualification.

My *Trio A* dealt with the "seeing" difficulty by dint of its continual and unremitting revelation of gestural detail that did *not* repeat itself, thereby focusing on the fact that the material could not easily be encompassed.

There is at least one circumstance that the chart does not include (because it does not relate to "minimization"), viz., the static singular object versus the object with interchangeable parts. The dance equivalent is the indeterminate performance that produces variations ranging from small details to a total image. Usually indeterminacy has been used to change the sequentialness—either phrases or larger sections—of a work, or to permute the details of a work. It has also been used with respect to timing. Where the duration of separate, simultaneous events is not prescribed exactly, variations in the relationship of these events occur. Such is the case with the trio I have been speaking about, in which small discrepancies in the tempo of individually executed phrases result in the three simultaneous performances constantly moving in and out of phase and in and out of synchronization. The overall look of it is constant from one performance to another, but the distribution of bodies in space at any given instant changes.

I am almost done. *Trio A* is the first section of *The Mind is a Muscle*. There are six people involved and four more sections. *Trio B* might be described as a VARIATION of *Trio A* in its use of unison with three people; they move in exact unison throughout. *Trio A*[1] is about the EFFORTS of two men and a woman in getting each other aloft in VARIOUS ways while REPEATING the same diagonal SPACE pattern throughout. In *Horses* the group travels about as a unit, recurrently REPEATING six different ACTIONS. *Lecture* is a solo that REPEATS the MOVEMENT series of *Trio A*. There will be at least three more sections.

There are many concerns in this dance. The concerns may appear to fall on my tidy chart as randomly dropped toothpicks might. However, I think there is sufficient separating-out in my work as well as that of certain of my contemporaries to justify an attempt at organizing those points of departure from previous work. Comparing the dance to Minimal Art provided a convenient method of organization. Omissions and overstatements are a hazard of any systematizing in art. I hope that some degree of redress will be offered by whatever clarification results from this essay.

Notes

This article was written before the final version of *The Mind is a Muscle* had been made. (*Mat, Stairs,* and *Film* are not discussed.)

1. In the case of Graham, it is hardly possible to relate her work to anything outside of theater, since it was usually dramatic and psychological necessity that determined it.

2. The term *phrase* must be distinguished from *phrasing.* A phrase is simply two or more consecutive movements, while phrasing, as noted previously, refers to the manner of execution.

3. I do not mean to imply that the demand of musical or metric phrasing makes dancing look effortless. What it produces is a different kind of effort, where the body looks more extended, "pulled up," highly energized, ready to go, etc. The dancer's "set" again.

THE MIND IS A MUSCLE
by
YVONNE RAINER

at the Anderson Theater April 11, 14, 15, 1968

with

Becky Arnold	William Davis	Harry De Dio
Gay Delanghe	David Gordon	Barbara Lloyd
Steve Paxton		Yvonne Rainer

The approximate running time of the evening is one hour 45 minutes.

interlude #1: Conversation *(Lucinda Childs, William Davis)*

1. Trio A . . . . .William Davis, David Gordon, Steve Paxton
2. Trio B . . . . .Becky Arnold, Gay Delanghe, Barbara Lloyd

interlude #2: Dimitri Tiomkin *(Dial M for Murder)*

3. Mat then . . . . Becky Arnold, William Davis
       Stairs . . . . David Gordon, Steve Paxton, Yvonne Rainer

interlude #3: Henry Mancini *(The Pink Panther)*

4. Act . . . . Harry De Dio
                Group

INTERMISSION

interludes #4: The Greenbriar Boys *(Amelia Earhart's Last Flight)*
          #5: Silence (6 minutes)
          #6: Frank Sinatra *(Strangers in the Night)*
          #7: Conversation (continued)

5. Trio A[1] . . . . William Davis, David Gordon, Steve Paxton
6. Horses . . . . .Group

interlude #8: John Giorno *(Pornographic Poem)*

7. Film . . . . Group
          Foot Film by Bud Wirtschafter; Hand Film by William Davis
8. Lecture . . . . Yvonne Rainer

interlude #9: Jefferson Airplane *(She Has Funny Cars)*

Facsimile of program of *The Mind is a Muscle* performed April 11–15, 1968 at the Anderson Theater.

Lighting Design .... Jennifer Tipton
Stage Manager................................. Peter Williams
Assistant Stage Manager .... Arthur Cohen
Projectionist ....Robert Cowan
Technical Assistant ....Keith Hollingworth
Sound Technician ....Ralph Flynn
Business Manager.................................Louis Lloyd

Special thanks to Christophe Thurman and Midsummer, Inc. and to those whose financial assistance made these programs possible:

SPONSORS

John de Menil
Foundation for Contemporary
   Performance Arts
Victor Ganz
Walter Gutman Foundation
Lena Robbins Foundation

Mr. and Mrs. Gilbert Hahn
Susan Morse Hilles
Lucy Jarvis
Philip Johnson
Vera List
New York State Council on
   the Arts

CONTRIBUTORS

Mr. and Mrs. Morton Hornick
Marion Javits
Joan Kron
Audrey Sabol

Extra special thanks to the performers of THE MIND IS A MUSCLE. Their good will and good spirits made the tasks lighter.

The polystyrene (.010 guage silver) was obtained from Coating Products, Incorporated, Englewood Cliffs, New Jersey.

STATEMENT

(It is not necessary to read this prior to observation.)

The choices in my work are predicated on my own peculiar resources – obsessions of imagination, you might say – and also on
an ongoing argument with, love of, and contempt for dancing. If my
rage at the impoverishment of ideas, narcissism, and disguised
sexual exhibitionism of most dancing can be considered puritan
moralizing, it is also true that I love the body – its actual weight,
mass, and unenhanced physicality. It is my overall concern to reveal people as they are engaged in various kinds of activities –
alone, with each other, with objects – and to weight the quality of
the human body toward that of objects and away from the super-
stylization of the dancer. Interaction and cooperation on the one hand;
substantiality and inertia on the other. Movement invention, i.e.
''dancing'' in a strict sense, is but one of the several factors in
the work.

Although the formal concerns vary in each section of THE
MIND IS A MUSCLE, a general statement can be made. I am often
involved with changes as they are played against one or more constants: Details executed in a context of a continuum of energy
(Trio A, Mat); phrases and combinations done in unison (Trio B);
interactive and mutually dependent movements done in a singular
floor pattern (Trio A^1); changing floor patterns and movement configurations carried out by a group moving as a single unit (Film,
Horses); changes in a group configuration occurring around a constant central area of focus (Act); and more obvious juxtapositions
that involve actual separations in space and time.

The condition for the making of my stuff lies in the continuation of my interest and energy. Just as ideological issues have no
bearing on the nature of the work, neither does the tenor of current
political and social conditions have any bearing on its execution.
The world disintegrates around me. My connection to the world-
in-crisis remains tenuous and remote. I can foresee a time when this
remoteness must necessarily end, though I cannot foresee exactly
when or how the relationship will change, or what circumstances will
incite me to a different kind of action. Perhaps nothing short of
universal female military conscription will affect my function (The
ipso facto physical fitness of dancers will make them the first
victims.); or a call for a world-wide cessation of individual functions,
to include the termination of genocide. This statement is not an

apology. It is a reflection of a state of mind that reacts with horror
and disbelief upon seeing a Vietnamese shot dead on TV — not *solely* at
the sight of death, however, but at the fact that the TV can be shut
off afterwards as after a bad Western. My body remains the enduring
reality.

Yvonne Rainer
March, 1968

Some Nonchronological Recollections of *The Mind is a Muscle*

Trio A was first performed at Judson Church, January 10, 1966, as *The Mind is a Muscle, Part 1.* My memories of rehearsing it for that particular performance have merged with other rehearsal memories, some very recent. At that time it was performed by Steve Paxton, David Gordon, and me. I remember showing it to David for the first time; he expressed doubts about being able to execute it in the proper style. Now I say anyone can master the style, or just about anyone. I didn't have a concept of that possibility in 1966. At one session something David was doing looked strange to me. I asked him what kind of imagery he was using. He said "I'm thinking of myself as a faun." I said "Try thinking of yourself as a barrel." More recently I had a similar experience with John Erdman, only at a different point in the dance. John had learned part of *Trio A* from Barbara Lloyd, who is the only person, to my knowledge, who was never officially "taught" *Trio A,* but, rather, picked it up entirely on her own by observing me, Steve, David, and Becky Arnold. On inquiring how Barbara had described a particular movement, John said "birdlike." I retaught it to him as "airplanelike."

The photo of that early performance shows wooden slats on the floor. They were hurled one at a time with metronomelike regularity from the balcony of the church for the duration of the dance (nine minutes, or *Trio A* done twice). They constituted the original "music" for *Trio A.* Audience members complained afterwards about the relentlessness of this "music." It may have been at this performance that a man sitting in the front row picked up a slat, attached a large white handkerchief to it, and waved it over his head. I retained the slats as an accompaniment for *Trio A* through the Anderson Theater performance (April 1968). Even before that *Trio A* had begun the first of its many transmogrifications. At Judson (May 24, 1966) it was done by David, Bill Davis, and me as the first section of a four-part *Mind is a Muscle.* The slats were reserved for the fourth section called *Lecture,* which was a special version of *Trio A* tailored to the balletic talents of Peter Saul. While teaching it to him, wherever possible I stuck in a pirouette or jump. Peter was unavailable for the Anderson show. I was stuck. I had grandiose fantasies of Jacques D'Amboise appearing at the end from nowhere to do a bravura *Trio A.* Next in line (in my fantasy dance) was Merce Cunningham. I became obsessed with this idea and eventually proposed it to him at a party. He laughingly declined. I finally did it myself in tap shoes (minus the balletic furbelows) with the slats shot in from a ladder in the wings, and with a wooden grid that filled the proscenium space descending in the middle of the solo. It stayed down for one minute, then ascended out of sight. I had the same ambivalence about decor I had about music: It shouldn't hang around too long, and the more grand the effect the briefer the appearance.

In the final version of *The Mind is a Muscle* the white motif appeared again: In each section a different person wore all white. Everyone had a chance to be a "star"—at least in appearance. Another carry-over from *Terrain* was the business of inactive performers watching—in view of the audience—the active performers. I hated the "magic" of entrances and exits, the nowhere or imaginary "somewhere" of the wings, or off-stage area. In *Terrain's Solo Section* the street barricade had provided an expedient and decorative observation post. At the Anderson Theater the inactive ones simply stood quietly at the back of the stage. I seem to have persisted with this device despite the complaints of my performers about "getting cold." Now we do a brief warm-up in view of the audience—those of us with dance training.

When I first began teaching *Trio A* to anyone who wanted to learn it —skilled, unskilled, professional, fat, old, sick, amateur—and gave tacit permission to anyone who wanted to teach it to teach it, I envisioned myself as a post-modern dance evangelist bringing movement to the masses, watching with Will Rogers–like benignity the slow, inevitable evisceration of my elitist creation. Well, I finally met a *Trio A* I didn't like. It was fifth generation, and I couldn't believe my eyes.

Trio A at the Anderson was for three men doing it simultaneously but not in unison. Behind them was a highly reflective wall of mylar stretching from wing to wing and floor to flies. It was "flown" halfway through *Trio B*. This was a hold-over from the Washington Now Festival performance (April 1966) for which I had had built an accordion-paneled wall of mirrors. Situated at the proper distance—rather close— one could observe simultaneously a performer walking from left to right and his multiple reflections—some of them walking in the same direction and some of them in the opposite direction. Seated two feet beyond this ideal vantage point, however, you saw absolutely nothing in the mirrors. Since the Now Festival took place in a roller skating rink, no one sat in the right place to benefit from the mirrors. And, of course, back in New York at the Anderson, the stage was elevated, so that particular mirror arrangement was out of the question. My first fiasco.

Trio B was a series of runs and athletic traveling movements performed in unison by three women—Becky, Gay Delanghe, and Barbara. At stage left, running up and down stage, were two three-foot-wide strips of bubble wrap and half-inch black rubber. This "decor" derived directly from my having performed in Steve Paxton's *Afternoon* of 1963, an outdoor piece that required us to execute difficult Cunningham-like movement in mushy soil. Though at the time I had been quite outraged by the difficulties posed, I later became fascinated with the idea. At the Anderson the different surfaces made for a change in the sound of the feet as well as a visible change in effort, depending on the particular movement. The bubbles in the bubble wrap popped delightfully. During the first part of this trio, which was all running, one of the performers counted aloud continuously to indicate the number of steps taken in any given direction.

Mat was a continuation of the *Trio A* aesthetic: two people doing the same sequence out of sync. It was a sequence that involved a four-by-eight-foot foam rubber mat and a twelve pound black dumbbell and incorporated various kinds of rolls, hand- and headstands, and repositionings of the body and dumbbell in relation to the mat—all executed in the same evenly paced, rhythmically uninflected dynamic. It was one of my favorite dances to do; there was something very satisfying about the constant return to the mat and the subtle adjustments of effort required in handling one's weight with and without the dumbbell. At the Anderson Theater it was performed by Becky and Bill.

For the record, *Mat* had an earlier debut: Bill and Becky did it as part of a Choreoconcert at the New School in September 1967. It was preceded by a tape of my voice reading a letter from a Denver doctor to a New York surgeon describing in technical medical terms the details of the gastrointestinal illness with which I was hospitalized at the time of this performance. It was one of many attempts to deal—via my profession—with the natural catastrophe that had befallen my body. It was using autobiography as a "found object" without any stylistic transformation. I don't think I could do that today, at least in an instance where the biographical details belonged so exclusively to my experience, as in the case of that particular letter.

Stairs had an unusual origin: I had gotten out of the hospital weak as a fly after the before-mentioned illness. Partly to keep busy I worked with Becky and Bill, having them "learn" my watery-legged movement as I shakily negotiated running, crawling, getting from a chair to a high stool and back down again. After the first session I got the idea of a staircase with two stairs the exact height of the chair and stool and wide enough to accommodate two people climbing at the same time. The next day a friend, June Ekman, told me about a dream she had in which she couldn't figure out why Becky, Bill, and I were having so much difficulty climbing a staircase with tiny steps. As a result I added two "tiny steps" at the top of my staircase, then later carpeted it and put it on wheels so that it could be moved around. This section had funny sexual references in it: David, Steve, and I took turns pulling or assisting each other up, down, and off the stairs by means of passing one hand through the other's legs and holding the crotch, or—in my case—they each placed a hand on a breast and so supported my torso as I jumped from the top step. I couldn't decide whether to perform this "fly-in-the-ointment" (in an otherwise formal and "dignified" sequence of maneuvers) in a nonchalant manner or underscore its eccentricity still further by some kind of facial response on the part of the person whose privates were touched. We tried various "responses"—from subtle to exaggerated—and finally we each did what seemed most comfortable: David and I responded less and less, while Steve continued to show a startled expression whenever it happened to him.

About *Act*: I had originally wanted a gymnast to offset the low-keyed imagery of our tableaux on the other side of the stage. I had actually auditioned an acrobat. It just didn't seem right. For one thing the duration of most gymnastic or acrobatic routines was much shorter than I required. Again I was involved with a kind of imagery—static and slow to change—that I felt required a certain amount of time to "register" on an audience. Harry De Dio and his magic act proved to be just the ticket as far as time went, and his facile manipulation of small objects was an unexpected foil for our careful repositioning of bodies, foam rubber mat, and two swings. My notes read: "Something is always happening—separated by momentary stillness—but only one thing at a time. It is like *Carriage Discreteness.* In the latter the hand of God changed the hugely dispersed configuration into a slightly different configuration. In *Act* the participants themselves rearrange the configuration, always returning to positions of neutrality, i.e., quietly observing a central focal point while at ease, but perfectly still, in a standing, sitting, or lying down posture, from which they can observe the rest of the configuration. Instructions are given improvisationally by each in a preset order to the rest of the group while the 'instructor' remains perfectly immobile. Eye movements are essential in order to maintain a look of attentiveness rather than self-absorption. This section is about changes in a configuration rather than about movement. The changes are made with quiet efficiency." Hand signals were given to the stage manager when an "instructor" wanted the level of the swings changed. It took awhile to figure out in rehearsal what this section was about, which—in view of my then premeditative working methods—was somewhat unusual for me. After repeated and disagreeable vetoing of the group's efforts at fulfilling my instructions, it finally dawned on me that I did not want intermittent movement "invention" but changes in static relationships of objects and people, which brought it into the realm of "tableau" and "task" rather than "dance."

Trio A[1]—originally for two men and one woman and later for three men—mainly involved traveling back and forth on a diagonal between two mattresses, also two people getting the third one aloft in various ways, some of them quite spectacular. I had dreams of flying then, as I had earlier momentarily in the no. 7 of *Diagonal* of *Terrain,* and later in the *Group Hoist* of *Continuous Project-Altered Daily.* It was definitely an extension—or inversion—of the ballerina fantasy. Later the women would again participate equally in getting the men into the air. It just took more than one to do it.

I don't remember much about *Film* except that it was very complicated to learn and made heavy demands on rote memory. It was all about traveling as a herd (as was the improvised *Horses* preceding it) with ten- and twenty-count halts, always behind a screen on which was projected a movie of legs from the knee down walking up to a volleyball. The projected image dominated the downstage center area, and when we were directly behind it our own legs, very small in comparison and from the hip down, appeared below the screen. Most of the traveling was on diagonals.

At a concert prior to the Anderson (Brandeis University, January 13, 1968) *The Mind is a Muscle* was presented in a slightly different order and without *Stairs.* Toward the end some audience members became quite unruly, almost abusive. There were others, some of whom later came to study and work with me, who said that *The Mind is a Muscle* changed their concept of dance. ("When we went out in the lobby and asked someone where the cafeteria was and he pointed, we all broke up.") Several even said it changed their lives.

Profile:

Interview by Lyn Blumenthal

In 1976 the late writer and video artist Lyn Blumenthal and artist Kate Horsfield founded the Video Data Bank at the School of the Art Institute of Chicago. Their original mission was to videotape in-depth interviews with visual artists. By the early '80s some of the interviews were being transcribed and published as pamphlets under the series title *Profile*. This one appeared in vol. 4, no. 6, fall 1984, transcribed from the original taped interview of June 1984. The interviewer is Lyn Blumenthal.

LB: Can you talk a little bit about your background? What were your early interests and what was your family like?

YR: My family was immigrants. My father had come to America from Italy just before the first World War. My mother was the daughter of Polish-Jewish immigrants. She was born in Brooklyn. My maternal grandfather had been a tinsmith in Warsaw. He was a socialist. So my mother and father met, according to the family mythology, in a raw food dining room in San Francisco. They were vegetarians. My father was an anarchist and a house painter. They were pretty unorthodox in many ways. We lived in a working class neighborhood in San Francisco—basically WASP. They were pretty isolated people. I mean, most of my father's friends were Italian and lived in another part of town.

It was a rather isolated, lonely existence. I studied piano for six months at the age of seven, and then I studied Hawaiian steel guitar for some reason. I think a salesman had come to the door. My mother was a potential stage mother. She put me through tap and acrobatic school, which didn't take. I was almost pathologically shy and finally persuaded her to let me discontinue the lessons.

I don't remember having any interests except excelling in school. I was very good, even into high school. I had one year of college at San Francisco City College. When I dropped out of college, I was involved with a kind of Bohemian, socialist, artistic milieu around North Beach. I was involved with painters and didn't aspire to do anything myself until I was about twenty, when I kind of accidently fell into an acting school. I realized I liked being in front of an audience. I had no idea what acting was all about, and performing.

LB: Apart from the ritual of going to different types of lessons, which you seemed to rebel against, what was interesting to you, what was interesting at school? How did you enter into this?

YR: I have a brother four years older than I am. I was interested in doing what my brother did. I had three years of Latin with the same teacher he studied with four years previously. That was important to me. My brother was my mentor pretty much. We read a lot of Italian and English novels. In grade school my interest was in playing on the streets after school. I was very athletic. And when I wasn't playing I was reading. I remember roaring through four Oz books in one weekend. The library was about ten blocks away, and I remember lugging these four heavy volumes of Frank Baum home.

It was a very depressed childhood. I can't remember having other interests except basic survival and avoidance of any embarrassing situations. It was like going from one embarrassing social situation to another.

LB: Well, how did you get a sense of whether or not the family was political or anarchist?

YR: It was not from my parents. It was from my brother's milieu, when he was about eighteen. Right after the second World War a group of Jewish anarchists came out from New York and there was this very heady mix of homosexual, artistic and radical people—and poets around Kenneth Rexroth. This social mix coalesced in weekly poetry meetings, readings and guest speakers at the Workman's Circle in San Francisco every Friday night. From the age of fifteen, maybe even earlier, I went to these meetings.

Of course, my brother got involved in this because there was anarchist literature around the house. My parents were definitely not intellectual, but they deplored the system, the Capitalist system—even though they were engaged in it. They owned their own house. This caused a lot of ambivalence which I acted out in rebelling against my parents when I was fifteen and sixteen.

Around 1952, I dropped out of school and went to Chicago. There I had my first steady, paying job. It was a very odd job. I was an order-filler for Hibbard, Spencer and Bartlett in Evanston, Illinois. It was a wholesaler of drygoods of every conceivable kind—household, sporting goods, toys. It was a warehouse about five blocks long. You had a quota to fill, and to meet and surpass this quota you wore roller skates and pushed this big wagon. The workers were mainly young, black women. I was the youngest and the only Caucasian, and they kind of adopted me as a mascot. It was hard work, but it was fun sometimes. I enjoyed the closeness to these women, and I enjoyed being independent. I enjoyed the feeling of being strong. But I only lived in Chicago for about six months.

LB: What did you find when you got home with your independence?

YR: I had grown up quite a bit, established that I could live economically and emotionally outside of my family's house. They pretty much let me do what I wanted.

LB: Is that when you became involved at the Theater Arts Colony?

YR: This friend of mine, one of the anarchist friends, had gone to this theater group to design costumes or sew. She was interested in theater in a peripheral way. I went with her, and the director of the theater asked me to audition for something. He set up a situation, and I came in and did something. And he said, well, I definitely see something there. Would you like a scholarship to the school? I said, sure. And I started taking classes.

This was a group that was established in this very beautiful old building called the Theater Arts Colony. At that time it was called that. I think it still functions as a little theater. They weren't doing Brecht, but they were talking about Epic theater. They did Americana and they did *All the King's Men*—I was in a crowd scene in *All the King's Men*. I loved being on the stage and I loved the whole ambiance of theater. So I studied acting.

The most important thing that happened to me there was the speech class. I had had a lisp since I had learned to talk. This speech teacher said, what other kind of *s* can you make? I said "s," and he said, what's wrong with that? I said, "Sounds funny to me." He said, "Well, it sounds alright to me." So I just slowed my speech for the next two weeks with everyone I spoke to. I was working for a fire insurance company. I spoke to my boss in very cadenced measures—and to my parents. No one seemed to notice I was speaking very slowly and carefully. And I acquired this new *s* which amazed me no end. It was like my first sense of achievement in transforming myself, in overcoming what I felt, and had been told, was a disability. So that was important.

The acting classes were somewhat frustrating. And meanwhile my New York friends were urging me to go to New York—"you really ought to get out of this slow town and go to New York." They were all settled with families and children. At that point I met the painter Al Held. He was in San Francisco temporarily. He went back and I followed him. In those first two years in New York, I took acting classes which were very frustrating and I took my first dance class which was totally exhilarating. And that is how I, again, kind of fell into dancing.

LB: When you first came to New York, what did you find there?

YR: I found this arena of fantasy and possibility. It was extremely heady and exhilarating.

LB: Did you have a sense of ambition?

YR: I wouldn't have called it ambition. It is only relatively recently that I have defined the energies that I discovered in myself as ambition. I mean, that was sort of a dirty word for someone coming from my background. It smacked of competition, aggression, and, I suppose, "unfeminine" things—although I didn't use that word either. In my head I was filled with an inchoate fantasy life, a sense of possibility and fulfillment, which I didn't dare to articulate for myself. And I was very much involved with the work of the man I was living with, Al Held.

Al had a retrospective several years ago at the Whitney and I attended the exhibition and suddenly came upon a painting dated 1959 that was more familiar than my own hand. I had stood in front of those paintings and memorized them. It was an abstract painting. I knew every stroke on this painting. And I have never been involved with painting to that degree since. So I guess I learned everything I know about painting from studying this man's work. So it was a kind of education. Whatever I was exposed to, this was my art school—New York. I went to 10th Street every Friday night for openings.

LB: So when you got to New York you were involved in the visual art world. But did you also continue a parallel interest in theater?

YR: I went to the Herbert Berghof school immediately and started taking regular classes in acting—technique, scene study. I think my very first teacher was Lee Grant who was blacklisted during that period from the McCarthy days, so was teaching. And as I recall, she told me I was too intellectual—I didn't feel it enough. That was a refrain I heard over and over. They could see me thinking up there. I wasn't really living it. Acting as it was taught in New York was strictly Method, Actor's Studio, Stanislavsky based and I never got the hang of it. And at that point I wasn't reading anything of the Russian formalists or those alternatives. Meyerhold was never mentioned of course.

So I lost interest in acting. I went to some auditions. They told me I was good for American Indian parts and there weren't many of those around. I had these very exotic dark looks so I couldn't get a job in *The Crucible* or *Picnic*. I think by about '58 I had stopped studying acting. I had begun going to dance concerts—Erick Hawkins' *Here and Now with Watchers* was a crucial work for me to see.

LB: What did it represent for you?

YR: Something I could do if I studied. It did not present an impossible challenge. Seeing that, plus already experiencing this excitement and exhilaration in dance class, pretty clearly showed me where I wanted to go. I hadn't encountered that kind of satisfaction in acting, either in the response of teachers or in my own experience of it. I was studying with Edith Stephan who ran this kind of eclectic, weekly dance class and during the summer took her company out to summer camps. She invited me to come along. We did improvisations. But meanwhile I was seeing a lot of different things including Martha Graham.

1958, '59, and '60 were pretty important years as far as my education went. Al and I had separated in '59 and I had been supporting myself by part-time office jobs and modeling for life classes in art schools. By that time I was 25. At that period it was still customary to think of the dancer's career as having to start very early, even in modern dance. If you didn't start early you didn't have much of a chance. It seemed pretty late for me to be starting. I didn't have a natural gift as far as body structure. I was not supple, but I was strong. I could leap and jump. At the Graham School they told me I should think of myself as more regal and less athletic—which I had trouble doing. So I figured if my mother could swing it—and she hadn't put me through college— that I better devote as much time as I could to dance classes, and stop this part-time work. So she supported me for the next few years. I took three classes a day and hung out in between classes at the Museum of Modern Art getting a film education in old movies. I saw a history of silent films, '20s and '30s American. I remember seeing mainly Buster Keaton and Chaplin. And I would hang out in the garden or the cafeteria and then go to my next class. Or I hung out at Horn and Hardart on 57th Street and Sixth Avenue.

LB: What kind of community were you forming for yourself at that time?

YR: I was still involved with the art community and went to loft parties and openings. I had very few contacts with dancers except at the schools, ballet classes. At that time I was seeing Cunningham, and I had begun to think that I would have to study with him at some point. But meanwhile I hadn't totally exhausted what I was getting out of the Graham situation. I remember seeing Merce at a WBAI benefit party, going up to him and telling him that I wanted to study with him but couldn't do it yet. I was still at the Martha Graham school. He smiled in his charming, sly way.

LB: What kind of ideas did he represent that you wanted to make that statement to him?

YR: He represented the avant-garde and the future. I wanted to get a classical training, and that began to include Graham. Even at that point when I was studying with her, I knew this was no longer modern—even though it was still called modern dance. And Cunningham was the first dancer who really stimulated me intellectually.

LB: How?

YR: The work did not deal with stories, with drama, with music. It seemed totally independent and freewheeling. It was difficult. It was ironic. There was something uncompromising in the way—although he had some funny dances—he was not pandering to the audience either through music or high drama or psychological atmosphere.

I'm trying to remember what I was reading in those days. I suppose art criticism. I wasn't aware of Clement Greenberg although he was talked about. I was still involved with theater. I read Beckett. By the early '60s, I was going to see—I guess they were pre-Happenings—things that were happening around Beverly Schmidt and the Bridge Theater.

Well, mainly the bridge for me between Graham and Cunningham was Simone Forti, who was then Simone Morris. I think I met her at the Graham School. She was taking a June course. I was finishing up there—I had been there a year, and was taking the advanced June course. She was taking the beginner's course. She had just come from working with Ann Halprin in San Francisco. She had come in '59, I think. And she was married to the sculptor Robert Morris.

I met Simone through Nancy Meehan who was the first dancer I became friends with, whose ambitions lay in dancing with Graham. Nancy Meehan had been at the Graham School a year or so. It turned out that she and I had come to New York in the same year and had lived and grown up ten blocks apart in San Francisco. I learned a lot about dance from her. She was a passionate modern dancer, a very beautiful, very talented dancer in her own right. I admired what she could do.

Nancy knew Simone from San Francisco, and she and Simone had wanted to start improvising together. Nancy invited me to come and I met Simone. So the three of us rented a studio that was then Dance Players on Sixth Avenue in the '40s—it has since been torn down. And then we later rented the Don Redlich studio. That was my introduction to jamming—fooling around with your body, with maybe a few rules or restrictions, and then embellishing and spontaneously elaborating on it.

LB: What ideas were you playing with or talking about in terms of your dancing?

YR: Spatial restrictions, I think. Like moving on the diagonal. Pretty much formal things. Or focusing on one part of the body. Or sometimes just totally free form. My memory of what the three of us did is very fuzzy, but I had an excess of energy. I remember just running around a lot, diving through people's legs and in very hypnotic slow motion going from one position to another. I have some small Polaroid photos from those sessions—there is Nancy, with her long legs, doing a huge leg lift; and there is me in some grotesque crouch position with shoulders askew and a very intense presence, an inward turning gaze. I was like in a trance.

Simone was going back to San Francisco that summer, which was 1960, to take Ann Halprin's summer workshop. She was really talking up that situation—she had actually performed with Ann for a number of years—and I got all excited from hearing her talk. So in July–August, she, Morris and I drove across the country. That was the first trip for me across the country by car. And I spent the summer there. Of course my brother and mother were still living in San Francisco.

It was at Ann Halprin's workshop that this whole world of ideas developed: chance procedures, improvisation, movement generated by everyday tasks, use of the voice while moving, playing with words. La-Monte Young was teaching a session. He came in every afternoon and we made sound scores. There was body work, and I remember being surprised about how Graham-oriented the technique was. Of course Halprin's relationship to the body at that time was still grounded in various kinds of stretches on the floor that seemed to me very related to

the contraction and release of the Graham technique. And that surprised me. But everything else was totally new. I didn't see any of Halprin's theatrical work and only gradually and later realized that, also to
my surprise, most of the things that she was doing in the workshop
were not the stuff of performance but were the point of departure for
transformation and theatricalization. So she still had ideas about the
transformation of these ideas, rather than their being a new form of
presentation.

Anyway, it was the people I met there who became my peers and
friends to this day: Trisha Brown, A. A. Leath, John Graham, June Eck-
man, who is an expert Alexander technique teacher and who I am now
studying with, Ruth Emerson, who became part of the Judson group,
and so it went.

This was simply a six-week course, very intensive, all day. You started
out about 9:00 in the morning, you worked on technique, and you
were expected to work by yourself. This was difficult for me because I
didn't have enough resources or background to know what to do, how
to spend those three hours. Then there was a lunch break. Then you
worked on structured projects for part of the afternoon and then with
LaMonte Young for part of the afternoon. The evening was totally devoted to improvisation, either free improvisation or setting up various
kinds of problem solving. It attests to our energies—everyone was in
their twenties, I guess—that we were still able to work on after a whole
day of very intense physical work. I remember myself in particular, in
the evening I had energy to burn. I was running around like a madwoman!

LB: So in 1961 you performed *Three Satie Spoons.* Was that your first
public performance?

YR: I returned to New York in the fall of 1960. Robert Dunn, who
was a disciple of John Cage and a composer, was starting a workshop in
the Cunningham studio, which was on the top floor of the building
leased by the Living Theater at Sixth Avenue and 14th Street. I had
been taking two June courses earlier that year, one with Cunningham
and one with Graham, one during the day and one at night. By the end
of June I knew I was through with Graham and that I would be studying full-time with Cunningham in the fall. In the fall I began taking a
ballet class during the day, Cunningham's class in the evening and then
once a week the Dunn workshop took place.

I knew I was ready to use whatever came my way. Simone, Bob Morris and I rented a studio, and I was going in there every day working on movement—short, eccentric phrases using gesture, technical leggy movement. I was becoming fairly competent in balletically based movement which, of course, was what the Cunningham technique vocabulary was based on—a combination of Graham and ballet. And then I guess there was some rebellious, exhibitionist fantasy life that took its form in my own movement invention which derived from eccentric bagwoman gestures and ordinary, everyday observations, friends on the street, etc. So I was working this out in these short, not organized movement phrases.

In his workshop, Bob Dunn was showing us John Cage's scores. We were discussing ways to adapt these scores to making dances. There were no assignments as such. He was simply presenting this material. Meanwhile, there were only about five people, and these people were bringing in their own ideas. Everyone was ready and willing to work, to talk, to share ideas, and Bob was the ideal person at that time to run something like this.

So it was in the fall of 1960 that I made my first solo dance, *Three Satie Spoons.* There were three sections, and I presented each section in the workshop as it was finished.

In 1961 more people came to join the workshop. Trisha, who had stayed in San Francisco, Ruth Emerson, Elaine Summers and Steve Paxton, who had been there the first semester. There were more people, maybe ten people. Judith Dunn came. Then, I made a second dance, a duet. It was natural to start adding people. Trisha was the second person. And again I used a piece of Satie. I called it *Satie for Two,* and it used the same system of organization.

LB: Was this performed in workshops, or was this performed at the Living Theater?

YR: My first public performance was in the summer, July of 1961 at the Living Theater.

Meanwhile I had started studying with James Waring, who had been operating in New York throughout the '50s. He was a great admirer of Cage and Cunningham and was ballet trained. I think for a brief period he and Ann Halprin had worked together. He came from the West Coast and he taught classes, basically ballet classes.

I started studying with Jimmy because I had seen the work of Aileen Passloff. She had a company and she also studied with Jimmy. She was totally ballet trained. And I had decided I wanted to dance with her. At that point I wanted some experience in dancing, and I thought I had to dance with somebody before I presented my own work. That was the usual way to go. So I started taking Jimmy's classes.

Then Jimmy asked me if I wanted to dance with him. He was doing a piece for an arts festival in Montreal. And I said, sure. So I started to rehearse with Jimmy in the spring of '61. At the end of the spring course of the Dunn workshop, we did a public workshop performance. We used the studio and I presented *Three Satie Spoons.* That was all I had done except for two solos, *Spoons* and another solo called *The Bells* which had no music. Jimmy was organizing a program of solos at the Living Theater on this tiny, pocket-size stage. He had seen the workshop performance and asked me if I wanted to perform, and I was utterly thrilled.

It's funny. I lived very much in the moment then. I had no idea of a career or where I was going to present these things. Showing the work in the workshop was sufficient for me at that time. It was very satisfying. I got a very good response. I had no further ambition. And it is funny, around the Cunningham studio, that word *ambition* did not come up. People were not involved with careerism as we know it today.

LB: But what about ambition in terms of the work?

YR: Well, that certainly showed itself by the amount of work that was done and by the intense involvement and concern people had for ideas of what was going on.

LB: When you say "ideas of what was going on," do you mean in terms of the art world essentially?

YR: Well, everything. It was as though the Cunningham situation was a center for me. It was only one thing. It was my direct showcase, you might say.

LB: So ideas were coming in from all over?

YR: From all over. Everyone involved in this situation was also going to happenings, to music concerts, to very odd events. This is a piece I shall never forget. I think it was around 1959 up at the York Theater—York Avenue in the 80s. I don't think anything has happened there since. It is a movie house. Someone named Stephen Tropp did an event which had two or three parts. One was simply lowering the battens with all the stage lights—it was a proscenium theater; the battens would go up and down, and the lights would fade on the stage and come up on the audience. So it was simply playing with the apparatus in the theater. Another thing he did was project, on an ordinary living room accordion screen, a film of the ocean.

There were polka dots painted on this screen, and someone in back of the screen was making a rapping sound. So there was this combination of nature, painting and sound.

LB: Is it also a time of questioning the autonomy of art?

YR: In what sense—autonomy?

LB: In terms of all the formal expectations of art? Was it a critique of pure art, with the happenings bringing in a synthesis of theater and fine art ideas?

YR: Yes. Well, that is of course what the happening represented. But it was for the most part being engaged in by painters and sculptors. Jim Dine and Claes Oldenburg were doing these things—and Red Grooms.

LB: But it was also bringing in different kinds of content. From ordinary activities, from street sounds, and things that generally weren't grist for the art mill.

YR: Yes. Using untrained performers, etc. But in the Dunn workshops we were using each other, for the most part people who were fairly skilled and trained in modern dancing and even ballet techniques.

LB: Were you thinking of yourself at this time as a performer and a choreographer?

YR: Yes. I was performing in other people's work. It was more about making oneself available to other people's ideas. Up to the point when James Waring asked me to be in his company, I thought, well, I am going to have to do my own work because I don't have these long graceful legs. It was very clear what kind of dancers the people around me, who were following the established format of the institutionalized companies, were using. They had a certain kind of body, a certain kind of accomplishment, and, even after I started performing Jimmy's work, it got back to me. People said, well, she can't do much, she doesn't have much technique, but she's a great performer.

So that is the way people separated out these qualities. Technique was still something highly valued if you wanted to be a professional dancer. Professionalism had to do with certain kinds of virtuoso skills. Of course Simone in '61 had totally overturned that with an evening of dance constructions where she made wood constructions and used whoever was around, dancers and nondancers, to negotiate and navigate on them—ropes, slantboards, task situations based on very simple instructions, all of which generated movement. And I was much more eclectic, because I was still involved in getting and improving technique.

I was still involved in this mind-set about what the dancer's body should be—pulled up, ready to go, more muscle tone than the average person. We still wore leotards and tights. I, in my early dances, was still involved in exhibiting the body—this idealized body—in a certain way, in that traditional way. The skintight nylon encasement for the body. Different colors—black, white, mauve, whatever. And in the early Judson work people were still wearing leotards and tights. Simone, in her work, did not require that kind of costume.

LB: I want to talk about that period. The first performance you did at Judson Church was *Ordinary Dance.* You did a long series of presentations or performances at Judson: *We Shall Run, Word Words, Terrain, Room Service, Shorter End of a Small Piece, Part of a Sextet,* the first version of *The Mind is a Muscle. The Mind is a Muscle* is the last piece you performed there?

YR: Yes, I think so. It was '66.

LB: Can you talk about the significance of the Judson Church in particular as it relates to the work you've done but also as it represented an energy center for lots of different art practices that were going on in terms of ideas.

YR: The church itself was a veritable boiler factory of activity, beginning in the late '50s, maybe '58 or '59. There was the Judson Poets Theater, there was the gallery, which did installations and happenings, and I think there were music concerts. Al Carmines came in the late '50s.

In '62, when the Bob Dunn workshop had completed a second semester, we realized we had a great deal of work and much of it was really first rate and important. We were ready to show it, to present ourselves to the world. We knew about the Judson activities, and there had been no dance program there, so we approached Al Carmines. Ruth Emerson, Bob Dunn, Steve Paxton, and I went down there and auditioned for him. I think I did *Three Satie Spoons* and Ruth and Steve each did solos. He was instantly more than interested. And in the summer of '62 we did the first concert. It was called *Concert of Dance.*

In the fall, because Bob was not doing the workshop, we still felt this need to meet, share ideas and show each other work. At that point I was sharing a studio with Aileen Passloff and Jimmy Waring. It was over the St. Mark's Theater on Second Avenue and St. Mark's Place. Jimmy taught there and we all rehearsed there. And so we started using that studio for the workshops, and then somehow got transferred to the Judson gym for weekly meetings. Out of these meetings came the body officially known as the Judson Dance Theater and the series of concerts that continued to be called Concerts of Dance—by number. They went from one to seventeen or eighteen, I think, in the middle of the '60s. The first one was in the summer of '62 where I did *Ordinary Dance.*

LB: How was the work received?

YR: Tumultuously—considering there was no air conditioning, it was a 90-degree day, and it was a three-hour concert. That audience hung in there with bated breath. I have attended very few events that can parallel those high spirits—their enthusiasm and our enthusiasm.

LB: What did success mean to you at that time?

YR: Exactly what I just described—mutual enthusiasm on the part of the performers. What excited me was that we had done it together. It was definitely a social and cooperative group event with a tremendous feeling of solidarity and *esprit de corps.* I think that must have communicated itself to the audience. There was no one person's work that was highlighted or dominated. Even small efforts could be incorporated; very short, modest pieces could be incorporated into this format and make a contribution. So it was a very unusual situation.

LB: Did this satisfy an anti-authority interest you had—the collective spirit?

YR: Yes. It certainly seemed an alternative to that single-minded social structure that fulfilled personal ambition and was a very isolated event—you rehearsed all year, hired the YMHA up on Lexington and 92nd Street and made this big presentation of everything once a year. It was like the once-a-year show. And here we had a situation that was available to us, that was ongoing. The workshops continued. We could show work informally, and, when there was a sufficient body of work, we could present it formally as a special event to the public.

LB: You felt not locked into that dominant structure?

YR: It was a very viable alternative to the structures that had been presented to us when we were students.

LB: How did your ideas develop during this period of time?

YR: Well, I went through a number of changes. I guess the range of my interests was quite a bit broader than was many other people's in the workshop. I mean just in terms of my personal performance and in terms of my choreographic work for a group. Like doing a dance that just consisted of running. That seems a very novel idea but, unlike Steve Paxton who did a dance that consisted only of walking, I was still wedded to or interested in undermining or making reference to certain kinds of theatricality that I was then becoming more and more in opposition to. I had to incorporate both strands into my work, the theatrical one and the oppositional, polemic, pedestrian one. So *We Shall Run,* a dance of running for ten or twelve people, also had highly dramatic, romantic music—Berlioz' *Requiem.* So you had this grandiloquence and inflation and nuance in the sound and in the music. In another era, Massine would have amassed an army of dancers in very complicated choreography for this kind of music; I juxtaposed this pedestrian, monotonic kind of movement.

LB: So you presented contradictions but also critiques.

YR: Yes. Within this juxtaposition was contained a critique of certain conventions—music, use of music and past use of music—which, of course, Cunningham was already doing in his own way. I was never attracted to the use of modern music. I either wanted to divorce the dance totally from music and use verbal text or silence, or use traditional romantic music to make ironic commentary.

LB: Can you talk a little bit about your use of language?

YR: That had started pretty early on. In fact, in my first solo. I had been exposed to language games and explorations with Ann and Simone. Simone did a number of improvisations where she would improvise a story or play with language while she was moving. In the last section, the third part of *Three Satie Spoons,* there were two sounds and one sentence. The sounds were *beep, beep, beep*—they came and went—ending with the sound *aaah oou.* And the sentence spoken was "the grass is greener when the sun is yellower; the grass is greener when the sun is yellow." That was the beginning of the use of this kind of material.

In *The Bells,* there was this very eccentric combination of standing on my tippy toes, facing the audience, while making this movement in front of my eyes and saying, "I told you everything would be alright, Harry." And this would reoccur. I was using these repetitive structures, the chance procedures. I would cough things up repeatedly, so that happened about three times in the dance.

Then I began to think about a more coherent kind of language, because I was dealing with movement that was not based on a theme and variations nor on a coherent progression or development. It was very fragmented. I began to think about a coexistence of a coherent storyline on one hand and these very cut up movement sequences on the other. So in 1963, that whole year, I worked on my first long dance called *Terrain.*

Terrain was presented as an evening-length work at Judson in the spring of '63. There were six people: Steve Paxton, myself, Trisha Brown, Judith Dunn, Al Reid, and Bill Davis. It contained a lot of language and a lot of different movements and movement situations. There were about five sections. One section was called the "Solo Section" because there were simultaneous solos. There were five solos; each person learned two; three could happen simultaneously. Two of them had the dancer reciting a story by Spencer Holst. They were two different stories. One was called "On Truth" and it was autobiographical. It was about how his grandfather came to Ohio, started the first newspaper in the nineteenth century and built a dam. He was a very community-oriented person, and he really got this small town on its feet. I guess he was an early entrepreneur, capitalist, progressive kind of individualist—eccentric individualist.

We learned the story independently and learned the sequence of movements, and I had no predetermined notion of where the movement would mesh with the image. There were lines like, "My father told me that his grandmother baked huge round cookies; and, whatever animal my father asked for, my great-grandfather could quickly bite the cookie into that shape." Of course, whatever shape the dancer's body was in then or traversing, you were immediately able to make this connection. With the coherence but also the diversity of detail in these stories, I had no doubt that there would be points of convergence that would make themselves manifest to the audience. Sure enough there were.

LB: Did you begin to feel any limitations from dance at this time?

YR: No. Not at this time. I continued to sense a field of opening up possibilities.

Also on that first Judson concert, I did this trio which had been performed earlier. Fred Herko and I had already made our debuts with choreography so we felt rather seasoned compared to the novices and younger people. I was by this time in my late twenties. Deborah Hay was only about twenty and Cindy Childs was twenty years old. Steve was also a kind of baby in the group. Trisha had presented her first solo in 1961 in a series at the Maidman Playhouse on West 42nd Street. Fred Herko and I shared a concert. I did everything I had made up to that date—five pieces; three solos, one duet, one trio. *Dance for Three People and Six Arms* was done at the Maidman—Bill Davis, Trisha, and I did it there. And at the Judson inauguration, Judith Dunn, Bill Davis and I did it.

Dance for Three People and Six Arms was predetermined movement, but the structure was indeterminate. The sequence was left up to the discretion of the performers. Certain movements had facial requirements or group requirements. If someone did the movement that had blam, blam, blam, blam in it, everyone had to join in. So there were always three people doing blam, blam, blam, blam. There were positions that had to be taken upstage or downstage, but for the most part you had about fifteen choices. So with three people and fifteen choices you have forty-five or more possibilities—I guess fifteen to the third power.

LB: I would like to skip ahead a little bit and talk about your work process—what you know about a piece before you begin. I was wondering if we could discuss *The Mind is a Muscle*. When you begin a piece, where do you draw your sources, what do you feel, etc.?

YR: Well, I'm sure it was quite different then than it is now. *The Mind is a Muscle, Part* I was *Trio A*—that was done two years before the final version.

LB: That was the first version?

YR: Yes. First there was *Trio A* which was done on a program with David Gordon and Steve Paxton in early '66. Then there was the short version of *The Mind is a Muscle* which consisted of maybe four sections with five people, also done at Judson. That was June of 1966. Then there was a longer version that was done out of town in early '68. And then the final version was done at the Anderson Theater in April of '68.

I worked for six months, I guess in late '65. At that point it was a solo, and I worked for about three hours every day. I allowed myself this latitude of time. I didn't really know what I was looking for except that each piece of movement would be very different from every other piece and nothing would repeat. I had been so involved with repetition of one kind or another. I wanted to make something that would have very discrete movements. I didn't know how I would link them up. I was not going to use chance procedures. And they would be strung together as I made them. I wouldn't reorganize it. And yet each would be different. It wasn't that one would grow out of the other. And it wouldn't be based on some kind of kinetic development—I've done this so the next one would be that. That, of course, is a more traditional modern dance way of moving or creating. Also I did not want to look at the audience. That was one of the very earliest ideas for that solo.

I had been criticized by Steve in particular for exploiting my own charisma. I had already made a solo where I blacked out my face. This was '65. It was called *Partially Improvised New Untitled Solo with Pink T-Shirt, Blue Bloomers, Red Ball, and Bach's Toccata and Fugue in D Minor.* I painted my face black to block out what I figured to be the main source of my presence and charisma. By 1965, the civil rights legislation and Supreme Court decision had been made. I didn't want to make any reference to that—racial or civil rights implications were totally absent from my thinking. When someone with Caucasian features paints their face black, the features are still there. Maybe today it would evoke that association but it certainly didn't then. For me or for that particular audience.

So I was still thinking, well, I am not going to pander to the audience or seduce them with my presence. I was very much aware and had even perhaps already written about the narcissistic involvement of the performer. I was aware of my own narcissistic pleasure certainly. Earlier you asked what was it like performing for the first time. It was as good as orgasm. I knew that was where I lived, that was where I belonged, doing that work and presenting myself physically to an audience. And that, of course, was part of the charisma. That is the urgency, and that pleasure in exhibiting oneself is part of the seduction of an audience. The performer has to experience that in order for the audience to get a sense of this presence or to be taken in by it.

So, this dialogue had begun. For Steve, it took a totally different form in his work. I was very indebted to him although it was very troublesome to me to be getting this as a critique. I was more successful as a performer than Steve was. I mean, people talked about his kind of uptight performance style. And Steve was thinking about, well, what is this convention of the gaze, this inward-looking gaze that the Judson performers have. They don't project it out. Where is it going? It is a sort of hypnotic thing. This was definitely a field for further investigation and discussion or argument. So I had done this thing where I blacked my face.

I was now going to make a solo called *The Mind is a Muscle* where I would never face the audience. It was not a proscenium situation. The audience was usually on one side, maybe three-quarters. (For most of the performances, I chose to have them on one side to get the advantage of the entire width of the performance space.) So every time the body would face the audience in this solo, the eyes were to be closed or I would avert my gaze, literally block it. Or the head would be involved in movement, turning or facing the ceiling or facing directly to the wings offstage. That was one prerequisite for this dance.

The opening move of the dance is facing away from the audience, looking behind myself, parallel feet, bent knees. I must have spent a couple of weeks working on what I could do to get out of that opening move. I would wheel around in a circle, lean into one hip, fall away in a kind of leap onto the right foot, bringing the left leg forward at the last minute, hunch my back and look at my foot. For some reason I just did this over and over again until I got the exact quality I wanted. And then I went on. It was a succession of leg-arm coordinations. Then I began to get a sense of the pacing and the dynamics. And I began to sense that what this dance was all about was not only discrete movements, which are what most of my solos are about, i.e., discrete movements with interruptions, but also a particular kind of transition. It would be about a kind of pacing where a pose is never struck. No sooner had the body arrived at the desired position than it would go immediately into the next move, not through momentum but through a very prosaic going on. And there would be very different moves—getting down on the floor, getting up. There would be this pedestrian dynamic that would suffuse and connect the whole thing. So the whole thing, though it would be composed of these fragments of movement unrelated both kinetically and positionally or shapewise, would look as though it were one long phrase. There would be no dramatic changes like leaps. There was a kind of folky step that had a rhythm to it and I worked a long time to get the syncopation out of it. In a way the opening *da, da, da, da* of the arms set the rhythm of the whole thing. There were exceptions to this rule, but this began to be the overall structure rhythmically and dynamically of this solo.

The title for *The Mind is a Muscle* had come to me early on. The alliteration of course appealed to me. Also it spoke about the life of the dancer—a life of work, dedication, of the mind requiring the same kind of daily work and stimulation as the dancer's muscle. There is a toughness to the title that I like. And it could cover almost anything that was going into this dance. I didn't know exactly what was to come—even then I called it *The Mind is a Muscle, Part 1.* This was the first part, and there would be other parts that would be of a totally different nature with more people.

For some reason it took six months to make a five-minute solo. I remember Steve telling me when he first saw it—I presented about two minutes of it at an informal workshop situation—that it was just very surprising, you had no way of predicting what would happen next.

Now, there has been so much postmodern dancing and so many ways of putting so many different things together. When I see the work of Wendy Perron, the way she sometimes puts things together, I think that has the same kind of weird, illogical, unpredictable, sequencing that was on my mind when I made *Trio A*. But it is very hard to see that in *Trio A* when you see it done today. I remember that that was the effect of it then, and that was on my mind when I was making it.

Anyway, it was finished, and I taught it to Steve and to David Gordon. We shared a concert together in January or February of '65 at Judson. It was a very unpopular concert. At that point the audiences at Judson were getting tired of some of the minimalist work. They were bored. The work was pretty dry. Some of Steve's work was pretty damn dry, austere, uningratiating. I was veering away from and trying to counter my charismatic, seductive presence—leaving the more eccentric street and madwoman incarnations. The only way out of Judson, if you were in the audience, was to walk across the performance space, and that is what happened at that concert. People trudged unhappily, disgruntledly, disconsolately across that space to get out. You had to be pretty disgusted—pretty unhappy to make a spectacle of yourself in that way.

LB: Did you feel limitations at this time?

YR: Do you mean did I take this as a critique of my own work when people did that?

LB: Yes.

YR: I was awfully excited about *Trio A*. I felt I had really done something difficult and new. Everyone learned the identical sequence. We began at slightly different times—like within ten seconds of each other. And each person had their own pace. That was another thing. In learning it, you had to find a pacing that created that look but that was appropriate for your body and your own way of hauling yourself around. So the phrases went in and out of phase. It was rarely completely unison movement. But the other thing was that I had these slats, the size of yardsticks, a whole stack of them, maybe two or three hundred of them. Someone in the balcony, in the loft of the church, flung these down one at a time in metronomic succession. And they formed a pile on one side of the space. At one performance, someone in the first row grabbed one that had fallen close to his feet, and he put his white handkerchief on it and flailed it in the air. Like saying, uncle, I have had enough of this. So it was not a very popular dance.

LB: You were talking before about the collective experience, all the ideas that come out of working with other people. Can you talk about Grand Union?

YR: Well, this is long after my tenure at Judson.

LB: Yes, we're skipping ahead.

YR: By '69 and '70 I had worked with the same group of people for several years. Of course I had known them much longer from workshops and classes in the Cunningham studio. Barbara Lloyd, Steve Paxton, David Gordon, Becky Arnold—from the middle '60s. They were an impressive group of performers and choreographers in their own right. I never thought of them as my company. They were people who made themselves available to me, and I made myself available to them and their work—Steve especially. But I was performing less and less frequently in other people's work. I was aware that I was not producing work fast enough to keep a coherent group together. Also I guess I had my own personal, psychological difficulties with being in that constant position of authority with these people whom I respected as peers and equals. I think the impetus actually came from Barbara Dilley (Barbara Lloyd).

We were going out on tour with *Continuous Project-Altered Daily* as Yvonne Rainer and Group. One of the things I had begun to do with this dance was introduce spontaneously into the performance props or situations that would require spontaneous decisions on the part of the performers. This had opened up a whole area of behavior, spontaneous behavior right in the performance, which I had not really explored before. There had been the so-called rule games, but this was structured indeterminate activity.

Around the same period I was thinking about introducing this actual behavior, rather than this professional mode of presentation—the distanced, cool style of performing something. Twyla Tharp had been videotaping rehearsals and then asking her people to learn what they saw on the videotape, including gestures, speech and the choreographic material. She was incorporating this into the final performance which made for very peculiar looking things. My way of handling that was to actually rehearse something as part of the performance—bring in new material to rehearse, bring in a prop that someone would put on for the first time that would elicit a certain kind of response.

For instance, in Kansas City, at the University of Missouri, I had brought along what I called a body adjunct. It was like a hump you put on under your shirt, and it made you look deformed, hunchback. One of the configurations required us to move very quickly using different modes of locomotion across this big space—it was a gym. And Barbara had put on this hump. I looked across at her and she was doing this movement as a hunchback, and it suddenly struck me as the most bizarre thing I had ever seen. I started to laugh as I was doing my movement, laugh uproariously. Then she saw I was getting off on her in this costume, and we went into hysterical laughter while doing this. That had never happened before. It wasn't that it was uncontrolled, and it wasn't hysterical in the sense of unprofessional behavior. But it was spontaneous response of extreme enjoyment of a certain everyday kind. So I was into eliciting this kind of thing—giving several people instructions that the other people didn't know about. They would come in and do something to interfere with what we were doing, and that would make for a certain kind of behavior.

At some point I was getting a lot of bookings from this New York Review booking agency and management company. We were going out on the road a lot and sharing rooms. We really felt high—we felt like a rock group. This creation of mine, called *Continuous Project-Altered Daily*, from its inception had incorporated the idea of continual change. Gradually I was letting go of my control, and Barbara was one of the instigators—well, why can't some of us bring in material?

At first it was difficult, and then at a certain point a momentum took over. And I saw my work literally being destroyed or overtaken, dispersed and diffused by the input of others. We began to think of ourselves as a cooperative, a collective. All of a sudden we were called Grand Union.

First the bookings came to me—Yvonne Rainer and the Grand Union, which created difficulties. Especially when people like Trisha and Douglas Dunn came into the group. Nancy Green came in at a certain point. Even though I would bend over backwards, send out publicity that was about this autonomous group, I would end up being the person who was paid the most attention. It was difficult for a while, but then at a certain point it really did become this autonomous group.

I lasted for a year in it. I wanted to do my own work. There were these psychological tensions in the group, and they were coming out in the performances in a way that I was very sensitive to. It was a group that would not rehearse together. They would just go out there cold and wing it. That I found more and more unsettling. It was just too much of a strain. So I realized the handwriting was on the wall for me. I mean, maybe I could have handled some other type of collective situation, but it had its own life. And I had a lot of ideas that required rehearsal, long rehearsal. I had to get out if I was going to go on. So I did a piece called *Grand Union Dreams*.

LB: *Grand Union Dreams* was your last work which was exclusively performance?

YR: Yes, without slides or film.

LB: However, it also contained cinematic devices such as fictional plot strategy and individual character development.

YR: Yes.

LB: So to what degree was *Grand Union Dreams* already the seed of a film?

YR: It contained the separation of performers into characters. That was the beginning of my film work. It had mortals, heroes, and gods. I had spent six weeks in India and was reading Jung when I came back. So the idea of using myths, legends, stories, and fragments of stories was very much on my mind. There was this ready-made group of people called Grand Union, and some of the material I used had actually come up in Grand Union performances. Some of the props that had been introduced in Grand Union performances I appropriated and used in *Grand Union Dreams.* Some of the material I had invented in Grand Union performances I used—like texts and activity.

I was getting into making relationships between people other than kinetic, dancelike relationships. In one section of *Grand Union Dreams* there were about ten mortals who donned these signs—words sewn onto felt aprons or bibs: father, mother, lover, friend, sister. People would take on these positions in *tableaux vivants.* At the foreground of the space there would be a trio of father, daughter, and lover sitting, standing, very simple in themselves. The positions didn't evoke anything in particular, but the combination, or the relationship made for a dramatic situation. I was looking for minimal means for suggesting melodrama.

LB: In a different way than when you had incorporated film and slides in other work?

YR: The early films were mostly about physical, athletic, dance situations. They were about juxtaposing ideas about scale—like a huge projection of legs from the knee down on a screen under which you could see normal size legs of people who came and went, who were dancing behind the screen. Ideas like that.

LB: Was this an area of confusion that you needed to separate out—at least two different kinds of ideas that were coming to the forefront?

YR: I wouldn't call it confusion, but I would call it a period of transition which never was completed. In my films today there are the same notions of scale and physical activity. It is just that notions of physical juxtaposition have been replaced by framing, dealing with the body as something that can be cropped.

This was my entry into narrative in a very general way, through costumes, props and character attribution. The main activities were physical. There was this staircase that was a holdover from *The Mind is a Muscle*. It was about forty-five inches high with steps of varying heights, on wheels so it could be rolled around. In *Grand Union Dreams* it was used for Mount Olympus. It was the stairway to heaven so to speak. The gods congregated around it. The five people who were then in Grand Union congregated around the stairs.

LB: What were some of the reasons that caused you to move away from dance into film?

YR: In the broad view, it was narrative. The conventions of cinematic narratives seemed to offer more possibilities, were more interesting to me to operate both within and against than were the conventions of dramatic theatrical narrative, i.e., the play dialogue and monologue format. In fact, I didn't even question it. There was no decision to make. I was already thinking in terms of framing and voice over.

I can't remember the very first ideas for *Lives of Performers*. There was a two-year gap between *Grand Union Dreams* and *Lives of Performers*. *Grand Union Dreams* was in 1970. In 1971, I did what was to be a precedent for this intermediary state between theater and film. It was just called *Performance*. It was done at the Whitney. I had received an NEA grant to do choreographic work. I also shot and rough cut a version of *Lives of Performers* that went into *Performance*. Dual versions were done simultaneously. The last section of *Lives of Performers* was presented as film on one side and *tableaux vivants* on the other.

Lives of Performers extended the character implications of *Grand Union Dreams*. Everyone had a name, albeit I used the names of the actual performers, and there were these fictional, romantic attributions made for them. So that first film was a combining of the factuality of my existence as a dancer, choreographer, and director and the performers' lives insofar as they were working with me. And then there was this whole fictional attribution about their romantic involvements while they were doing this work.

LB: I know you were using film in some of your other dances. What caused you to drop that mixed-media form?

YR: Film just seemed much more pliable and less static. Cutting could be fast, could be slow, could be static. And you could get instant transformations of the field—closeup, wide-shot, all these variations.

I guess, somewhat instinctually, this became clear to me when feminist film theory began to be articulated—the implications of the look as duplicated and multiplied in the spectator's look, the character's look, the camera's look, the director's look. All these interfacings of the gaze were contained in cinema. And I had already begun to explore this in live performance beginning with my own condition of being looked at, a woman who finds satisfaction and fulfillment as a performer who is looked at. So this was something that carried over into film, not totally articulated by me at the time. Hindsight gives me a much clearer perspective of this.

LB: So it seemed to be a very seamless transition for you from dance to film.

YR: Well, it was not without traumatic aspects. There was a critical moment—my last public performance at the Walker Art Center in 1975. It was a piece called *Kristina (for a . . . Opera)*, and it was about this lion tamer that I had actually seen in Germany. And there were photos of her. I had made a skimpy costume, a green-sequined two-piece brassiere and trunks, that I performed in. Again I incorporated early dances, *Three Satie Spoons,* into the first version of this multimedia piece. There were slides but no film.

I had already devised this plot—a European, Jewish refugee comes to America, gives up lion taming, and takes up choreography. John Erdman and I were the performers, and it contained this kind of mock autobiographical element. It began with John getting up and pretending to be the director of this piece but paying homage to me, Yvonne, for having taught him everything he knew! He did this long introduction, and then I came out and there were various scenes between us. It had some curious things in it considering it was my swan song to live performance.

The performance did contain some things that I didn't think about transposing to film, that were interesting as performance. One was that I played this music, I think it was Offenbach, a cello sonata. And John had told me a story about a very interesting grandmother of his, in her eighties, who still drove back and forth from New York City to Florida and was still a very adventurous person.

I had taped this story. Then John read the transcript, but he had to relearn it note by note, by listening to the tape. He had learned it like a song. Rather than reinterpreting the script, he had memorized the nuance and pitch, pauses and pacing of the original. So it had this peculiar, regurgitated quality about it. We had a record player on the stage in front of us playing this Offenbach record. Gradually, as he began to read the script, I turned up the volume which drowned him out. He and I began to talk, and then we got into this mock fight like we were disagreeing. But by the time that this was happening, the volume was so high that you couldn't hear anything he and I were saying. So there was this transformation of a somewhat formalized situation into a melodrama, a psychodrama.

Then I performed; again I showed him my dance. I was still the main performer in my performance. But I was not in very good shape. I hadn't rehearsed the dance. I had thought to myself, "Well, I'll do an improvisation. I'll wing it." I have this book on Mary Wigman with photos. I'm going to take this book on Mary Wigman out on stage with me and do an improvisation based on the photos.

Babette Mangolte had come along, and I wanted her to film it, thinking that it would later go into the film. And there was also someone there videotaping it—a dancer who lived in Minneapolis. This is 1975. It was truly a swan song.

When I saw the footage several weeks later, I looked at it and said, that's it. This is not interesting. That is not a person who should be dancing as though that is the best that she can do. This person is not enjoying being there, she is not inspired to do an improvisation. "If you're not going to work at this anymore," I said to myself, "give it up." And I did.

I was not happy in my physical condition. I was unhappy with being looked at, with that whole thing. Although there were certain things about the performance I liked, my own condition of performing was no longer satisfactory. And I was ready to move on. It was not an easy transition, but there was only one period where that unhappiness or conflict was visible publicly.

LB: One thing that you brought up had to do with an understanding or reading of feminist film theory. I don't know if I should use the word *formal,* but during your introduction into filmmaking, there was sort of a male-identified, avant-garde film practice typified by maybe Michael Snow, Hollis Frampton, George Landow. I am wondering how you made a synthesis and a location for yourself in that.

YR: Stan Brakhage, Kenneth Anger, etc. I had followed all this work in the '60s, of course. I first saw a Maya Deren film at the Living Theater around 1960–61. I followed much of this work to keep up. The ideas didn't really turn me on in a way that Cage's ideas in music and '60s art practices had turned me on. Godard was someone I followed out of interest but not a passionate interest—Pop culture aspects of Godard. The pretty people and the degree to which he was breaching or violating those traditions were a little too subtle for me at the time. *Breathless* didn't have much meaning for me. However, by 1970 three Hollis Frampton films were really a turn-on for me: *Hapax Legomena: Nostalgia, Poetic Justice,* and *Critical Mass.* I would say they were very influential.

As far as feminism goes, I didn't care whether these filmmakers were guys or little green monsters or transvestites. There wasn't a certain point where I was suddenly inspired by feminism. It was a slow, evolving set of problems for me. I remember reading *Sisterhood is Powerful* more or less when it came out. But I was reading it in a reactive rage having to do with the breakup of a long relationship.

By '73 when I was working on *This is a story of a woman who . . . ,* I was aware that the latest feminist groundswell was giving me permission to deal with myself and psychological issues from my own point of view. I mean, my autobiographical interests and experience as a woman were converging and being given support by this background of feminist writing and thinking. But as far as models for formal strategies, these had been forged in the male-dominated art world. They were strategies that I did not question and that continued to be productive and useful to me. As you know, I took issue with the *Camera Obscura* feminists who came to interview me around 1975. These ideas of counter-strategy are useful to feminism as they are useful to any resistant discourse, I would say. And there is nothing essentially male or female in language. I think it is how you use it, and what you bring it to bear upon. So yes, these strategies were dominated by men, and they were absorbed and exploited by me in my work.

LB: Let me ask you one question here. There is already, in the subtitle of *Lives of Performers (a melodrama),* the seed of oppositional thought to this dominant avant-garde stripping away of formal practices.

YR: Yes, sure. A key event in my work around 1970 was the introduction of narrative-type objects or objects that lent themselves to a certain kind of narrative. I pointed out how the stairs, which had been purely a gymnastic device, a surrealistic stairway leading nowhere carpeted on wheels in *The Mind is a Muscle,* became Olympus in *Grand Union Dreams.* Also in *Grand Union Dreams* there were other props, e.g., a suitcase. Then I got turned on by the Pabst film with Louise Brooks, *Pandora's Box.* In '71, *Lives of Performers* ends with these *tableaux vivants,* and there is a gun. I'm reenacting the series of published production stills from a scenario of *Pandora's Box.* So these artifacts of melodrama are being introduced into my work, and I am aware of a whole new set of connotations that I am not totally prepared to pursue. But the mere introduction of these artifacts suggested melodrama to me.

I was aware then that there was a certain amount of irony in calling this stripped down narrative with the barest hints of a story, a melodrama. But in terms of where I had come from, these were very loaded terms to introduce: a murder, a woman's rage, the other woman, the femme fatale, the gun, the suitcase. I had done this in dance with loaded objects—the mattresses in *Parts of Some Sextets.* I chose those mattresses for their multiple dramatic and psychological connotations. They were not sofa pillows, they were mattresses with the striped mattress ticking. So they suggested everything from a derelict flophouse to a hospital, sex, sleep, and dreams; and I felt I had to add nothing to make this point. The very presence of these objects provided as much as I wanted in terms of directing the attention to these references.

As to the political implications of calling this a melodrama and beginning to refer to women's issues, I wasn't so aware of how '40s melodrama in film contained submerged mythologies about women and the ways in which the conventions of narrative filmmaking constrain, limit, or degrade women. Of course none of that writing had happened yet.

LB: In the introduction of *Film About a Woman Who . . .* , there is a statement which says, "This is the poetically licensed story of a woman who finds it difficult to reconcile certain external facts with her image of her own perfection. It is also the same woman's story if we say she can't reconcile these facts with her image of her own deformity . . . Not that it is a matter of victims and oppressors. She simply can't find alternatives to being inside with her fear or standing in the rain with her self-contempt." Can you talk about that?

YR: I can't really talk about what I was thinking then. Certainly now it seems I was torn between the idea of myself as a victim and an alternative that seemed to be a suffragette—the big woman to me. That is why I found calling myself a feminist not accurate at that time. Because to me a feminist was someone who was politically active or making documentaries with a lot of facts and statistics. My films, I did not feel were overtly political.

LB: But at the same time you were investigating an entirely new form. So that the interpretation that you had of feminism was an overview, or a version of what ought to be your job in terms of feminist analysis. No?

YR: I was not making a feminist analysis. I was making an art based on various kinds of resistance, which now seems a highly political enterprise. At the time, I thought of the feminist as a much more active, out-in-the-world person. Now, of course, I see the political and feminist implications of that early work, and of my dancing too, which has evolved into incorporating more precisely or concretely political and theoretical issues.

LB: Well, in terms of *This is a story of a woman who . . .* and your previous statement about making an art that was in resistance or in opposition—in resistance to what, in opposition to what?

YR: Smug assumptions about what art should be—idealization of the dancer for instance. The idea that the dancer had to be regal or goddess-like, the idea of modern dance pioneers as matriarchs—which carried over once they were institutionalized and the vocabularies were codified as means for training the body—seemed so stultifying and limited. So these ideas were very much in keeping with the thrust of Pop art and Minimal art, ideas of incorporating debris, noise, silence, these low, so-called degraded art forms into the work. The introduction of pedestrian movement was in keeping with this impetus.

LB: When you completed *Film About a Woman Who . . . ,* how did it fit in with other kinds of avant-garde film that was going on at that time?

YR: What is more interesting to me is the question of how the earlier film, *Lives of Performers,* appeared in the general film context when it came out. I seemed very isolated. I remember telling Annette Michelson, this is a very flawed film. Well, it seemed so crude. It is crude technically. It doesn't flow together; it is very episodic; it stops and starts; it is against these white blank walls. And of course, parts of it were totally calculated. Like the way it is a big, bare loft space and there isn't even a decent couch. I didn't even own a couch at that time. There is a pile of material with a bedspread over it, a wooden chair. The camera pulls back and you see lights. It was very strange. So I thought of it almost as crude. I had almost overdone it.

I had sat down one day and just typed up this weird script: "And then Valda says, and then they go to, and so-and-so leaves, and then, and then, and then, and here Valda says." Mainly it was like captions for choreographic comings together, groupings and regroupings, interpreting and extending the implications of groupings and regroupings. In this case there was a very small number of people, basically about four people.

I had deliberately mixed up the names. If you tried to follow the plot, who was involved with whom, it was very confusing—especially since John Erdman became ill. When we made the soundtrack we tried to assign various pages of the script with instructions: read this, Valda; you could paraphrase this, Fernando here; read this; I want that sentence read. John's voice is nowhere to be found even though his image is there. So there are these peculiar discrepancies and ambiguities. You cannot follow the story although a very loaded set of circumstances begins to emerge—of infidelity, emotional entanglement, sexual conflict, etc.

LB: Your work always has those layers—density and contradictions.

YR: Deceptions. My films always were meant to confound in a certain way. You can get involved with them up to a point, and then you have to start over. The spectators themselves have to figure out their position, their relation in it.

LB: Well, you play a lot with the audience expectations.

YR: Yes. Right.

LB: You talked about *Lives of Performers* and this idea of sexual conflict and emotional risk taking, putting out one's emotional self to threat rather than presenting as traditional Hollywood films do—the idea of physical danger. I guess I want to get back to *This is the story of a woman who . . .* in terms of the representation of the central female character.

YR: Who is now called "she," right? She has no name.

LB: Right. Can you talk about the expectations of the audience? You're always confounding and presenting contradictions to the audience.

YR: At the level of narrative?

LB: At the level of narrative, but also at a psychological level. The audience falls into a level of narrative and then is asked to move back into a psychological interpretation, involving themselves more closely than traditional film requires now.

YR: Oh, that is complicated.

LB: So can you talk about the presentation of the female as a victim, maybe even a perfect victim, in *Film About a Woman Who . . .* ? In the disrobing scene, you have this presentation of extreme sexual fantasy and extreme vulnerability. Then you have this mediated media representation of Angela Davis. So there is the contradiction between someone who is following something and does herself in, in terms of the sexual fantasy, and then the way the social structure does in Angela Davis.

YR: I never thought of it that way. This business of victimization begins in *Lives of Performers,* of course, with the melodrama at the end, the reference to the film *Pandora's Box* in which, of course, Lulu is stabbed by Jack the Ripper. In *Film About a Woman Who . . . . ,* this theme is repeated—and this connection is totally unconscious on my part—in the *Psycho* stills. It is about a woman who gets stabbed in the tub. When that was pointed out to me I was really blown away. I was interested in Hitchcock and cutting, and the woman getting stabbed seemed to me to be secondary. But obviously my artistic unconscious is always in there. The return of the repressed, yes.

In *Film About a Woman Who . . . ,* there is the sexual fantasy enacted where the two figures, a man and a woman, disrobe Renfreu Neff; and it is sort of at her bidding. She seems a victim in that she is being exposed and revealed for the camera; but also it is her fantasy and she is calling the moves, so to speak. She presents her foot when she wants her shoe removed; she presents her arm when she wants her bracelet removed. And she prevents the man from untying her waistband. This whole scene is rather excruciating because it is so slow and complete. She is very sumptuously dressed, and every last garment is removed.

The final garment to be removed is her underwear, and this is done in a separate shot. It is a ten-minute take where the camera moves back as the underpants are slowly lowered by Dempster Leech; and as they are raised, the camera moves in. From a very tight shot it becomes a wider shot with Shirley and me on either side of the sofa. And I have these peculiar things pasted on my face. The camera moves in, it veers off of Renfreu's pubic area as the underwear is pulled up, closes in on my face—extreme closeup to the point where these texts on my face can be read. They were cut from newspapers. I made a strategic error cutting exactly on the columns, so that it looks like it was maybe typed. You cannot really tell that it was newsprint. I should have made a ragged edge around it to show other columns. I wanted these texts to be seen as coming from a public tabloid.

We move in and we read these peculiar, very privatized expressions of passion by a woman for a man—"I love you, my husband." There are four of these: on my forehead, either cheek, and on the chin. The final one reveals, "I love you more than ever, George Jackson, my husband. Forever, I love you forever." My point was that there was this woman, Angela Davis, with this public persona of being a radical, a militant, a Marxist whose most private diaries are being revealed in court to be used by the prosecution to establish her connection to George Jackson in this conspiratorial situation. So we've moved from the staged enacted victimization where the woman with the sexual fantasy is in collusion herself. I mean, her very innermost fantasies are involved with a certain exhibition, narcissism and psychological collusion. And now we're at this actual public arena of social collusion. The audience certainly has a lot of time to think about this, but I don't know whether it connects in the way in which I've articulated it—you've helped me to articulate it.

I was thinking about the theme of sexual passion running through my films and here is another example of it. Also of course, I wasn't sure whether I myself wasn't exploiting Angela Davis in simply using this material. So it is very complicated. But it was something very powerful for me at the time and continues to be. It points out all the problems that are involved in dealing with the idea of a victim. Do you make the woman a victim all over again in the cinema, with the camera by using her as a stripped away object, objectifying her this way? In my next film, although there are two scenes with sexualized women, the main female character is present only as voice-over. And I am still pursuing this reaction to my work over ten years later. This problem is being addressed by women filmmakers in all kinds of ways. The latest one is Bette Gordon's *Variety.*

LB: Well, in what way in your films do you see emotional risk rather than physical danger being one of the main activities, and physical presentation, physical action being replaced by text—words and language?

YR: Ruby Rich has made that analogy. The arena of the action film has been replaced by psychological risk. That was never too clear for me. Certainly action has been replaced by speaking and by words, by language in all of its manifestations: print, speaking, monologue, recitation, voice-over. That still interests me. It is sort of part and parcel of low-budget filmmaking, but also there is for me a moral and political dimension that continues to be vital and useful. The action film is certainly the opposite of a contemplative film. I make films which may drive viewers to distraction, but also provide this arena where they have room, plenty of space and time to contemplate issues or their own place and position within certain issues. You may say that the way in which I use this very slow pacing and extended time, repetitive framing, long shots and shots of long duration derives from the music concert of the '60s—LaMonte Young and John Cage—where you listen and your mind starts going away. You think about yourself; you think about what you had for breakfast. There is that type of possibility or hazard in making these kinds of films. But it is something that continues to attract me as an alternative to what I call the thralldom of traditional narrative cinema where your mind gets taken away by these strategies of identification and vicarious, voyeuristic action and enactment.

LB: In *Kristina Talking Pictures,* the central character—or characters, because they are played by more than one person—seems to represent the embodiment of a paradox of the public persona. Can you talk about that in terms of all the different syntheses that you make—what you read, what you see in documentary type extrapolations as well as autobiography?

YR: Well, there has always been this interest in the overlapping areas of public and private, how one exhibits oneself in terms of everyday life and also for the special occasion, the party, the stage. What one chooses to reveal or conceal. It is not exactly a paradox but in film I eschew action and prefer stasis, prefer to put all the action into speaking, into language; whereas the live performances were all based on activity, and even where there was stillness there was still a physicality suggested that was more akin to action than to the language-oriented strategies of my films. People literally sit in bed in *Kristina Talking Pictures* and yap for forty minutes. Annette Michelson who plays the patient in *Journeys from Berlin/1971* sits all but strapped to that chair and talks of sex, of being in the world, of other people who have been in the world in a very active way—women who followed their husbands to Siberia, literally walked to Siberia. So there is this discrepancy between my means and the images that are evoked. I wouldn't dream of intercutting a photo or a reenactment in any form of a woman following her husband to Siberia. And where I do choose to show action, it is again done almost as this bare arena into which is introduced some trace of an environment or situation. Like the architectural backdrop in *Journeys from Berlin* in front of which a man and a woman repeatedly walk. Their paths intersect through the editing strategies, while the soundtrack is these highly detailed, elaborated narratives of terrorist, so-called terrorist, *attentats.*

LB: So you have set up various different situations. I would like to ask you at this point, to what degree does the paradox reflect you and your equivocations?

YR: Well all the way down the line. Just in the way the camera seems to reveal and yet doesn't. The way photography suggests truth and reality, and yet constantly comes up against a world of appearances. The ideology of beliefs and belief systems. I guess at any given moment I'm interested in having these things collide. The politics of representation—which not only refer to things outside the film, like social constructs, but to the strategies of the film itself. So my films differ and probably will continue to differ from films "across the Rubicon" of narrative cinema. I may begin to get a little disjointed here, in the way that I speak of these things, because I haven't resolved them.

And it is why it has taken me so long to come out with another film. I have felt myself beginning to cross this frontier of narrative. I'm scratching at the frontier. You might say that a lot of people have been scratching at this frontier for a number of years and now have crossed it. I will continue to scratch, I think—which means that a narrative line will only be pursued for a limited duration in any given film; but the ways in which I will gainsay and violate the very thing I set up will continue to be of interest to me as strategic operations.

LB: So we are not talking full-blown narrative here when you say scratching?

YR: Well, we are talking now about my current project where we follow a man, or two performers who play a male character. We actually will follow them around quite a bit in a realistic situation. But the voice-over and the introduction of documentary material, which doesn't directly deal with this man's physical, fictionalized situation, has to do with the environment in which the woman on the soundtrack, his ex-lover, has placed herself. So these two very separate fields will be colliding constantly I think. There will be a somewhat coherent narrative strand, but it's going to be intercut between soundtrack and image. At this point it is still pretty rough. A lot of it will be worked out on the editing table.

However I describe it, I still think of narrative being of interest only to the degree to which I can establish it and undermine it almost simultaneously—which, of course, is what people like Peter Wollen and Laura Mulvey have attempted to do in various ways. I will do it in another way. Films like, you might call them New Wave films, don't seem to worry about this anymore. Like the films of Michael Oblowitz, Bette Gordon's new film, and Lizzie Borden's *Born in Flames*.

LB: So you are saying they are more a celebration of narrative.

YR: Or more accepting of a direct relation to narrative.

LB: You said that with film you could feel more connected with your audience, and that that gives you great comfort.

YR: At a certain point, I just felt I had broadened the field. However I presented myself as a dancer, I was still this object of fascination which provided this voyeuristic escape for an audience. I was the dancing lady no matter what I did. Now, with all these multifarious narrative and non-narrative strategies, something else is at work. I'm not providing the spectator with this image that can either repel or fascinate. I'm really interested in getting away from that.

In this next film I run a risk with this man—of course, it doesn't have to be a woman; it can be a man. How will I create this male character without this same operation coming into play? I don't know whether or not I can do it, but it is challenging. I don't want to make a man you love to hate, or a man who would be a new man. In terms of my project I don't know what the correct procedure will be. But I'm going to have to work it out and face that very selfsame problem. It cannot be avoided, but everyone must deal with it fresh with every film.

LB: Do you feel that you came into your own as a director with *Journeys From Berlin?*

YR: No. Not necessarily. In a way, it is my most ambitious film, but I don't know that it is the best. I mean, it has its own problems in terms of politics.

LB: I was thinking of the more traditional stuff that goes into filmmaking—location, working with actors and actresses, etc. I see your films as being hybrid, as being something very much defined and developed, as not finding a neat little niche to fit into. So in this film you have to take on the role of formal director. I was thinking in particular of the scene with Annette which you referred to before, which seemed to me to be this master performance on her part.

YR: A *tour de force.* That virtuoso performance happens because she has mastered, so to speak, this very elaborate language, which came first. I was not thinking, of course, of a virtuoso performance. I thought of her landing on a dime and taking off into something totally different, or like talking very rhetorically and then talking very intimately, changing the sentence structure midway, doing these non sequitur reconstructions of coherent language and description, kind of hit and run with subject matter.

LB: Sort of as it unfolds to her shrink?

YR: Right. Which could be interpreted as stream of consciousness. But, of course, as one shrink who saw it said, that is not the way patients speak. Of course it's not. In the way it runs on and in the way that it is directed at one person, even though that person changes form from boy to woman to man, it can be interpreted as an analytic session because nowhere else is talking so obsessive, and talking so obsessively so important. The film puts this in a very artificial situation where you might say the unconscious is enacted in the background by these big shadowy movements of people walking, sitting, and engaged in task activities like rolling out a carpet, etc. So yes, I run the risk there of making her into a new object of fascination, but in the way that my presentation of myself in dances did earlier. I think that aspect of it is subservient to the language. She becomes a character, but she remains the servant of the language, of the writing.

LB: It is interesting when you say she becomes this object of fascination but has this incredible ability to dominate through language. In a way, instead of someone who is sitting there to be looked at and taken up, the language comes back and represents itself as a phallus almost.

YR: Why phallus?

LB: Because of her control.

YR: Are you saying that language is necessarily male?

LB: No. When a woman is set up to be looked at, the idea is that we are in a male-defined structure. When a woman puts it back, she is appropriating strategies.

YR: So she is simultaneously male and female. That is an interesting solution to the problem. I hadn't thought of it that way.

LB: How does your interest in psychoanalysis contribute to the major themes in your work: ambiguity and power, interpersonal relationships, sexuality, male/female dichotomies?

YR: My interest in psychoanalysis, unlike many feminist theories today, came out of my own involvement with psychotherapy for many years, which provided various points of departure for aesthetic choices and investigations. So, the autobiographical component here is inextricable from that history of introspection, that examination of my own psychic operations. I owe a great deal to my own therapy. Now, the theoretical aspects of it are somewhat secondary and of course very interesting; they overlap and repeat a lot of my own insights. That is what intrigues me and often bothers me about a great deal of this work based on a psychoanalytic Lacanian model that seems very divorced from actual experience. My films do come out of a very concrete experience which is both their limitation and their power. I refer to this whole notion of the look, and the woman operating in the social constraints of the look in patriarchic structures. As we have discussed, I was involved with this theory long before it was articulated. And it comes out in a very concrete and precise way in my films, in a way that I think is in some ways more accessible to a general audience than in the more theoretically based films that came later.

Then there is another argument, also from feminist quarters. My films have been attacked for their elitist strategies that came out of the avant-garde art world context. But they are this mix of nonpopulist aesthetic strategies and accessible content and subject matter—sexual conflict, ambivalence, personal crisis, feminine rage, etc. That is what has made *Film About a Woman Who . . .* the most popular of my films. The interest lies in that convergence of very specific experience and authentic voice with these so-called avant-garde strategies.

LB: In terms of the visual pleasure that women traditionally provide to a film audience and the absence of visual pleasure from your films, can you talk about choices made in the film that you are working on now with the absence of a female central character?

YR: Well, as it has been pointed out to me, there are other pleasures than the female body in this life, and in cinema. The mantelpiece in *Journeys* is a great source of pleasure for many people—this changing, intimate landscape of objects, references, images, etc. There is very often an animal in my films, a dog or cat. There is humor in *Film About a Woman Who . . .* though maybe it doesn't happen often enough. Many people who have seen *Journeys* a second time say to me that the first time they are busy trying to figure it out, but the second time they realize it is awfully funny. There are a great many small jokes in it if you relax—which is a problem. How do you make a complex film but also one that doesn't require a second viewing to find enjoyment?

I don't do a Straub-Huillet kind of film where it is all education and no play. I am interested in different kinds of playfulness, or interjections of materials that offer relief from something that has gone on too long or is too static. In *Film About a Woman Who . . .* , there is that subway train shot. Shirley and Dempster are facing the camera, and I am sitting perpendicular to them on another seat. I hand Shirley a piece of paper and she starts reading it and bursts into hilarious laughter. Then *I* start laughing because she is laughing. I'm so delighted that she is laughing. Then she looks at me laughing so hard and it makes her laugh even harder. I think it is very enjoyable to watch people engaged in that kind of very spontaneous enjoyment. That is a vicarious pleasure, but it is genuinely infectious also. There could be more of that, more slapstick in my films. I haven't quite figured that one out. In this new film I'm thinking about a seduction scene that might be very funny using critical theory as dialogue.

LB: As the language of seduction?

YR: Right. The capacity and the use of this massive body of theory for seduction has not been explored—the way in which it is used by individuals or at conferences, even on the printed page.

LB: In what way are you victim to that kind of seduction?

YR: Victim?

LB: Susceptible.

YR: Not vulnerable, but susceptible. I have noticed it. Sometimes reading Stephen Heath is a turn-on. I can't account for it—my fascination with that theory. Even though it has never become a language in which I am comfortable. I often make an ass of myself trying to speak theoretical language, but reading it I'm quite fascinated. At various periods I read it quite intensively. Of course, it becomes problematic when I have to teach it, speak it, and explain it. I can't break it down. It becomes very difficult. But this business of seductive properties of language is interesting to think about.

LB: In what ways would you define your work to be a search?

YR: In every way. In every conceivable way. That is what it is about. That is why it continues to be interesting. Search may not be the right word. Exploration. A search implies there is a final closure of some kind, as if you can find the pot of gold or ultimate solution. I think of art as an ongoing exploration rather than a search for a conclusion, an ongoing set of questions, finding new ways to ask the questions, and visual answers. At any point you deal with a question by presenting, if not a resolution, a treatment or a way of addressing a question. So it is not a search for answers. I guess the overall question is how do we understand the world in which we live? And how do we resist other people's answers?

LB: I have one last question. How would you define success for yourself?

YR: I can see it in the questions raised for me by other people's work. It is very hard to see it in relation to my own work. Where they've been looking for certainty, I have presented a temporary interpretation and the notion that there is more to be said. I hate the idea of any representation indicating a correct politics or a correct way to think about things. I don't mean to disclaim what I'm doing. *Journeys from Berlin* has obvious limitations; it doesn't ask enough questions for one thing. And I always run the risk of getting too involved in the subjective and personal experiences. That is probably what my later films try to address, not as successfully as the earlier films, the idea of presenting the personal aspect of experience or social life.

So I don't know if I feel that any of my work is successful. Success obviously is where your work continues to stimulate people, provide a field for discussion, and provide people with energy to go on making things or doing things. I used to be concerned about this mass audience and I am not anymore. There are many overlapping circles of activity. It doesn't matter what the volume is. What matters is that films affect these circles that are not sealed off from each other—that they affect each other. And I think that is happening now.

In a way, it is an exciting time even though the world around us seems to be going to hell on roller skates. I see enough people engaged in these questions of cinema and artmaking that it seems a vital time. It seems a time in which it is important to make art—and to go on asking questions and taking risks in art.

Looking Myself in the Mouth

This essay, which appeared in *October,* no. 17 (Summer 1981), constitutes a phase of my ongoing (interior) dialogue with John Cage, culminating—at least to all the intents and purposes of the present volume—in a Commencement Address delivered at the School of the Museum of Fine Arts in Boston in 1997. (See p. 130) May he rest in peace. Having been privileged to know him, however, I doubt if he would want to.

> Sliding Out of Narrative and Lurching
> Back In, Not Once but . . .
> Is the "New Talkie" Something
> to Chirp About?
> From Fiction to Theory
> (Kicking and Screaming)
> Death of the Maiden, I Mean Author, I
> Mean Artist . . . No, I Mean Character
> A Revisionist Narrativization of/with
> Myself as Subject (Still Kicking) via
> John Cage's Ample Back

I. *A Likely Story: What I Know and What I Think I Feel*

She says, "Yes, I was talking with Joan Braderman about the subject in signifying practice, and she brought up the idea that everything is fiction except theory."

Hard as she tries to focus on this most intriguing idea, she finds herself distracted by the recognition of an annoying habit to which she reverts whenever discussing theory, viz., a tendency to transform theory into narrative by interpolating what she calls "concrete experience" in the form of a first-person pronoun and progressive verb, such as "Yes, I was talking with . . ." or "I've been reading this book by . . ." or, even worse, "Yesterday as I was walking down Broadway, I was thinking . . ." The obvious motive might be to bolster or support her own argument by referring to known and respected figures who have advanced similar arguments, or to make an analogy that might illuminate the issue at hand. There is, however, another way to describe the phenomenon which points to either a conflict or a contradiction—depending on how one looks at it.

(Artist as Exemplary Sufferer)

(Artist as Self-Absorbed Individualist)

(Artist as Changer of the Subject)

She knows that the content of her thoughts consists entirely of what she's read, heard, spoken, dreamt, and thought about what she's read, heard, spoken, dreamt. She knows that thought is not something privileged, autonomous, originative, and that the formulation "Cogito ergo sum" is, to say the least, inaccurate. She knows, too, that her notion of "concrete experience" is an idealized, fictional site where contradictions can be resolved, "personhood" demonstrated, and desire fulfilled forever. Yet all the same the magical, seductive, narrative properties of "Yes, I was talking . . ." draw her with an inevitability that makes her slightly dizzy. She stands trembling between fascination and skepticism. She moves obstinately between the two.

"Yes, I am constructed in language," she thinks. "And no, I don't think I've ever really advocated a 'restored integrity of the self.'" She pauses, bites at a cuticle, and finally—in a burst of sheer exasperation—faces the camera squarely and blurts, "But when I say, 'Yes, I was thinking . . . ,' you'd just better believe me!"

> Linguistically, the author is never more than the instance writing, just as *I* is nothing other than the instance saying *I*: language knows a 'subject', not a 'person', and this subject, empty outside of the very enunciation which defines it, suffices to make language 'hold together', suffices, that is to say, to exhaust it.

Roland Barthes[1]

(Artist as Medium)

(Artist as Ventriloquist)

II. *The Cagean Knot*

In the late 1950s and early 1960s the ongoing modernist assault took as its targets certain assumptions by then codified in the institution of American modern dance: the necessity of musical accompaniment; the inadmissability—and necessity of transformation—of everyday movement; the rigid and inviolable separations between humorous, tragic, dramatic, and lyrical forms; the existence of rules governing sequence, climax, development of movement ("theme and variations"), and the relationship of movement to music, clichéd notions of coherence and unity, and exact conditions under which "dissonance" might replace "harmony" (as in "modern" themes of "alienation"). You heard a lot of Bartók at dance concerts in those days.

The forerunners of this assault were Merce Cunningham and John Cage.

(Artist as Innovator)

In mutual determination they succeeded in opening a veritable Pandora's Box, an act that launched in due course a thousand dancers', composers', writers', and performance artists' ships, to say nothing of the swarms of salubriously nasty ideas it loosed upon an increasingly general populace, ideas which are apparent even today in fluxus-like punk performances. I would venture to say that by now the "Cagean effect" is almost as endemic as the encounter group. I say "Cagean" and not "Cunninghamian" because it is Cage who has articulated and published the concepts which I shall be addressing here and which have been especially problematic in my own development. It is not my intention to force the lid shut on John's Box, but rather to examine certain troubling implications of his ideas even as they continue to lend themselves to amplification in art-making.

Only a man born with a sunny disposition could have said:

> This play, however, is an affirmation of life, not an attempt to bring order out of chaos nor to suggest improvements on creation, but simply a way of waking up to the very life we're living which is so excellent once one gets one's mind and one's desires out of its way and lets it act of its own accord.

John Cage[2]

(Artist as Consumer)

Let's not come down too heavily on the goofy naiveté of such an utterance, on its invocation of J. J. Rousseau, on Cage's adherence to the messianic ideas of Bucky Fuller some years back, with their total ignoring of worldwide struggles for liberation and the realities of imperialist politics, on the suppression of the question, "*Whose* life is so excellent and at what cost to others?" Let's focus on the means by which we will awaken to this excellent life: by getting our minds and desires out of the way, by making way for an art of indeterminacy to be practiced by everyone, an art existing in the gap between life and art. All this and more has been stated hundreds of times in more ways than one.

Who am I and what is my debt to John Cage? My early dances (1960–62) employed chance procedures or improvisation to determine sequences of choreographed movement phrases. At that point, for some of us who performed at Judson Church in New York City, repetition, indeterminate sequencing, sequence arrived at by aleatory methods, and ordinary/untransformed movement were a slap in the face to the old order, and, dimly beknownst to us, reached straight

(Artist as Transgressor)

back to the surrealists via the expatriated Duchamp. Our own rationales were clear, on the offensive, and confident. We were "opening up possibilities" and "thwarting expectations and preconceptions." A frequent response to the bafflement of the uninitiated was "Why not?" We were received with horror and enthusiasm. I can't beguile myself into thinking that the world has not been the same since.

What is John Cage's gift to some of us who make art? This: the relaying of conceptual precedents for methods of nonhierarchical, indeterminate organization which can be used with a critical intelligence, that is, selectively and productively, not, however, so we may awaken to this excellent life; on the contrary, so we may the more readily awaken to the ways in which we have been led to believe that this life is so excellent, just, and right.

The reintroduction of selectivity and control, however, is totally antithetical to the Cagean philosophy, and it is selectivity and control that I have always intuitively—by this I mean without question—brought to bear on Cagean devices in my own work. In the light of semiological analysis I have found vindication of those intuitions. In the same light it is possible to see Cage's decentering—or violation of the unity—of the "speaking subject" as more apparent than real.

Before going on I wish to say that it makes me mad that, as important a figure as he is to any discussion of American modernism, John Cage has not to my knowledge been examined within the framework of the various reworkings of Freudian and Marxist theory that have been accumulating with such impressive results over the past two decades. In France and England this is in part attributable to the fact that such theoretical writings have concentrated on literature and film to the exclusion of music. Not that the French—with their tendency to romanticize American "irrationalism"—could do him justice at this point. The English know little about him, and the Germans zeroed in on him too early to make use of French critical theory. I am ignorant of writings on him that may have appeared in other countries in which he has performed and lectured extensively, such as Sweden and Denmark. In America I tend to blame the avant-garde critical establishment for its neglect of this most influential man. So whom does that leave? Me?! Well, sometimes artists rush in where critics refuse to tread. In

(Artist as Failed Primitive)

(Artist as Failed Intellectual)

the noisy silence that surrounds the man, I shall produce a few semiotic chirps.

III. *Five-Hundred-Pound Canary*

What are the implications of the Cagean abdication of principles for assigning importance and significance? A method for making indeterminate, or for randomizing, a sequence of signifiers produces a concomitant arbitrariness in the relation of signifier to signified, a situation characterized not by an effacement of signifiers by signified as in *Gone with the Wind,* nor by a shifting relationship of signifier to signified whereby the signifier itself, or the act of signifying, by being foregrounded, becomes problematic, but by a denial and suppression of a relationship altogether.

What is this but an attempt to deny the very function of language and, by extension, the signifying subject, which is, according to Lacan's definition, dependent on and constructed through and in systems of signification, i.e., language?

> *A signifying practice . . .* is a complex process which assumes a (speaking) subject admitting of mutations, loss of infinitization, discernable in the modifications of his discourse but remaining irreducible to its formality alone, since they refer back on the one hand to unconscious-instinctual processes and, on the other, to the socio-historical constraints under which the practice in question is carried on.

Julia Kristeva[3]

The highest purpose is to have no purpose at all.

John Cage

For Cage, either to problematize, i.e., call into question, a "purposive" subject, or to grant admission to a "mutating," finite one, would have been to risk becoming reentangled in those hated measurements of genius and inspiration

(Artist as Shaman)

(Artist as Visionary)

that particularly infested the world of music, and in those "ambiguities, hidden meanings (which require interpretation), . . . silent purposes and obscure contents (which give rise to commentary)."[4] Cage's solution was to throw out the baby with the bathwater. In the absence of a signifying subject, not only "modifications of discourse" become untenable, but also the concept of an unconscious which manifests itself in the heterogeneity and contradictions of the subject as it is positioned in relationships of identity and difference by "socio-historical constraints," not the least of which is the patriarchal order itself. Trying to operate outside of these processes, a Cagean "nonsignifying practice" sees itself as existing in a realm of pure idea, anterior to language—without mind, without desire, without differentiation, without finitude. In a word, that realm of idealism which so much of our capricious, wavering, flawed, lurching twentieth-century art has similarly failed—while being so committed—to violate.

> Surrealism, unable to accord language a supreme place (language being a system and the aim of the movement being, romantically, a direct subversion of codes—itself moreover illusory: a code cannot be destroyed, only 'played off'), contributed to the desacrilization of the image of the Author by ceaselessly recommending the abrupt disappointment of expectations of meaning.

Roland Barthes[5]

From the standpoint of consumption, if meaning is constantly being subverted before a practice that refuses to make or break signs, if the avowed goal of a work is a succession of "nonsignifying signifiers," one is left with an impenetrable web of undifferentiated events set in motion by and referring back to the original flamboyant artist-gesture, in this case the abandonment of personal taste. The work thus places an audience in the "mindless" (sensual?) position of appreciating a manifestation of yet one more

Artist as Transcendental Ego

and excludes it from participation in the forming of the meanings of that manifestation just as surely as any monolithic, unassailable, and properly validated masterpiece. John Cage can now—and perhaps always could—be safely taught in any high school music appreciation course. His genius is beyond question; the product of that genius beyond ambiguity.

> What was it actually that made me choose music rather than painting? Just because they said nicer things about my music than they did about my paintings? But I don't have absolute pitch. I can't keep a tune. In fact, I have no talent for music. The last time I saw her, Aunt Phoebe said, "You're in the wrong profession."

John Cage[6]

(Artist as Misfit)

I was telling some of my students at the Whitney Independent Study Program that ten years ago I had been invited there to conduct a seminar. I had begun by playing a record of Billie Holiday singing "The Way You Look Tonight," repeatedly lifting and replacing the arm of the record player as, with increasing difficulty and embarrassment, I tried to learn the melody. I couldn't get it and had at length to give it up. At this point in the story Marty Winn said, "So they hired you!"

IV. *Bang the Tale Slowly*

> After I had been studying with him for two years, Schoenberg said, "In order to write music you must have a feeling for harmony." I then explained to him that I had no feeling for harmony. He then said that I would always encounter an obstacle, that it would be as though I came to a wall through which I could not pass. I said, "In that case I will devote my life to beating my head against that wall."

John Cage[7]

I was just beginning to congratulate myself for having finally triumphed, in *Journeys from Berlin/1971,* over the tyranny of narrative. I didn't need it anymore, I told myself. The distinct parts of that film never come together in a spaciotemporal continuity. From this point of view, narrative seemed no longer to be an issue. If the film made any effort toward integrating the separate "speakers," it was at the level of another kind of discourse, propelled not by narrative, but by a heterogeneous interweaving of verbal texts acting on/against/in relation to images. What a thrilling idea: to be free of the compelling and detested domination of cinematic narrativity with its unseen, unspoken codes for arranging images and language with a "coherence, integrity, fullness, and closure," so lacking in the imperfect reality it purports to mirror.

Upon closer examination, however, it becomes clear that a particular aspect of narrative, namely character, is a consistent presence in *Journeys from Berlin/1971* as it is—often by dint of its conspicuous absence—in my three previous films. It was, in fact, a decisive factor in a move from dance to film in the early '70s. Upon closer examination it seems to me that I am going to be banging my head against narrative for a long time to come.

> But once we have been alerted to the intimate relationship that Hegel suggests exists between law, historicality, and narrativity, we cannot but be struck by the frequency with which narrativity, whether of the fictional or the factual sort, presupposes the existence of a legal system against or on behalf of which the typical agents of a narrative account militate.

Hayden White[8]

"Language knows a 'subject,' not a 'person,'" says Barthes. A central presumption of narrativity is that "subject" may become synonymous with "Authority of the Law" in an unseen leap that is implicit in every instance of narrative discourse. In literature it has traditionally been the author-conflated-with-narrator that has occupied this position of authority. In mainstream cinema a more encompassing illusionism tends to suppress the presence of the writer/director to a greater degree. As a consequence, authorial status is assumed exclusively by a "character," a designation which—with all of its implicit compounding of self-contained narrator, "person," "persona," and legal/psychological existence—blocks the intrusion of an anterior authorship, at once embodying the representation of, and unseen leap between, subject and legal system.

Godard was probably the first director working within the illusionist narrative film tradition to "meddle" with the integrity of this usually singular speaking position. He accomplished this by having a given character speak from different authorial positions, including that of performer, but also by introducing the presence—usually in voiceover—of another authorship, a commentator neither sufficiently "filled in" to be a character, nor sufficiently "omniscient" to be a narrator, nor identifiable with any conclusiveness as speaking the opinions of the director/writer himself, even when it is unquestionably the voice of the director that we hear. The tension attendant on this splitting of authorship among character, performer, commentator, and director/ writer produces fissures and contradictions which the viewer must consciously register in order to "get" anything from the film.

> Who *speaks* (in the narrative) is not *who writes* (in real life) and *who writes* is not *who is.*

Roland Barthes

The thing that pushed me toward narrative and ultimately into cinema was "emotional life." I wished not exactly to "express" emotion, certainly not to mimic it, and I wasn't sure whether a recognizable social context would play a part. I knew little more than that its means of presentation would be largely language, and that when spoken, it would be spoken by someone. Not that I hadn't used spoken texts before. In every case, however, either disjunction between movement and speech or the separation inherent in dance presentation between what is performed and the person performing it had prevented the speech from being received as "belonging to" the performer uttering it. Upon taking up film, I would perforce be dealing with an entirely different register of relationship between "spoken" and "speaker." The problem would be not so much in getting them together as tearing them apart.

I was not only entering a new medium, but was jettisoning a whole lexicon of formalized movement and behavior, realizing instinctively that certain concessions to "lifelikeness" would have to be made. For the most part my speaking performers would be doing what people, or characters, so often do in "the movies": sit around, eat, walk down the street, ride bicycles, look at things, etc. If they danced in my early films, I gave them good reason by assigning them the occupation "dancer."

From the beginning I used a loose, paratactic, nondramatic construction, more narrative in feeling than fact. My primary "mission," as I see it now, was to avoid narrative contextualizing that would require synchronized, "naturalized" speech to continue for very long in any given series of shots. I could never quite satisfactorily account—publicly—for the necessity of my particular alternatives to conventional narrative films. I veered unsettlingly close to formalist generalizations ("It hasn't been done; it's there to do; it's another 'possibility'") to the point of almost denying altogether that my enterprise had any significance as social criticism, or that it was an "intervention" against illusionist cinema. Or I about-faced and took up the cudgels of the illusionist-cinema-produces-passive-viewer argument. I felt inadequate to the task of advancing a more pertinent argument to support my aversion to the "acting" and "acting out" required by the narratological character.

As recently as the summer of 1980 I find myself saying in *Millennium Film Journal*:

> Previously I used whatever interested me. I was able to absorb and arrange most materials under some sliding rule of thumb governing formal juxtaposition. Everything was subsumed under the kinds of collage strategies that had characterized my dancing, and could even include a kind of mechanistic, or quasi-psychological narrative.[9]

Still laboring under long-standing Cagean habits of thought about what I'd done—and here I'm talking literally about doing one thing and describing it as another—I was willing to annex my labors to that segment of the surrealist tradition which, from Schwitters to Cage to Rauschenberg, has used "collage strategies" to equalize and suppress hierarchical differentiations of meaning. On another face of it, my work can be, and has been, read as a kind of reductivism coming out of '60s Minimal art, a view which I myself held when I was making dances. It still seems that the refusal to invest my film performers with the full stature and authority of characters shares at some level the same impulse that substituted "running" for "dancing" many years ago. What marks this refusal in the medium of film as not simply an obsolescent holdover from an earlier way of doing things is that from the very outset it was brought to bear against a full-blown institution and manifested itself in specific, pertinent, and contesting strategies.

Speaking of the medieval annals, an early form of European historiography, Hayden White writes:

> For the annalist, there is no need to claim the authority to narrate events since there is nothing problematical about their status as manifestations of a reality that is being contested. Since there is no "contest," there is nothing to narrativize. . . . It is necessary only to record them in the order that they come to notice, for since there is no contest, there is no story to tell.[10]

The implied narrator of the annalist's account is the "Lord," whose supreme authority has subsumed all human need to change "the order [in which things] come to notice." Here we can discover the story of John Cage come full circle. For all of John's Buddhist leanings and egalitarian espousals, for all of his objections to hierarchies and consequent seeming to operate in the space left by the absence of God, his ideas lead inevitably back to the "no contest" of White's early historian. We can't have it both ways: no desire and no God. To have no desire—for "improvements on creation"—is necessarily coequal to having no quarrel with—God-given—manifestations of reality. Any such dispassionate stance in turn obviates the necessity of "retelling" the way things have been given. The converse of this situation is a state of affairs which Cage—rightfully—most feared: we are surrounded by manifestations of reality that are not God-given but all fucked up by human society and that must be contested and reordered by a human "Narrativizing Authority" which, by so representing them, will impart to events an integrity and coherence cut to the measure of all-too-human desire.

Maybe I'm being simple-minded when I say the problem (not the solution) is clear: to track down the Narrativizing Authority where it currently lives and wallop the daylights out of it. And where does it now live? The battle zone is not a serene plane of indeterminacy outside of the overdeterminations of narrative, nor, as I put it in 1973, "somewhere between the excessive specificity of the story and the emotional unspecificity of object-oriented permutations,"[11] thinking it would be something like steering between the narrativity of Scylla and the formalism of Charybdis.

(Is *who speaks* [in the essay] *The Artist*
[in real life] and is *The Artist who is?*)

In cinema the battleground is neither between nor outside. The battleground is narrativity itself, both its constructs/images and the means by which they are constructed; both its signs and its signifiers.

V. *In the N.A.'s Lair*

The reluctance to declare its codes characterizes bourgeois society and the mass culture issuing from it: both demand signs which do not look like signs.

Roland Barthes[12]

By refusing to assign a 'secret', an ultimate meaning, to the text (and to the world as text), [writing] liberates what may be called an anti-theological activity, an activity that is truly revolutionary since to refuse to fix meaning is, in the end, to refuse God and his hypostases—reason, science, law.

Roland Barthes[13]

Arguing with Douglas Beer about Dan Walworth's film, *A House by the River: The Wrong Shape,* stirred up some thoughts. There are a number of clues in this film pointing to the instability of the narrative, I mean a fragility in the relationship of speech to speaker, action to actor. This instability in turn tells us that we are to listen to the verbal text, a historical critique of the bourgeois family, in its own right, at least not to judge it primarily and absolutely from the standpoint of its having emanated from the lips of a "bad actor" or a particular character, in this case a seventeen- or eighteen-year-old student. True, recognition of the character: "student," and situation: "presentation of paper," does affect our reception of the text. Whatever one's initial impulse, however, to discredit or be inattentive because "it's only a student's term paper" is quickly mitigated by a number of factors. In this kind of film the various representations of social reality do not have, necessarily, equivalent relations to their referents with respect to meaning. The "classroom" is stable as a signified insofar as it consistently illustrates those parts of the text that deal with school. The "student," on the other hand, is not. What with the prolongation of the classroom shot, the formality of its fixed framing, and the density and duration of the student's reading, our "reading" of the performance moves back and forth from "character" to "agent-for-transmitting-a-text." The effect of this movement is to put both the representation and the verbal text into a precarious balance: the characterization constantly dissolves and reforms—the signifier-performer alternately exposed and covered over—and at the same time the unstable signified- "student" spills over as a kind of metaphor, rather than identity, informing the spoken text as being other than authorial, as being in a state of flux, in process, to be scrutinized by the artist-filmmaker and "audience-filmmaker." The audience, rather than moving from perception/recognition to identification/repulsion now passes from recognition to critical attention.

Do I seem to be paraphrasing Brecht? Yes and no. I'm not mentioning knowledge/understanding. You can lead a horse to water; you cannot make it drink.

This text has been concerned with the necessity for problematizing a fixed relation of signifier to signified, the notion of a unified subject, and, specifically, within the codes of narrative film practice, the integrity of the narratological character. Any such problematizing, calling into question, or "playing off " of the terms of signification of necessity involves an "unfixing" of meaning, a venturing into ambiguity, an exposing of the signs that constitute and promulgate social inequities.

I have also analyzed the contradictions in John Cage's concepts of indeterminacy. It is important that Cage's efforts to *eliminate and suppress* meaning should in no way be confused with the refusal to *fix* meaning of which Barthes speaks. Cage's *refusal of meaning* is an abandonment, an appeal to a Higher Authority. The refusal that has been of more concern to me is a confrontation with—and within—authorial signifying codes. I wouldn't go so far as Barthes in calling such confrontation a revolutionary activity, at least not at this point in time. Nevertheless, insofar as it involves a certain amount of risk and struggle, it is an important and necessary activity.

A last paraphrase on the battleground of cinematic narrativity: As the character dies it is not inconceivable that some members of the audience will come to their senses. And I don't mean Aristotle.

Notes

1. "The Death of the Author." In *Image-Music-Text,* trans. Stephen Heath (New York: Hill and Wang, 1977), p. 145.

2. Quoted in Richard Barnes, "Our Distinguished Dropout." In *John Cage,* ed. Richard Kostelanetz (New York: Praeger, 1970), p. 51.

3. "The Subject in Signifying Practice," *Semiotext(e),* no. 3 (1975), p. 19.

4. Michel Foucault, "What Is an Author?" *Screen* 20, no. 1 (Spring 1979), p. 17.

5. "Death of the Author," p. 144.

6. *A Year from Monday* (Middletown: Wesleyan University Press, 1967), p. 118.

7. Ibid., p. 114.

8. "The Value of Narrativity in the Representation of Reality," *Critical Inquiry* 7, no. 1 (Autumn 1980), p. 17.

9. Noel Carroll, "Interview with a Woman Who . . . ," *Millennium Film Journal,* nos. 7–9 (Fall–Winter 1980–81), p. 44.

10. "The Value of Narrativity," p. 22.

11. *Work 1961–73* (Halifax: The Press of the Nova Scotia College of Art and Design and New York: New York University Press, 1974), p. 244.

12. "Introduction to the Structural Analysis of Narratives," *Image-Music-Text,* p. 116.

13. "Death of the Author," p. 147.

Letter to Arlene Croce

In her *New Yorker* column of June 30, 1980, dance critic Arlene Croce claimed that Robert Wilson "as a writer and director of esoteric visionary plays and as a teacher of movement has been the biggest influence, after Cunningham, on choreographers working today." The performance art magazine *Live* (published by PAJ Publications) printed letters of protest from Meredith Monk, Kenneth King, and me in its issue number 4 (1980). After looking over my shoulder and reading the above, my girlfriend remarked that this kind of heated interchange doesn't seem to happen anymore. If such is the case, what has changed? I was just going to write that cultural critics no longer take polemical positions, that the Christian Coalition's attempts at suppression notwithstanding (*vide* the hysterical uproars around Serrano and Mapplethorpe), the post-Rauschenbergian era for the most part accommodates every gesture, from the beautiful to the scabrous to the confessional. But then I was reminded of Croce's more recent curmudgeonly diatribe, in which she trashed a work of Bill T. Jones as "victim art" without having attended the event. (Would a program note characterizing the piece as "survivor art" have affected her view of it?) Certainly one thing that has changed is that very few artists today construe their work as having an adversarial relation to the past. This may not be a bad thing, though it is worth noting that at a particular historical "moment"—namely, the decade of the '60s—such embattled positioning was productive of a livelier cultural climate than has been seen at any point since. But I have to admit to a generational bias here.

July 18, 1980

Arlene Croce
The New Yorker
25 West 43rd Street
New York, N.Y. 10036

Dear Arlene:

May I add my two-cents plain to the brouhaha accruing from your article of June 30? Insofar as Kenneth King has done so admirable a job (and one with which I largely concur) on the Monk-King-Dean-Wilson-Glass connections, let me confine my remarks to my own peers. For this purpose I am enclosing a crudely drawn—and vastly oversimplified—genealogy chart which adds several wrinkles to your revisionist sense of history. Mainly, I have enlarged your oddly reduced number of fountainheads, thus opening up the patterns of lineage. I have also given the poor bastard—our esteemed mutual friend, David Gordon—a proper parentage worthy of his name and have ejected Trisha Brown from the ranks of the "Mercerians." (I so much prefer this term to your "Mercists." After all, while we're at it why not call forth the whole imperial baggage—what Kenneth King calls the "bankrupt monarch model"—and use a term lying closer to "Caesarian" and Caesar?)

Even *my* name gets absorbed into this model in your hands. You say "The whole post-modern movement from Yvonne Rainer onwards" as though at a given point in time my work formed an apex from which everyone else descended. I fervently wish you Sunday historians might acquire a sense of history based on something other than a sequence of one-man/woman epiphanies. Things are always more complicated than that. True, Cunningham/Cage were doing their thing thirty years ago. But why was their influence in the dance world not felt in any visible degree until 1960? Clearly it required a convergence of a number of people from different areas of art-making to manifest the ideas that in the intervening ten years had lain fallow. And to further muddy the metaphor, the harvest ultimately yielded bears in many instances no relation to the original association. Hence, to call Steve Paxton's Contact Improvisation Mercerian is like calling Morris/Judd Smithsonian simply because David Smith's work immediately preceded theirs. Much of the work that developed in the Judson Dance Workshop was in *opposition* to Cunningham's then-perceived elegance and classicism. Things like walking, running, and quotidian activity performed in varying repetitive modes have never been of much interest to Cunningham, and the term *austerity* frequently used to connect the two generations, is a cliché more obfuscating of differences than revealing of similarities.

This suggests that a good deal of the work of Paxton, Childs, Hay, and Rainer might be shunted off to another corner of the yard (I don't think I'm too far off in describing your enterprise in these "railroading" terms). As for Trisha Brown, she hardly studied with Cunningham at all. Although she participated in the Robert Dunn workshop, her real roots come straight out of the Halprin/Forti axis, e.g., her equipment pieces early on in her career and her highly personal—and, I agree, untheatricalized—approach to movement exploration more recently.

You're right in making a distinction between Childs and Dean. However, I prefer to articulate it as the difference between task and trance. Despite Childs' recent predilection for dancing on the beat, her emphasis on floor patterns and the stiff, slightly awkward, almost parodistic relation to balletic steps thrusts her work more in the direction of children's games than toward the transformational and ritualistic atmosphere of Wilson and Dean. In this respect Childs is true to her Judson origins.

Perhaps a whole new set of categories is called for: Cagists, Warevers, Judsonians, West Coastites, Halprinians, Literarians, Paslovians, Fortitudians, and post-any of the above. And what about Artworldlians? Thus I would qualify as former Paslovian-Fortitudian-Judsonian Cagist and lapsed Artworldlian Mercist and new Literarian Cinemist. If my chart provides Rainer with a more complex input than any of the others, that is merely the result of knowing my own history best.

One last exhortation: Let's stop blaming everything on Cunningham, for heaven's sake, and—if I were you—I wouldn't blame *anything* on Wilson!

> Yours in felicity and art,
> Yvonne Rainer

P.S. Preferences from the standpoint of taste are no justification for the rewriting of history.

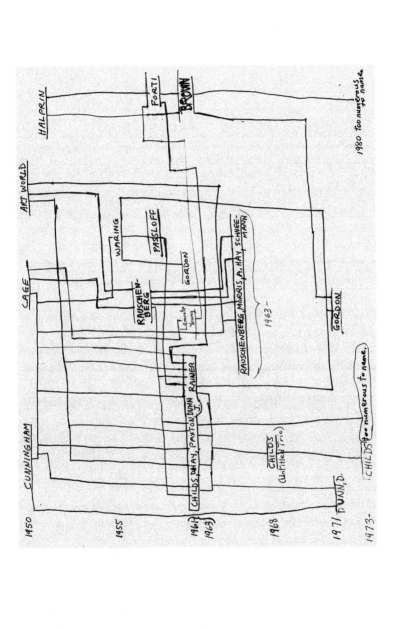

Revisiting the Question

of Transgression

The following is a paper delivered on April 14, 1989, as part of a symposium called *Strategies of Performance Art 1960–1989,* which took place at the Maryland Institute College of Art, Baltimore. It was organized by Maurice Berger, who also moderated the panel called "The Aesthetics of Production and Dissent: The 1960s," on which appeared, besides myself, Jill Johnston, Brian Wallis, and Dan Graham.

Paul Willemen, the British film historian, in a summation of the concept of Third Cinema put forth by Latin American filmmakers Fernando Solanas and Octavio Getino, has cited "its flexibility, its status as research and experimentation, a cinema forever in need of adaptation to the shifting dynamics at work in social struggles."[1]

The term *social struggles* seems a good point of departure for looking—yet again—at certain cultural activity that took place in the 1960s. Having lately returned from the largest mass demonstration in the country's history—600,000 people marching for abortion rights in Washington D.C.—I am struck by how the boundaries and definitions that constitute radicality and transgression shift from decade to decade. The former radicals of the '60s who fought for legalized abortion now find themselves the defenders of the status quo, while the Right-to-Lifers set the agendas of front-line embattlement with the law.

Art-making of the 1960s can be said to have shared with institutionalized law the idea of clearly demarcated zones of transgression and compliance. If these boundaries—in the art context, at least—have blurred in the intervening thirty years, it is due more to the voraciousness of "postmodernist" consumerism than to the disappearance of sites of cultural struggle. For me, during this same period, the notion of transgression has shifted from art history and its embattled aesthetics to the interaction of specific social struggles with the means and conditions of representing them. Although there were artists in the '60s who were attempting to integrate social criticism and formal concerns (as there have been in every historical period), for the most part something else was going on. To illustrate the "legalistic," abstracted-from-social-reality frame of mind that dominated much of the thinking about art at that time, let me quote a fragment of my own writing that attempted to carve out some new axioms for sculptural and choreographic practice (heavily influenced by the "fundamentalist" writings of Robert Morris, Barbara Rose, and Donald Judd).

What I celebrated as ripe for elimination from sculptural and choreographic practice were "the role of the artist's hand, phrasing, hierarchical relationship of parts, development and climax, texture, variation in rhythm, shape and dynamics, figure reference, character, illusionism, performance, complexity and detail, variety in phrases and the spatial field, monumentality, and the virtuosic movement feat and the fully-extended body." What were to be substituted for these outdated graces were "factory fabrication, energy equality and 'found' movement, unitary forms, modules, equality of parts, uninterrupted surface, repetition or discrete events, nonreferential forms, neutral performance, literalness, task or task-like activity, simplicity, singular action, event or tone, and human scale."[2]

Since—twenty-five years later—all this sounds like patent cant, I feel obliged to attempt a salvage operation, however minimal, to give some idea of the degree to which passions—yes, real passion and desperate fervor—were expended on art-making and theorizing as autonomous and self-perpetuating exercises. Change for its own sake—its predominant reference and highest aspiration being the toppling and discrediting of what immediately preceded it—was the sacrament and dominating ethos of the time. Swept along on a tide of moral/aesthetic outrage, many of us saw abstract expressionism, modern dance, and the symphony orchestra as the triple-headed hydra of a depleted legacy. Inflated with their self-importance and success in the most respected quarters of their respective citadels, these cultural leviathans, as we perceived them, were fair game for the most iconoclastic challenges. And never has a decade seen so many challenges to honored precepts of "connoisseurialized" art.

From Nam June Paik's smashing of his violin, to Simone Forti's "Huddle," Wolf Vostell's burial of a console TV set, John Cage's four minutes and thirty-three seconds of silence, and Warhol's *EAT* and

KISS, the '60s were awash in gestures of resistance and refusal—refusal to please, refusal to soothe, refusal to inspire, refusal to make fine distinctions, refusal to reassure, refusal to entertain, refusal to comply with and cater to all previous voyeuristic, aesthetic, and professional expectations. All of this was no mere matter of stylistic change; it was an unconditional revolt against the very idea of style and nuance.

Unlike the gestures of the earlier Dadaists and Surrealists, the sounds and acts and objects of the most well-known Fluxists, Minimalists, and Popists were, for the most part, not surrounded by a rhetoric of social revolution. You did not hear or read many discussions interpreting this work as a stand against social inequities, imperialism, or the bourgeoisie. For most of the '60s the cold war continued to exert its stranglehold, muting such debates in the art world. (Not until the late '60s and early '70s did artists become active against the Vietnam War.) And under the extraordinary influence of John Cage's mixture of Duchamp and Zen Buddhism, a new generation of artists—without judgment, heedless of social stratifications outside of their own sphere of activity, responding primarily to the narrow hegemony of the cultural institutions that directly affected their activity—set about discovering the wonders of those phenomena previously excluded from the canons of high art: walking, ordinary people, silence, coughing, comic strips, electric chairs, grey boxes, corporate logos.

In the mid-'60s a reviewer of one of my dance concerts stated, "Her work represents the view that everything in the world is equally uninteresting." I countered with the—equally questionable—Cagean view that "everything in the world is equally interesting." The dictates of the new canon governing the "new (or newest) and interesting" could be fulfilled by the—to use Susan Sontag's term—"radical juxtaposition" of elements and conditions previously perceived as totally incompatible. One result was an insistence on a value-free equivalency. We see this simplistic phenomenologism rampant in the art and avant-garde media world of today. "Adversarial culture," another Sontag formulation, was, in the '60s, readily and irreverently produced. (To quote from yet another review, this one titled, "The Avant-Garde Is At It Again": "[Her group] performed last night in sloppy street clothes—mostly jeans and sneakers, without benefit of hair brush or make-up, sets, wing curtains or music. And the choreography consisted mainly of walking or running, aimless repetition, without grace, logic, style, sequence, virtuosity, or meaning."[3] Today, nourished and validated by institutionalized funding, exhibition, and distribution, adversarial culture is readily and *reverently* produced. I am not sure that the difference is a substantial one.

Getting back to a cinema of "flexibility . . . research and experimentation, a cinema forever in need of adaptation to the shifting dynamics at work in social struggles"—the question must be asked: What can be salvaged from the socially deficient avant-gardes of the past that might invigorate the social struggles of the present and future? To name a few of those struggles: the struggles for autonomy and visibility of racial and sexual constituencies whose voices have been consistently excluded from white-administered cultural venues; the struggle against the decline of the dignity of labor; the struggle against the marauding self-interest of U.S. corporate profiteering throughout the world; the struggle against the world-wide weapons trade; the struggle against nuclear proliferation; the struggles against the depredations of real estate interests; the struggles for abortion rights and low-cost housing and medical care. And from the immediacy of a current preoccupation of my own: the struggle to understand the intricacies of a social privilege that has, at least in part, assured the visibility of my work from the '60s to the present. (At a recent "Town Meeting" on "Cultural Participation," organized by Group Material in New York, a consensus was arrived at whereby those present agreed to demand that every panel on which they might subsequently be invited to speak include people of color. One reason I "forgot" to do this on being invited to this panel was that there were virtually no artists of color who were recognized within the race- and class-bound limits of the '60s avant-garde. Aside from the flamboyant Nam June Paik, who, subsequent to his violin-smashing, was to become the father of video art, the only people I can remember as even marginally recognized are two painters—David Diao and Emilio Cruz—and Ralph Ortiz, who, in the mid-sixties, made happenings in which he beat live chickens to death against the harp of an eviscerated grand piano. I should have suggested that at least one of them be here today. The rarity in that period of women artists—and the virtual invisibility of women artists of color—now seems truly shocking.)

In conclusion I offer, not another manifesto, but a plea for utilizing, and not dumping, our cultural past. Gestures of refusal and dissent are still needed, not, however, in the service of refusing previous art, but rather to point to—and protest—existing social inequities. Had Ralph Ortiz not thrown out the chicken along with that symbol of classical cultural hegemony, the guts of the baby grand, might he not possibly—

as a case in point—have drawn attention to the plight of the migrant worker? The documentary, realist tradition is not the only means for representing social issues, and the gesture of savage rage need not displace all thought of a social referent. (As one [black female] character in my current script says to the [white female] other, "So please, get your ass back in there; there's more work to be done!") The avant-garde tradition has much to offer if its formal and aesthetically iconoclastic propensities are engaged for a broader purpose. Experimentation and research were a large part of what the '60s were all about. Now it is time, once more, to bring that spirit of investigation to bear on "the shifting dynamics at work in social struggles." So that the heading "The Avant-Garde Is At It Again" might take on a different meaning, one that is socially progressive rather than culturally hermetic.

Notes

1. Paul Willemen, "The Third Cinema Question: Notes and Reflections," *Framework*, no. 34 (1987), p. 17.

2. Yvonne Rainer, "A Quasi Survey of Some 'Minimalist' Tendencies in the Quantitatively Minimal Dance Activity Midst the Plethora, or an Analysis of *Trio A.*" In *Minimal Art: A Critical Anthology*, ed. Gregory Battcock (New York: E. P. Dutton, 1968), pp. 263–73. Reprinted in Yvonne Rainer: *Work 1961–73* (Halifax: Nova Scotia College of Art and Design and New York: New York University Press, 1974), pp. 63–69; in Richard Kostelanetz, *Esthetics Contemporary* (Buffalo: Prometheus Books), pp. 315–18; and in *The Twentieth-Century Performance Reader*, ed. Michael Huxley and Noel Witts (New York: Routledge, 1996).

3. Frances Herridge, "The Avant-Garde Is At It Again." *New York Post*, February 7, 1969.

Letters to Judith Mayne

The first of these two letters followed my return home to New York from a screening of *Privilege* at Ohio State University in Columbus, where Judith teaches film and women's studies. The second needs no introduction! Both can be seen as the beginning of an ongoing investigation into the politics of sexual identity, which is wrestled with in *Working Round the L-Word,* historicized in *Skirting,* and dramatized in *MURDER and murder.*

November 5, 1990

Dear Judith:

Just off the plane, grabbed a sandwich, made a negligible dent in pile of mail, turned on the Mac. What I could have said, what I should have said, about sexual identity in response to the question "Why were the people of color and the lesbian peripheral to white heterosexual Jenny's story; why didn't you make Jenny a lesbian?" woke me in the middle of last night and has been energizing me ever since. I remember pausing for quite a while after my response. I knew it was all wrong but couldn't think on my feet quickly enough to set things right—or in motion—and didn't realize until the middle of the night that once again "autobiography" had short-circuited my synapses. To express slightly differently something you brought up at breakfast: autobiography and theory are not the most congenial bedfellows.

Or confession and theory. "I am not black and I am not a lesbian." Why is the first an obvious fact and the second a confession, the first a foregone conclusion and the second necessitating all kinds of qualifications? What I *should* have said: "Jenny, or, more accurately, Jenny's past, represents that part of my experience, the predominant part, I might

add, that can be characterized as—to use Monique Wittig's phrase—
'the straight mind.' " I am still involved in investigating my own
straightness, and it is still around this vantage point that my films re-
volve. In fact, all of my films, to some degree or another, can be seen as
an interrogation and critique of straightness in its broadest and most
confining sense: Straightness as a bulwark, as a protection, as a punish-
ing code against all kinds of difference, not only sexual, what Trinh
Minh-ha has described as "the apartheid type of difference." The earlier
films scream and the later ones examine. I might also describe Jenny as
the straight mind in disarray, still thrashing around in her paper bags,
much more so than the Trisha character in *The Man Who Envied Women*.
But then Trisha (in *TMWEW*) has not yet dealt with her aging.

Getting back to the beginning of that "performed lecture" I was
telling you about, I'll quote it again: "I am a single, white, menopausal
heterosexual; I am a political lesbian; and, to borrow a phrase from the
medical professionals, I am sexually inactive." I think what I'm currently going through is both a (private) reawakening of sexual desire (a
natural aftermath of incredibly intense work on the film) and a (public) struggle with the restrictive nomenclature that defines desire, i.e.,
"heterosexual, homosexual, bisexual," and sometimes I get the two
stances mixed up, as I did the other night. Whatever my sexual preference, living arrangements, fantasy life evolves (or doesn't evolve) into, I
do believe that it is necessary to start mixing up the terms that place us
so implacably as dominant or marginal.

There is no denying that coming out as a lesbian can often be politically expedient. *I wish I could do it,* if only for that reason. Under the
circumstances, however, given that I've had a total of three sexual experiences with two women in my whole life(!), my feelings of solidarity,
admiration, and affection have to be expressed in other ways. One way
is to (publicly) blur the boundaries, imperatives, and possibilities of
what has hitherto been known as heterosexuality. So far I've come up
with "a-woman" as a gender designation and "lapsed heterosexual" and
"political lesbian" to describe my current celibate status. If I ever have
sex with a man again, I could say I am a provisional heterosexual, or a
makeshift hetero. These imply sleeping with a man until the right
woman comes along, or sleeping with a man but dreaming of women.
How about "heterofluxual" or contingent hetero, or *nonessential* hetero? All of this may sound trivializing, but there is reason here. If I'm
going to continue to investigate sexual straightness in a (de)contestable
or problematic way (which *TMWEW* does more effectively than *Privi-*

lege, now that I'm thinking about it, simply by focusing so heavily on a straight *man*) I have to not only think of characters but also of new language that will interrogate and comment on those characters. And of course it is challenging to start thinking of a character, an a-woman and political lesbian: . . . Is she black? Is she 60? Is she going to be middle class again? (*Privilege 2?*) How does she deal with the garbage coming into her ears as she walks down the street: "She is a woman who was never attractive to men, that's why she's a lesbian. Some of my best friends are lesbians. She's single and old, so she turned to women. She's too old to attract a man, that's why she's single. She's a dried up old maid. She failed with men, so . . . She can't hold a man."

OR, do I try to make a lesbian protagonist? Frankly, Judith, I don't think I could do it right. Happily, I'm a long way from the agonizing that that part of my process will entail. I'm still coasting and free-associating. Thanks again for your part in a stimulating two days. If you're interested I could send you a copy of the lecture I did in Australia. It's sixteen pages. Can't wait to read your book.

Very best,
Yvonne

Jan. 6, 1991

Dear Judith:

My letter of Nov. 5 can now be relegated not to the dust heap (let's retrieve everything around sexual i.d.!) but to some fictional annal à la Borges or my next film. I am out. small *o.* You never knOw until it happens, I guess. An end tO a particular periOd of ambiguity. On to the next. I said tO her "I feel like a fraud." She (whO's been out fOr Over 20 years) respOnded, "SO dO I."

LOve,
Yvonne

Working Round the L-Word

Originally delivered as a lecture at the Lookout Lesbian and Gay Television Festival at Downtown Community Television, New York City, October 13, 1991, this essay appeared in *Queer Looks: Perspectives on Lesbian and Gay Film and Video* edited by Martha Gever, John Greyson, and Prathiba Parmar (New York: Routledge, 1993).

These musings began to take shape over a year ago in a lecture called "Narrative in the (Dis)Service of Identity: Fragments toward a performed lecture dealing with menopause, race, gender and other uneasy bedfellows in the cinematic sheets. Or: How do you begin to think of yourself as white when you've finally gotten used to thinking of yourself as an 'a-woman'?"

I subsequently—a deceptively simple way to say it is: I subsequently became a lesbian, and accordingly revised both paper and title. Let me quote the revised title and beginning of the revised paper: "Narrative in the (Dis)Service of Identity: Fragments toward a performed lecture dealing with menopause, race, gender and other uneasy bedfellows in the cinematic sheets, Or: How do you begin to think of yourself as a lesbian—and white—when you had just about gotten used to the idea of being an 'a-woman'?"

"A young, white, artist-activist in New York City named Gregg Bordowitz begins a lecture on AIDS and safe sex with the words: 'I am gay; I am HIV-antibody positive; I like having sex with men.'

"Bordowitz inspires me to lay it—or something not quite like it—on the line: I am a white, menopausal lesbian, and, after many years of celibacy following decades of a heterosexual identity, I am once again—to borrow a phrase from the medical professionals—sexually active. You

110

may well ask what prompts (what some might call) these embarrassing confessions, or why my sexual preference or sexual activity is anyone's business. Who wants to know? Not any of you, certainly, or, if you do, I feel under no obligation to reward such prurient curiosity. And why should I even mention the words 'white' and 'menopausal' in one breath as though they might in some way be equivalent, when in fact they denote contradictory relations to social privilege, and it is blatantly obvious that I am a middle-aged Caucasian? And if it is not so obvious that I am a lesbian (notwithstanding the short hair and lack of makeup that in some quarters might signify 'butch'), why is it necessary to state my sexual status so baldly?

"If you know anything at all about gay culture in the United States, you can conclude quite correctly from the foregoing that I am a novice at all this, an *arriviste,* newly 'come out,' not from the closet, however, but from the sanctuary of heterosexuality, that hallowed site legitimated and regulated by the institutions of patriarchy, not the least of which is the family. Upon learning about my newly launched romantic attachment, a member of my family responded, 'It's wonderful that you're with someone, but you don't have to call yourself a lesbian.' An entire history of disavowal, repression, and persecution is contained in that simple declaration. 'You don't have to call yourself a lesbian.'

"So what does it mean to 'call yourself a lesbian' for the first time at the age of fifty-six? Outside of the usual requests on passport and bank account applications for age, gender, race, and citizenship, I never had to 'call' myself anything but dancer, choreographer, filmmaker, or teacher. I can even remember a time when I didn't question the benefits I enjoyed from being young, white, and middle-class, or the disadvantages that accrued from being female. As recently as six months ago I could describe myself as engaged in a struggle with the reductive nomenclature that defines desire, i.e., *heterosexual, homosexual, bisexual,* believing that by mixing up the terms that position us so implacably as dominant or marginal, privileged or unprivileged, protected or endangered, I could somehow invent a new position for myself, something along the lines of a *lapsed heterosexual* or *political lesbian,* or even a utopian *a-woman,* the last derived from Monique Wittig's declaration in her 1978 essay, 'The Straight Mind,' that 'Lesbians are not women.' If lesbians are not women, I persuaded myself, then I too could renounce the culture-debased designation, *woman. A-woman* was the alternative I came up with. *A-womanly. A-womanliness.*

"But then, the first time I kissed my female lover on the street, I knew I was into a whole new ball game and that my previous wordplay had been a charade keeping me from acknowledging that—however dormant my sexual drive had been—I had been living in the safe house of heterosexuality, under the illusion that I was benefiting from all the security and legitimation that such habitation could offer, and not realizing that it is a protection system that does not serve everyone equally, especially women. One of the spoken house rules is that after a certain age women have to move out; you're on your own. Many of us try to pass as young in order to prolong our residency. But the day of reckoning inevitably comes.

"Following from my new sexual status, to 'call myself' a lesbian is not only a statement of sexual preference, it is a way of pointing to where I—and others like me, for the same, also different, reasons—live: outside the safe house, on the edge, in the social margin. As a lesbian and aging woman, I reside in this margin. In contrast, as a Caucasian and successful artist, I reside in what Audre Lorde has called the *mythical norm,* that place in the United States usually reserved for those who are 'white, thin, male, young, heterosexual, Christian, and financially secure.'[1] As you see, I am still about forty percent safe."

In this context, if I'm going to distill out my lesbianism from those other markers of social status that comprise a heterogeneous identity, including lapsed heterosexual, political lesbian, and a-woman, it might be worthwhile to start from scratch and ask, "What is a lesbian?" If calling myself a "political lesbian" was an attempt to declare solidarity, it was also an effort to challenge the notion of a fixed and closed sexual category. However, once my sexual life had undergone change, I was more than willing to embrace the category, come what may, to indicate my sexual preference. I welcomed and carefully noted every opportunity for formally or casually declaring my new sexual status. "Oh yes, my girlfriend lives near there," or "I'll either be here or at my girlfriend's house; here's the number," or "Now that I'm a lesbian . . . ," and so on. I've already noted the family response. Most people congratulated me on my newfound felicity, but I was amazed to learn that in some quarters lesbians would, like my family members but for different reasons, be reluctant to accord me *lesbian* status. You may be sleeping with a woman, but you're not a lesbian.

Hey! what is this? A club or something? I eat pussy just like you. Just 'cause you've been doing it longer does that make you more of a lezzy

than me? Well, evidently. Unlike the term *gay man,* the word *lesbian*—
at least to some who identify as such—carries more than a sexual meaning. A man comes out, and no one questions his credentials as gay. If
you're out and a man and have sex with men, then you're gay. But a
woman doesn't necessarily become a lesbian by changing the gender of
her sleeping companion. In those quarters you have to earn your
stripes, have been on the barricades, taken shit, and certainly you must
have foresworn men as sexual partners.

OK, OK. I'm not the pushy type. I'm perfectly happy with my neol-
ogisms, for the time being, anyway. And I have a strong survival sense:
while trying to get into the club I didn't burn my bridges; I didn't give
up my identity of a-woman, lapsed heterosexual, and political lesbian.
So next year I'll simply reapply. After all, my résumé does contain some
impressive data—I marched in the Gay Pride Parade before ever applying for admission to the club, and some of my best friends are lesbians.
As for pussy-eating, you'll have to take my word for it.

Yes, I mean to be a bit silly here; forgive me if I strike the wrong
note. One thing I find unsettling is that in the gay and lesbian public
sphere I am being paid attention to as a lesbian *before* doing any work
that identifies me as one. It's not that I wish to preserve privacy, far
from it, but as a former member of the dominant sexual category I can
still see it as odd that the gender of the person one has sex with is a determining factor in public recognition. This, of course, is a view that a
gay person can afford to sustain only in the best of all possible visions
of a world. In the world we know, where same-sex preference is a signal
for exclusion, ridicule, persecution and neglect from individuals and institutions that don't have to name their sexual bias, only point to ours,
our relegation to weirdo-freak-queer marginality if we do name ourselves still demands that we exceed the bounds of polite address and
scream our name. Fundamentalism and essentialism aside, I therefore
call myself a lesbian, present myself as a lesbian, and represent myself as
a lesbian. This is not to say that it is the last word in my self-definition.
"Lesbian" defines not only a sexual identity but also the social "calling,"
or resistance, made necessary by present societal inequities. I must keep
in mind that "white" and "aging woman," as markers of both social
privilege and social stigma, form other parts of this identity, and that
my status as aging lesbian, however stigmatized in daily life, is not
equivalent to the experience of people of color.

On the other hand, whatever my sister-in-law or I or other lesbians call or don't call me, the dominant culture is definitely going to call me a lesbian. The specific negative consequences of this have yet to make their appearance. So far, my life as a lesbian has been filled with satisfying work and unpredicted pleasures. I find myself, however, suddenly in a unique position from which to examine the social benefits I have derived from being a heterosexual for so many years. There is no doubt in my mind that the extent to which I can currently be called a successful artist can be directly traced to a life as a white heterosexual. I doubt if Jill Johnston's championship of my dance work in the early sixties would have been a sufficient impetus to my career without the influence of the white, male artists who also supported it. It is interesting to note that at that time I knew of only two lesbians connected with the Judson Dance Theater, where many of my early performances took place, and their relationship was an object of destructive gossip or detachment on the part of the straight women, and outright harassment by male artists. It is also interesting to speculate about how my career might have fared if the content of my work—both dance and films—had focused on lesbian subjects and subject matter throughout the '60s and '70s.

Yes, I have to say that I enter the arena of lesbian sex with less risk than I might have twenty-five years ago. Besides the career factor there is also the consideration of my age. Because older women are not relevant to dominant sexuality, they can become lesbians with less fear of discrimination. To paraphrase one of the interviewees in *Privilege,* we don't have to please straight men anymore.

It's time to talk more directly about representation. Much has been said to me about Brenda, the lesbian character in *Privilege.* First of all, she is played by a straight woman, one who I belatedly discovered was somewhat homophobic. When we first meet her in the film she has no name because Jenny, the narrator, has forgotten it. She is the object of a sexual assault and is therefore required to speak generally *for women* and not specifically for lesbians. Later she articulates a questionable psychoanalytic theory aligning people of color and women as victims, which, though contested by the African American documentary filmmaker Yvonne Washington, puts Brenda in the position of crackpot theorist. In her last appearance she is seated on the other side of the desk of an assistant district attorney, confronting him with a quote from Joan Nestle's *A Restricted Country* about an erotic interaction between two women. It is a powerful moment—the DA is dumbfounded—but it is yet another instance of the lesbian character's not being allowed to be seen *in her own life, as a lesbian.* The justification might be that Brenda is a peripheral character seen through the eyes of Jenny, the straight protagonist. But so were the African American and Puerto Rican characters in the film, and yet I managed to place *them* both within the story and outside as commentators on their respective social conditions. This, in fact, was the whole point of the flashback. Unlike these characters, the only opportunity given to Brenda to detach herself from the diegesis and address the camera is her recitation of a short poem by Judy Grahn. I now think that, coming at the end of an intense interaction with her alleged attacker, this was too brief a moment to establish an autonomy and savviness comparable to that of the other characters.

After seeing the film, Geeta Patel, who teaches Indian literature at the University of Iowa, said, "I was impressed by certain omissions, particularly the omission of the lesbian's subjectivity. It suggests that one subjectivity, or its representation, always excludes another." Admittedly, there is a trade-off of subjectivities operating in *Privilege,* but I don't think it need necessarily be the case.

And I don't think one has to be a lesbian to make a film about lesbians. The question arises: How—let alone why—should one speak the struggles of those with whom one does not have precisely the same things at stake? Stated so baldly, the why part of it seems almost like a dumb question, one that must be put into perspective by further questions: if you are no longer of reproductive age, do you drop out of the fight for abortion rights? If you are a man, do you not speak out for women's right to control their bodies? If you are not HIV-positive do you not take a stand against the government's foot-dragging policies around AIDS? If you are white do you not express your revulsion at the neoconservative defense of white racist behavior on university campuses parading under the First Amendment?

The answers to the above are self-evident to anyone who sees her- or himself as a progressive. The ticklish part is when those in more advantageous positions—white, First World, with more money, behind the camera, rewarded, institutionally legitimized—represent the "struggles of others." The debates around documentary and ethnographic film have amply delineated the problems inherent in the invisibility and supposed neutrality or objectivity of the filmmaker, who is *ipso facto* empowered. As for fictional scenarios, it has become painfully clear to me that when peripheral fictional characters are used to represent people who are also peripheral in white-dominated society, those characters must be given their day in court. Overall, this is not news to me. As I indicated before, I have been more than theoretically aware of the dangers in using marginalized people casually, that is, without making reference to their particular marginalized positions. In response to criticism about Brenda that followed screenings I attended before becoming a lesbian, I would agree on the specifics, but then justified her characterization on the basis of her *feminism*. I maintained that she spoke for both feminists *and* lesbians. This would have been fine if her lesbianism had had a more complete airing *vis à vis* scenes in which she would not have had to be *accountable to heterosexuals*. As things now stand in the film, Brenda is the patsy. The mistake is telling: Jenny, the straight, white protagonist, is concerned about her racism, not about her homophobia. Her last line is a portent of things to come in the life of her creator, namely me. When Yvonne Washington asks her if she ever "made it with Brenda," Jenny replies, "Hell no, I was terrified of women."

So, on to new cultural work. In closing I shall relay some scenes and notations for a new film that as yet has no story.

Possible opening: An almost-deserted beach, maybe Coney Island, slightly garbage-strewn, very wide shot. The theme music from Jaws *is heard. Steadi-cam begins to meander toward two figures who cannot at first be identified as the focal point of the shot. Two white women in their early sixties are seated in the sand, leaning against a sea wall (San Francisco?) or against a support under the boardwalk. One is huddled under a blanket, speaking while the other listens. As we approach we begin to hear their conversation.*

WOMAN #1: So what's it like?

WOMAN #2: What's *what* like?

WOMAN #1: (*laughing*): Whadya mean "what?" Sex of course.

We are now in close-up on WOMAN #2*'s face, which is in three-quarter or complete profile.*

WOMAN #2 (*after thinking for a bit she delivers line with a cunning smile*): You know something? Never in my wildest dreams, my most far-out fantasies, did I ever come close to imagining that I would one day be able to say—with the utmost conviction—*"I love eating pussy."*

My mother, far into her dotage, was looking at a photo of Marilyn Monroe. She said, "What beautiful breasts she has." My then husband later remarked—in disbelief—"She sounded just like a man!"

Conversation between two WHITE WOMEN *in their seventies:*

#1: . . . and they had this wonderful old dog named Emma . . . Emma . . . G, begins with a G . . .

#2: Goldman.

#1: Emma Goldman. And she had this great trick. She had two . . . two . . . she would fetch a blue or red . . . (gesticulating wildly)

#2: What?

#1: She would fetch . . . what you throw in the air . . . you know . . . (gesticulating)

#2: frisbee!

#1: Yes! frisbee!

LESBIANS #1 *and* #2 *are lying nude at opposite ends of a bed. One lies with her feet resting on the breasts of the other. Her toes play with her lover's nipples. They are engaged in a serio-comic discussion around "What constitutes a lesbian?"*

#1: Well, *your* credentials as a bona-fide lesbian have never been in question.

#2: No, that's not true. My old girl friend always said I wasn't the real thing because I had been married. . . . Not only that but I'd had sex with men.

#1: You mean she never fucked a man, even once? That's pretty extreme, isn't it?

#2: I'd say it's fairly common.

#1: Oh Christ, then they'll never let *me* in, after my lifetime of copulation. And here I had thought all I had to do was give up wearing two earrings. But I don't even know if I *want* to be in the club! I don't want to be a professional lesbian.

#2: I don't know about the professional part, but really, do you have a choice? You're a lesbian, like it or not.

#1: How do you *know?*

#2: I don't sleep with straight women.

#1: I was straight when you first got involved with me.

#2: No you weren't. A straight woman wouldn't have behaved the way you did.

#1: You mean, at the Clit Club? How did I behave? Tell me again, my love. Tell me about the rabbits and the chickens.

#2: (*laughing*): The way you came on to me. Only a lesbian would have behaved like that.

#1: OK, I'm a lesbian. I'll take your word for it . . . for now.

C'S STORY: I fell in love with a woman in Australia. I had always known it was a possibility. I was there for six weeks. She was wonderful. Then when I came home I let her come visit me, and it was a dreadful mistake. I couldn't stand the social thing. As a heterosexual I don't have to say I'm heterosexual or be known as something special, but as a lesbian I would be put into this category, and I couldn't stand it.

N'S STORY: After my divorce seven years ago, which was very ugly and nightmarish, I vowed I would never get involved in something like that again. So I've been pretty much alone since then. In feminism it's a big problem here [Germany]. Lesbians have their own conferences and culture. Feminist conferences include lesbians, but the differences are never talked about. And much of the organizing wouldn't happen without the lesbians because they are the most active and energetic and advanced in their thinking.

Notes

1. Audre Lorde, "Age, Race, Class, and Sex: Women Redefining Difference," in *Out There: Marginalization and Contemporary Cultures,* Russell Ferguson et al. eds. (Cambridge/New York: MIT Press/The New Museum, 1990), p. 282.

Skirting

This essay was written for *The Feminist Memoir Project: Voices from Women's Liberation,* edited by Rachel Blau DuPlessis and Ann Snitow (New York: Crown, 1998).

It must have been sometime in 1985 that I bragged to a friend "I'm no longer afraid of men." I hadn't trucked sexually with "them" for at least four years—I was fifty years old—and it would be another five years before I would venture into intimacy with a woman, although I had already begun to call myself a "political lesbian." The question continues to vex me as to why I spent so many years fooling around with what now seem to have been preordained doomed heterosexual partnerships. The answers are as numerous as the day is long: (1) I didn't possess foresight and couldn't make use of a constantly unraveling hindsight. (2) The prospect of "working at" the relationships with the help of a succession of professionals always held out the possibility of imminent "success." (3) Until the late '80s I was more attuned to heterosexual feminism than to the gay rights movement and therefore was not given, or could not give myself, permission to tune in to another level of desire. (4) Compulsory heterosexuality.

But it hadn't always been that way. My first "liberation" came at age eighteen when I moved out of my parents' house across the bay to Berkeley. While browsing in a bookstore, the most beautiful woman I had ever seen struck up a conversation with me. Tim was twenty-five, a graduate student in psychology at UC Berkeley, and "bisexual." She took me to her house, told me her life story, talked about her conquests. I fell in love. Tim was worldly-wise, wore Navajo jewelry, had studied modern dance, could discuss anything and everything, had an IQ of 165 (so she said) and long flowing black hair (I had chopped off

my hair bowl-fashion shortly after falling in with some socialist Zion-
ists from Hashomer Hatzair in my third year in high school). Although
we slept in the same bed, she refused to make love to me, her reason being that she didn't want the responsibility. I confided to her that the
woman in my sexual fantasies looked like Marilyn Monroe or Jayne
Mansfield. She said that a woman like that would probably want someone more butch than me. It was 1953.

The foregoing anecdote can be situated in its proper historical context when I confess that shortly thereafter I got myself picked up by an
ex-GI in a North Beach bar, thereby unwittingly launching a life of
compul*sive* (rather than compul*sory*) heterosexuality. This may sound
like a harsh judgment, a view through the spiky gauze of aging, a
change in sexual preference, and breast cancer (I had a mastectomy over
a year ago). Yet it cannot be said often enough that for a young woman
in 1953 everything in the culture militated toward pleasing men. I suspect that my bisexual mentor was no exception. Tim's bisexuality may
have served as a refuge when she became too uncomfortable in the lesbian underground. As for me, the heterosexual assumptions of the
dominant culture coupled with a lion's share of traumatic (so what else
is new?) deprivations in early childhood guaranteed a scenario wherein
a docile Goody-Two-Shoes compulsively (and impulsively) falls into
bed with every Big or Little Daddy that comes along. Insofar as the '50s
sanctified virginity as a way of preparing women for lifelong monoga-
mous bedlock, my scenario was not as unexpected as you might think.

My parents were totally unfit to raise children in a reasonable way (in
fact, they farmed me and my older brother out to various foster homes
until we were seven and eleven, but that's another story). In the 1920s,
as anarchists and vegetarians, opposed with equal fervor to the evils of
the State and carnivorism, they had been social rebels, but by the time
I was an adolescent in the late '40s, their latent puritanism surfaced to
mesh with the sexual conservatism of the era. It was only a matter of
time before I would transform the terms of their former radicalism, acting out in the bedroom a rebellion against both social prohibitions and
parents while seeking through compliance with the sexual expectations
of men the love I had been denied as a child. (A shrink I consulted in
the late '50s said I was the most compliant person he had ever met.
And, of course, far be it from him to steer me in the direction of a
differently gendered sexual partner!)

So it transpired that I conveniently "forgot" the implications of my
lesbian desires. Libidinal amnesia was subsequently compounded by

prolonged exposure to psychotherapeutic revelations of my mother's insufficiencies, with the—happily, temporary—consequence of a deepening distrust of women. The return of a women's movement in the early '70s coincided, in my case, with the disintegration of an emotional house of cards. Busy with "my brilliant career" of dancer and choreographer, I had hardly taken notice of the gathering tumult of feminist voices. A white, unconsciously ambitious artist, oblivious to art world sexism and racism, ensconced in the profession of dancing (a socially acceptable female pursuit), protected from the reality of my ambitions by skulking in the shadows of male artists, I started reading *Sisterhood is Powerful* in 1971 as a seven-year relationship blew up in my face, necessitating a long haul—aided and abetted, and in some respects impeded, by feminist essays—out of the ashes of an almost-successful suicide attempt. Shulamith Firestone and Valerie Solanas figured prominently in my enraged demise and recovery.

I had never thought of myself as belonging to an inferior class, especially as I began to achieve recognition in my field. Hadn't I gotten a Guggenheim before he did? Wasn't he always encouraging me and taking pride in my success? Hadn't he said that he hated "false modesty" when I tried to claim I wasn't ambitious?

Excerpts from Firestone's analysis of romantic love in "The Dialectics of Sex" still read with a burning clarity:

> Thus "falling in love" is no more than the process of alteration of male vision—idealization, mystification, glorification—that renders void the woman's class inferiority.
>
> However, the woman knows that this idealization, which she works so hard to produce, is a lie, and that it is only a matter of time before he "sees through her." Her life is a hell, vacillating between an all-consuming need for male love and approval to raise her from her class subjection, to persistent feelings of inauthenticity when she does achieve his love. Thus her whole identity hangs in the balance of her love life. She is allowed to love herself only if a man finds her worthy of love.

Yes, it was the light from *his* eyes as I described the making of *Trio A*—the dance that was to become my signature piece—that first illuminated my achievement. This may have taken place in Monte's, or maybe the San Remo, in the Village, over double vodka martinis in the winter of 1965. I watched his expression change from polite attention to intense appreciation, even wonderment, as I described the details of creation. I was saved.

In a male-run society that defines women as an inferior and parasitical class, a woman who does not achieve male approval in some form is doomed. To legitimate her existence, a woman must be *more* than woman, she must continually search for an out from her inferior definition.

I extracted what I needed to fuel my woman-scorned fury. The corruption of love by power inequities in the "sex class system" produces the proverbial song and dance:

> . . . while men may love, they usually "fall in love"—with their own projected image. . . . It is dangerous to feel sorry for one's oppressor—women are especially prone to this failing—but I am tempted to do it in this case. Being unable to love is hell . . . as soon as the man feels any pressure from the other partner to commit himself, he panics. . . . He may rush out and screw ten other women to prove that the first woman has no hold over him . . . for him to feel safely the kind of total response he first felt for his mother, which was rejected, he must degrade this woman so as to distinguish her from the mother.

Hot stuff! But Firestone's recasting of Freud and Marx and Solanas's apocalyptic vision did more than fuel my outrage. Their writings—and those of a welter of other feminists—gave me permission to begin examining my experience as a woman, as an intelligible and intelligent participant in culture and society rather than the overdetermined outcome of a lousy childhood that had previously dominated my self-perception. I began to come of age reading this stuff. Change, of course, comes with greater difficulty than the reading of a couple of books. The struggle to throw off the status of unknowing collaborator in victimization—at both ends of the domination scale—is uneven and ongoing. But after 1971 my work began to reflect with ever more confidence the details of daily life and implications of "being a woman" in western culture.

By the mid-'70s women in the New York art world were flirting and dancing with each other at parties. It was as though the women's movement had heaved a cornucopia of same-sex sexual fantasies into the face of heterosexual propriety. While real-life lesbians were battling for recognition at NOW conferences, we ladies of illusion were riding a backlash of resentment at our real and imagined oppressors, indicting our failed straight love affairs in displays of wanton—if not libidinous—abandon. Maybe some of us ended up in bed. Not me. I was all show and no go.

"The movement" had penetrated, but I still wasn't calling myself a feminist. It was hard to shake off those received notions of feminists as upper-class women from the '20s and '30s who wore plus fours and rode horses, like Vita Sackville-West or Nancy Cook and Marion Dickerman, the gals with whom Eleanor Roosevelt hung out. (Clearly, a tacit homophobia was operating here. Marilyn and Jayne's departure from the center stage of my fantasy life had occurred with some consequence; it had opened the door to a very specific mistrust.) Furthermore, I thought to be a feminist you had to be politically active, and I wasn't, at least not in that arena. It wasn't until 1975, when Mimi Schapiro convinced me that feminism is as much a state of mind as a matter of activist alliances, that I dared to use the term self-referentially.

At that point I had made two feature films, *Lives of Performers* and *Film About a Woman Who . . .*, both of which dealt in an elliptical fashion with aspects of my own real-life melodramas. With one foot in a quasi minimalist verité and the other in soap opera, I was struggling toward some hybrid form that I hoped would encapsulate and redound with everything from catharsis to pathos to irony to bathos, give or take the baby and the bathwater. My subject matter, for the most part, was heterosexual romance and conflict from a woman's point of view, and the form issued from the broadest definition of narrative: There was no beginning, middle, or closure, no climax, no denouement, no character development, no plot. But there was lots of language which dealt with the trials and tribulations of a she, a she who was here to stay and would have her say.

Some people have called those early films "prepolitical" or "prefeminist." In any case, *Film About a Woman Who . . .* became a focal point for more than one brouhaha among feminist film theorists over issues of positive versus negative imaging of women, avant-garde versus Hollywood, strategies of distanciation versus traditional conventions of "suture," elitism versus populism, documentary versus fiction, and so forth. The debates go on, but in more muted fashion with regard to feminism, as theoretical center stage has been preempted by postcolonial and queer theory, both of which concerns, I should add, were woeful omissions in straight white middle-class feminist discourse in the 1970s and early '80s. Another reason the feminist film wars have somewhat subsided is that as the sheer volume of women's output in film and video began to accrete, it became apparent there are almost as many styles, strategies, and tactical choices manifest in women's work as there are women producers. Progressive feminism does not reside exclusively in any one mode of representation.

But fifteen and twenty years ago the debates over formal procedures were heated and, in several instances, a bit nasty. If my films have become more "accessible" in the sense of availability, it is because I found a distributor who pegged my work as marketable and acted accordingly. As for accessibility in the sense of intelligibility, I still believe in the necessity of certain kinds of narrative "distanciation," a belief that may lack the polemical fervor that characterized my espousals of ten years ago, but which nevertheless continues to inflect many of my decisions. The goals remain the same: to jar the spectator out of comfortable identification (or repulsion) into critical detachment, to complicate and compound the spectator's relation to the immediate scene with additional information, analysis, or emotional affect, and to provide comic relief.

I could now write about relationships with "my last men" and the ten-year gathering of courage and need that propelled me toward a particular woman—not only to "women." I would have to give credit to the examples of younger lesbian and gay friends, their courage and determination and high spirits. I would have to describe getting caught up in Gay Pride marches, getting tired of loneliness, and, most important, inviting Jayne and Marilyn back into my living room from the back porch to which they had been banished for so many years.

I've always looked at women's bodies. Everyone knows that women ogle each others' bodies. We used to be told that we look in order to compare, to see what attracts men. It was a competitive gaze, we were told. Uh-uh. We look because we like them, because women's bodies please us, and it pleases us to look.

Toward the end of the Stonewall 25 march, my lover Martha and I sit down on a railing in Central Park near three women in their late 50s and early 60s. I shall call them Constance, Doris, and Alice. (Not being a journalist, I neglect to ask their names.) They are carrying signs that identify them as NOW activists from Vermont and New Hampshire. We chat about this and that. Finally I muster my nerve and say, "Could I ask you ladies some nosey questions? I'm a filmmaker doing research on aging and sexuality. . . . Did you come out late in life or have you been out for a long time?" Alice instantly retorts, "What makes you think we're out?" I gulp. Does she mean they're not out or that they're not lesbians? I say, "Well, you're *here!*" Alice explains that they're here to support gay and lesbian rights as twenty-year activists in NOW. Doris and Martha exclaim in one voice, "It wasn't always that way!" Alice is quick to add that they're all "just good friends." "But you never know," Constance interjects, "life is full of surprises."

The Avant-garde Humpty Dumpty

This essay was published in the *X-Factor Virtual Conference* on America Online in November 1996 along with other responses to a manifesto sent out by a group of San Francisco media artists.

At the outset I would like to point out the way in which I am not present at this conference. As an ongoing technophobe (only recently—and grudgingly—acquiring a fax machine) who can barely handle word processing, I don't own a modem and therefore cannot participate as "virtually" as most of you.

That said (and casting virtue to the winds), I wish to address certain contradictions in X-Factor's manifesto. It is clear at the beginning that you set out to define the new priorities and classifications being laid out by the cultural bureaucracies, but by the end you have elaborated them to the point of giving the impression that these categories have validity and substance for avant-garde practice. It seems to me that by setting up an "us-and-them" polarization that sees "them" as producing "social service" that aspires to revealing and curing social ills ("short-term palliative triumphs") and "us" as "promoting new categories of informed engagement . . . [for the] long term emancipation of the viewer," the manifesto concludes that we can make clear-cut assumptions about the effect of media on viewers. The palliative effects of social documentaries can no more be anticipated or assessed than "emancipation" from a screening (or ten screenings) of *Wavelength*. (I went to the bathroom during the 1967 screening and missed the bit of drama in the middle.) And we're not even touching the "entertainment" film, as though there is no social value here at all. Yet it was recently noted that *Schindler's List* has to some extent been responsible for the revival of interest in Jewish culture—if not of Jewish culture itself—in parts of Poland.

Another point: I don't think you meant it, but X-Factor comes perilously close to suggesting that "topicality," which the cultural agencies currently favor, cannot be addressed in an innovative or experimental mode, or that experimental media is only concerned with "resistance . . . within the arena of convention." One has only to think about *Two or Three Things I Know About Her* or *Man With a Movie Camera* or *Killer of Sheep* or Tracey Moffat's *Night Cries* to know that this is patently untrue. And at the expense of modesty, I must point to my own efforts of the last fifteen years that have dealt with such topicalities as German politics, New York real estate, U.S. imperialism, and racism, while offering various kinds of resistance to documentary and fictional conventions.

So what *is* the value of an avant-garde cine-video practice? And why is it seen more and more as irrelevant? I'm not sure I have anything new to say about the former. Someone I know (another "last Marxist"?) recently called the avant-garde "a tick in the armpit of the masses." I used to counter charges of elitism with the metaphor of the single stone thrown in the pond. I used to (and still, at the drop of a hat) fulminate against the manipulations of dominant media, against the passivity of the spectator created by the seductions of narrative, against the kind of cinema that "sends the mind away." I was always ambivalent, however, even in my most polemical moments. I'm now more uncertain than ever about what kind of film creates what kind of spectator. I'm not sure what it means if 25 people see a given film rather than 1,000. (My most "famous" dance work, *The Mind is a Muscle,* was seen by no more than 250 people in the course of four performances.) I do know that, like John Cage in relation to harmony, I must "devote my life to beating my head against that wall." In my case the wall is cinematic narrative.

Why that particular head-beating and others like it should be supported by taxpayers' money is another story. There is no doubt that the NEA and other public agencies are scared shitless of the angrier members of our constituency. The NEA's current guidelines are mind-boggling in bending every which way to create weird and absurd categories of social value. They have made it impossible for any self-respecting artist to comply with a straight face; in fact they have made it impossible to apply as an individual, period.

However, I can't be entirely pessimistic about the "current climate" where art is concerned. The mean-spirited shift in economic policies and withdrawal of resources from welfare agencies will have a calamitous effect on people in the lower part of the economic pyramid, but young—mostly middle-class—artists have always found some underground in which to operate, witness the—and I'm now talking as a New Yorker—"it's all moving to Williamsburg" phenomenon. Film, however, because it requires heavier funding than the other arts, and more expensive exhibition trappings, is already suffering.

The mainstream has always beckoned. If you carpet with music, get "better" or more glamorous actors (preferably young), up your production values, add some plot twists, add a murder or two, make it ninety minutes (for theatrical distribution) or fifty-eight and a half (for TV), and tack on an upbeat ending, you may "make it." Between 1975 and 1990—and again I'm talking about New York—you could find an exhibition space and an audience, albeit a small one, either by flouting or ignoring the above requirements. Not only that, but you could sometimes get a pretty interesting discussion going about art and politics. Today, in contrast, the attrition in funding and venues has created a situation in which specialized annual festivals, like Lesbian and Gay Film Festivals, the Mix Festival, and the Asian-American Film Festival have absorbed the energies and interests of young cine-video artists who don't want to be isolated at Anthology or Millennium, which are seen as the last desperate bastions of the avant-garde. An ongoing scene of vigorous all-year-round exhibition of and attendance at film classics and new work just doesn't exist anymore. It is therefore understandable that young cine-videomakers, in the absence of ongoing dialogue about, with, and around experimental cine-video, its antecedents, its viewers, and its venues, look to the economic and aesthetic imperatives of the marketplace. Add more music, get "better" or more glamorous . . . etc., etc.

All this groaning simply means I miss the Collective for Living Cinema. I miss the Millennium before it started to reek of mildew. I miss the events at the Whitney Museum. I miss feeling part of a community. Festivals don't provide that. Although I'm one of the lucky ones—I've managed to keep working—and, for many reasons (generational for one), have so far been insulated from the current grimness, I see the handwriting on the wall. The days of public and foundation funding for fiction features are over, for me at least (the big ones, Wexner and MacArthur, that enabled me to complete my last film, *MURDER and murder,* are once-in-a-lifetime). And from the standpoint of the marketplace, it may be over if I insist on banging my head against that wall. The fact remains, you can't make an avant-garde omelette without breaking some eggs. And the lines are drawn, in every quarter, as to the number of eggs you can break.

A last addendum: According to a buzz that reached me at this year's Toronto Film Festival, the definition of "independent" is a film that opens in less than 500 theaters! What's the world coming to?

Commencement Address

This address was delivered at the School of the Museum of Fine Arts, Boston, May 16, 1997.

Some years ago I saw Trisha Brown perform a dance in which she recounted how she had addressed a graduating class at her old high school in Aberdeen, Washington. She had urged the girls to keep up the good fight and told the boys they were doing all right.

I'd like, for the moment, to override this opportunity for comparable inspirational exhortations and face several facts: (1) You can make art out of anything (I mean, who could have imagined a fragment of a commencement address becoming part of a dance!), and (2) I don't envy you and wouldn't like to be in your shoes.

Call this a kind of performative play between the joys and terrors of both art-making and what may turn out to be some presumptuous projections into your futures as working artists. Let me illustrate my first point: Whether you raid the ice box of art history or ransack the daily paper or your own refrigerator, a potential goldmine lies in wait. Not a literal goldmine, mind you; after all, the alchemical era of the '80s art world, when shit could be transmuted into gold by young and living artists, came to an end quite awhile ago. I am talking about the cornucopia, the "world-is-my-oyster" mode of thinking in which artists may find themselves as they search for subject matter and representational formats.

Such a cornucopia beckoned to composers, dancers, and visual artists of my generation as we entered the 1960s. By the early '60s the ongoing modernist assault took as its targets certain practices that had become accepted and downright respectable in critical circles. In music it was Schönberg and the twelve-tone row; in dance it was Graham and

Humphrey and the exalted transformation of the performer; in the visual arts it was the Abstract Expressionists and their heroic gestures. All of this was grist for the mills of the followers of Marcel Duchamp, Merce Cunningham, and John Cage. There ensued a period of exuberant productivity in which dancers walked and ran, painters and sculptors made dances, and composers sat at pianos doing nothing in particular while the audience coughed. And yet, and yet, for all the wealth and euphoria of ideas, there were devastating omissions and neglectfulness.

John Cage characterized his aleatory methods of composition as "an affirmation of life, not an attempt to bring order out of chaos nor to suggest improvements on creation, but simply a way of waking up to the very life we're living, which is so excellent once one gets one's mind and one's desires out of its way and lets it act of its own accord." And the means by which we were to awaken to this excellent life? By getting our minds and desires out of the way, by making way for an art of indeterminacy, existing in the gap between life and art, to be practiced by everyone.

Let's not come down too heavily on what may now seem, in its combination of J. J. Rousseau and Zen Buddhism, like a goofy naiveté that totally ignored worldwide struggles for self-determination, the destructive effects of profit-geared economic policies, and, most significantly, the question, "*Whose* life is so excellent and at what cost to others?" After all, Cage's widespread influence occurred sometime before the art world was ready to listen to the disruptive voices of women, people of color, and lesbians and gays, all clamoring for recognition and legitimation. I will even suggest that Cage's notions about democratizing art helped pave the way to the airing of all those issues around race, gender, sexuality, and class that have since burst through the palace gates of high white culture. Even in the '60s the debates around Warhol could not resolve whether his soup cans were a celebration of unfettered capitalism or a critique of commodity fetishism.

Today, in a time of mounting pressures from the Religious Right and a deteriorating quality of life for the poor and those unable to cash in on the stock market or information economy, in a time of embattlement for those who continue to be marginalized or excluded from public life and its representations, art-making still lures us with the possibility of being for a few moments in charge of our lives, our bodies, our imaginations—in a nutshell, in charge of the show. At the same time the intricacies of identity politics have created new minefields wherein artists at every stage of their development, if you are in the least bit critical, are confronted with a conflict. You may feel you have to choose between focusing your practice on the politics of a singular aspect of cultural/racial identity and the temptation to do something more idiosyncratic, cross-cultural, or abstract. This dilemma would seem to apply to many of you—both men and women—as you embark on your careers, but let me assure you that it is just as relevant to someone who's been around as long as I have.

Following the '60s controversies surrounding Cage and Warhol (and Johns and Judd, etc., etc.) '70s feminism challenged what was perceived as the new male-dominated canon with images from women's experience, the domestic and public spheres, the body. Hallowed biological and social assumptions were thrown with great gusto through the window and against the wall by the likes of Martha Rosier, Nancy Spero, Miriam Schapiro, Vito Acconci, and others. The work of these artists (and, incidentally, my own work) was in turn implicitly called into question by the emergence of the art of African Americans, Latinos, and Asians, or, more accurately, by the newly raised consciousness of curators who began to realize what was out there. By the early '80s I, for one, became enamored of the work of Charles Burnett, Julie Dash, Carrie Mae Weems, and Faith Ringgold.

Which brings me back to my second point made at the beginning of this talk: I don't envy you and wouldn't want to be in your shoes. The big question is: What with the cost of living and the general climate of backlash and vindictiveness toward affirmative action, assistance to the poor and old, and subsidy of the arts, how does a young artist today get a career foothold or simply maintain minimal conditions for productivity? When I started out, art-making was a way out of social conditions that fostered a severely repressive conformity, and for the first eight years of my life as a choreographer there was no such thing as government support. Those were the days when a two-and-a-half-room apartment cost $40 a month, and you could get a spaghetti dinner and a glass of wine for 99¢ and live on a part-time job. Only later, with the advent of arts funding and increased enrollment in art schools, did it become apparent that art-making could also be a way out of poverty.

But now what? Arts subsidies are drying up, a two-and-a-half-room apartment costs $1,500 a month, and a spaghetti dinner costs $25. Everyone is scared. Dinner conversation, once enlivened by arguments about aesthetic strategies and politics, now revolves leadenly around academic positions and real estate. And for all the twenty-five years of agitation for broader cultural inclusion in museum shows, the latest mailing from the Guerrilla Girls tells us that out of seventy-one artists in an upcoming show at MOMA, there are only three white women, one woman of color, and no men of color. I can add a dismal statistic from my own field: The last New York Film Festival included thirty male directors and three women. When I confronted one of the (all-male) panelists about this he whined, "One can't select a film just because it's made by a woman." For a moment I thought I had been thrust back to the '70s when there were also a few token females present, like Agnes Varda and Marguarite Duras. Of course, *they* were French, a probable mitigating factor in their selection.

Now who's whining? I must remind myself—while reminding you— that as artists we are not necessarily entitled. Period. As a dancer I knew that the rewards would only be commensurate with the effort, and at that time my expectation was simply more work as a reward for work done. In this day and age it is a little quaint, even downright utopian, to harbor such a notion. So I will not leave it at that. If you want to survive as artists, you must take advantage of all available systems—like networking, sending out slides, shmoozing, making formal applications for grants, etc. A young woman I know who now edits a small art journal told me some years ago that at parties she became aware that the guys were networking, sharing information, and hustling, while the gals were getting drunk, dancing, and having fun. OK ladies, GET SERIOUS. And this applies to you gents as well: If you're disillusioned with exhibition opportunities, band together and create your own, and it doesn't have to be with your own gender. Collaborate, organize, agitate. It won't come to you on a platter.

Let me end with some provocative questions that pertain to my own situation and may border on yours: You wanna bet that Madonna will be hitchhiking, nude on that highway, with purse and plastic heels and scarred abdomen and aching hip joints and single breast when she's sixty? I'll lay you odds. You wanna bet that before the year 2000 we'll see a romantic mainstream film about two 60-year-old black lesbians? You wanna bet that the postmenopausal female protagonist will become a mainstay of drama and film without having to have a nervous breakdown or die of cancer in the process? Will an audience that hungers for cultural products that reflect something other than the consummation of young love be created in larger numbers as the U.S. population ages? Will the demographics of immune deficiency disorders that are raising infant mortality rates throughout the western hemisphere, afflicting more and more people between the ages of twenty-five and forty-four, wiping out whole villages in Africa, and decimating and demoralizing the former Soviet Union, result in a greater interest in representations of the experiences of old ladies, queers, and the indigent? Is someone making—will someone please make—a theater or film or video work, avant-garde or otherwise, about the grim legacy of nuclear power—civilian no less than military—that we have inherited and of which we must now bear the consequences in unequal measure regardless of race, economic class, sexual preference, gender, or age? And will these representations be dismissed as "victim art" or will they be heralded as "survivor art?"

Yes, you can make art out of anything if you put your mind to it. I urge all of you to keep up the good fight and not be afraid of trying on other people's shoes. If they pinch, I'm sure you'll find some way to represent that. I also wish every one of you all the luck in the world.

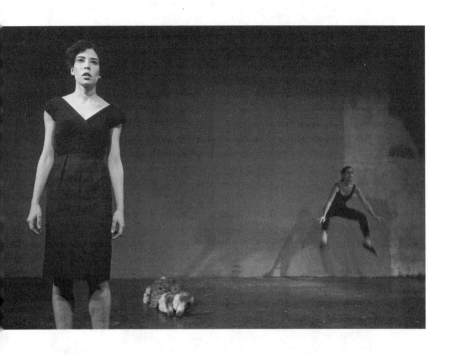

Deborah Hay, Lucinda Childs, and Yvonne Rainer in *Dialogues* at
Stage 73, New York City, February 9, 1964. Photo by Peter Moore.

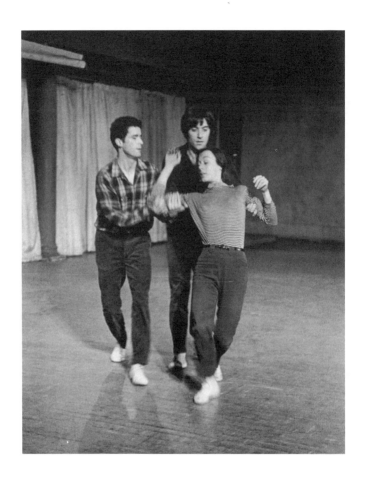

William Davis, David Gordon, and Yvonne Rainer in *Trio A¹* from the first version of *The Mind is a Muscle,* performed at Judson Church, May 24, 1966. Photo by Peter Moore.

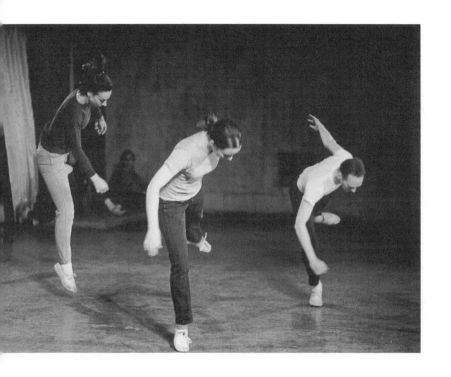

Becky Arnold, Barbara Dilley, Peter Saul in *Trio B* from the first
version of *The Mind is a Muscle* at Judson Church. Photo by
Peter Moore.

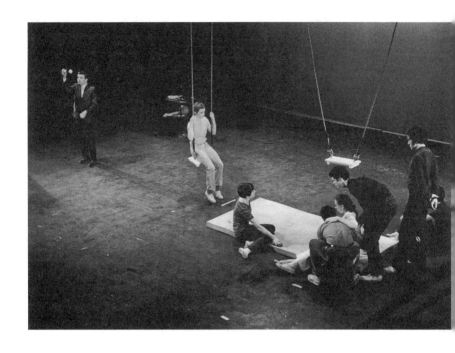

Harry De Dio, Barbara Dilley, Gay Delanghe, Steve Paxton, Becky Arnold, William Davis, David Gordon, and Yvonne Rainer in *Act* from *The Mind is a Muscle,* performed at the Anderson Theater in New York City, April 11, 1968. Photo by Peter Moore.

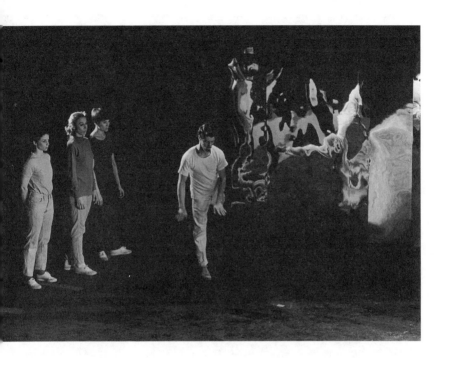

Barbara Dilley, Becky Arnold, and Gay Delanghe watch Steve
Paxton perform *Trio A* during *The Mind is a Muscle* at the Anderson
Theater. Photo by Peter Moore.

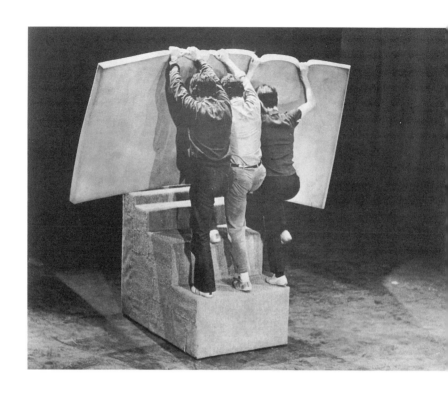

David Gordon, Steve Paxton, and Yvonne Rainer in *Stairs* from *The Mind is a Muscle* at the Anderson Theater. Photo by Julie Abeles.

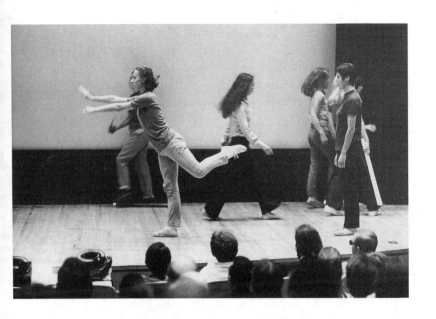

Yvonne Rainer teaches Becky Arnold *Trio A* during *Performance Demonstration* at the Performing Arts Library, Lincoln Center, September 16, 1968. Photo by Peter Moore.

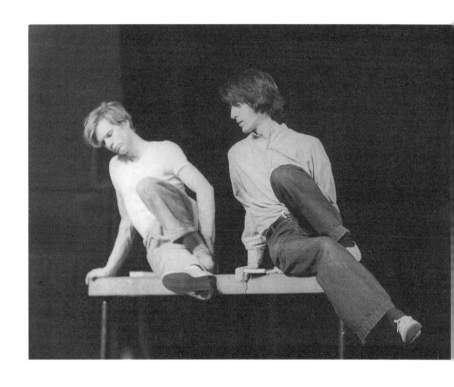

Douglas Dunn and Frederic J. Lehrman in *North East Passing* (choreographed in 1968), performed at the Billy Rose Theater, February 6, 1969. Photo by Peter Moore.

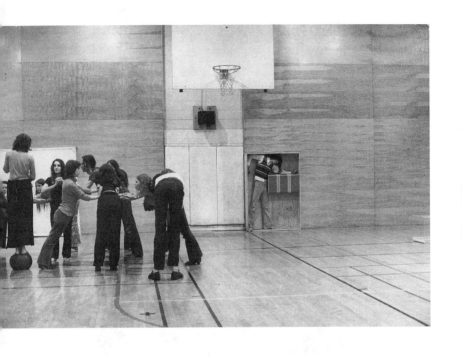

Grand Union Dreams at the 14th St. YM-YWHA, New York City,
May 16, 1971. Photo by Susan Horwitz.

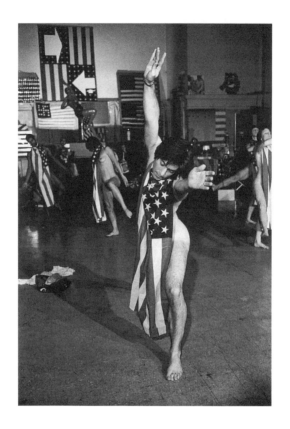

Trio A, performed in the People's Flag Show at Judson Church, November 9, 1970. David Gordon in foreground. Photo by Peter Moore.

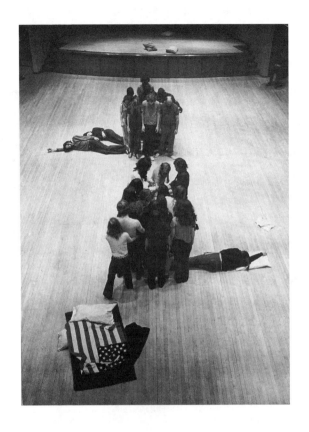

War at Loeb Student Center, New York University, November 22, 1970. Photo by Peter Moore.

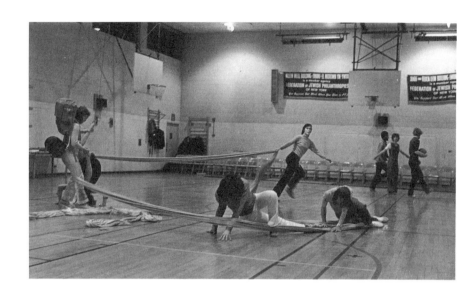

The Grand Union at the 14th St. YM-YWHA, New York City, Spring 1971. Photo by James Klosty.

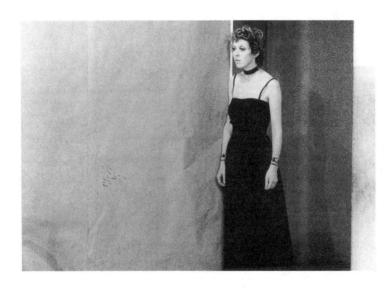

Valda Setterfield in *Lives of Performers* (1972).

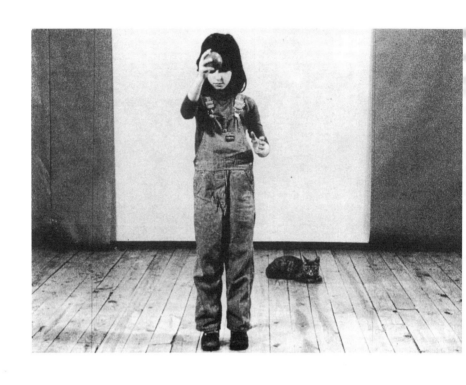

Sarah Soffer in *Lives of Performers* (1972).

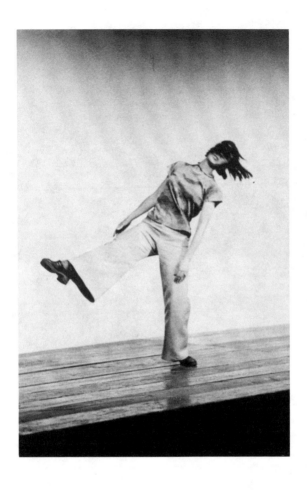

Yvonne Rainer performing *Trio A* at the Portland Center for the Visual Arts, Spring 1973.

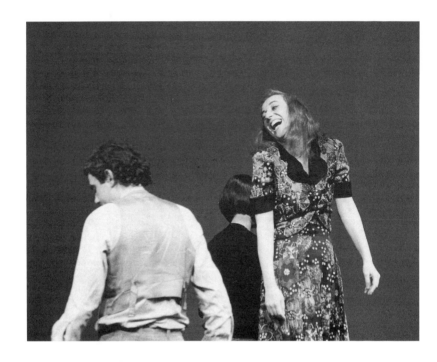

John Erdman, Yvonne Rainer, and Shirley Soffer in *This is the story of a woman who . . .* performed at the Theater for the New City (Fall 1973). Photo by Babette Mangolte.

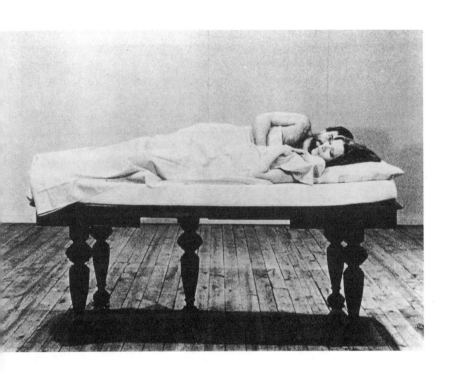

Dempster Leach and Renfreu Neff in *Film About a Woman Who . . .*
(1974). Production still by Babette Mangolte.

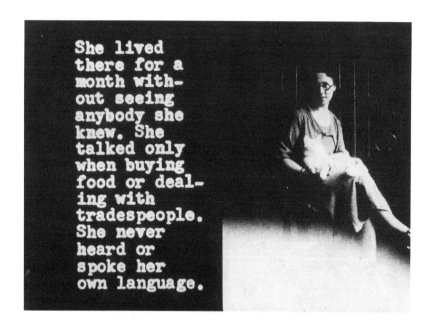

She lived there for a month without seeing anybody she knew. She talked only when buying food or dealing with tradespeople. She never heard or spoke her own language.

Frame enlargement from *Film About a Woman Who . . .*

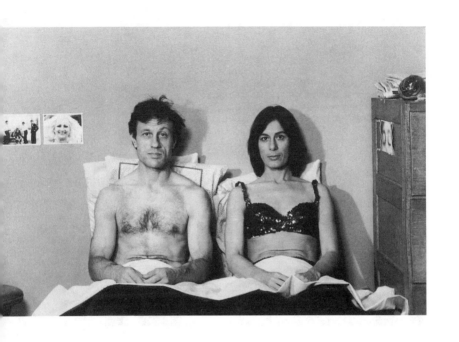

Ivan Rainer and Yvonne Rainer in *Kristina Talking Pictures* (1976).
Production still by Babette Mangolte.

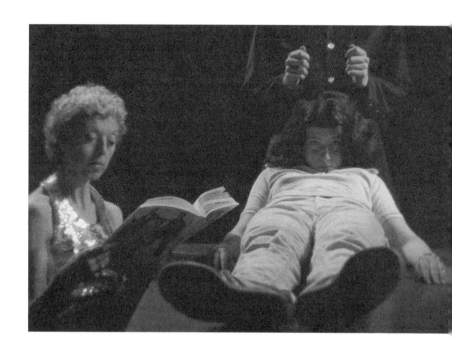

Valda Setterfield and Sarah Soffer in *Kristina Talking Pictures*.

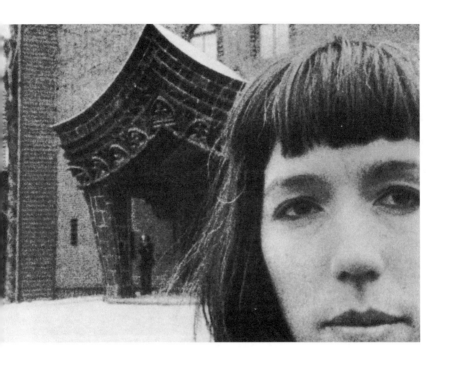

Cynthia Beatt in *Journeys from Berlin/1971* (1980).

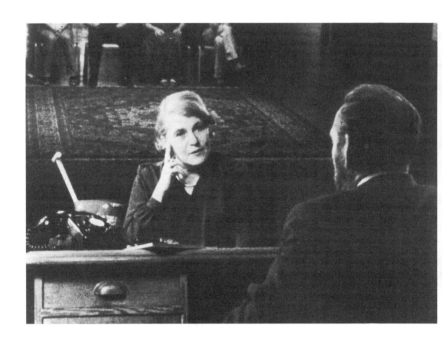

Annette Michelson and Gabor Vernon in *Journeys from Berlin/1971.*

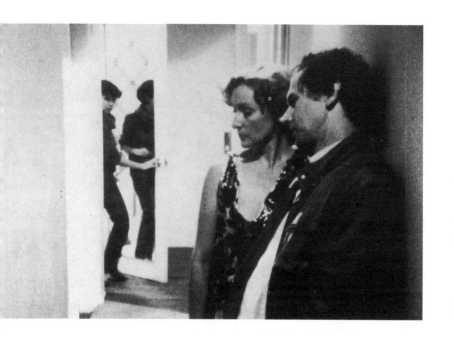

Melody London, Jackie Raynal, and William Raymond in *The Man Who Envied Women* (1985).

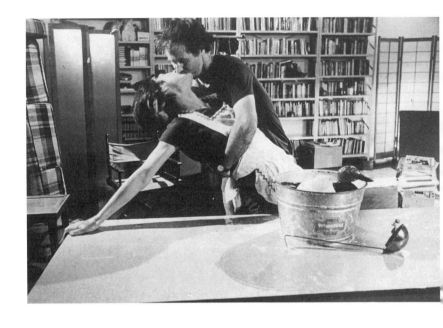

Yvonne Rainer and William Raymond in *The Man Who Envied Women.*

The most rem thing was the silence emaated from friends an famil regarding the details of ny single middleage. Whn I was younger, my sex life had been the object of all kinds of questioning, from prurient curiosity to solicitous concern. Now that I did not appear to be looking for a man, the state of desires seemed of no interest to anyone.

Frame enlargement from *Privilege* (1990).

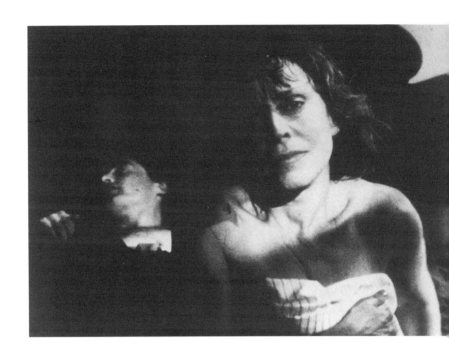

Dan Berkey and Alice Spivak in *Privilege.*

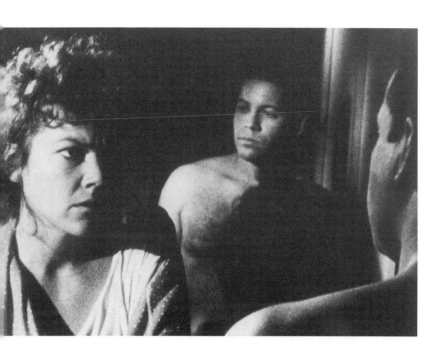

Blaire Baron and Rico Elias in *Privilege.*

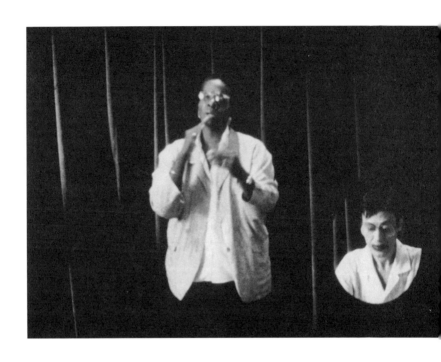

Claudia Gregory and Yvonne Rainer in *Privilege.*

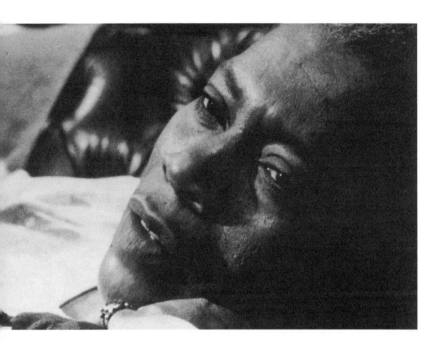

Novella Nelson in *Privilege.*

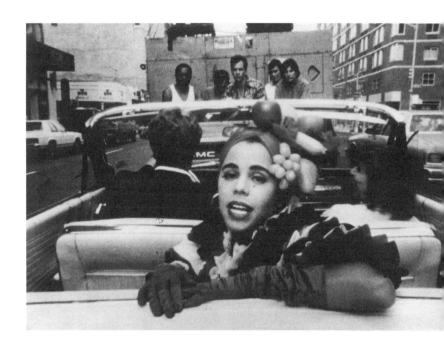

Gabriella Farrar in *Privilege.*

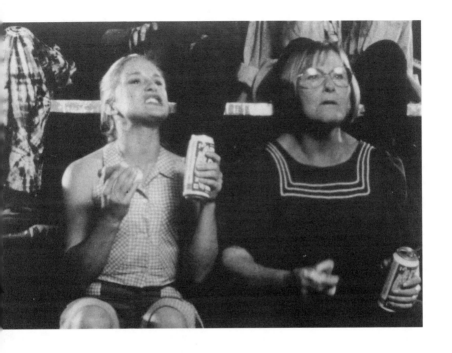

Catherine Kellner and Isa Thomas at the boxing match in *MURDER and murder* (1996).

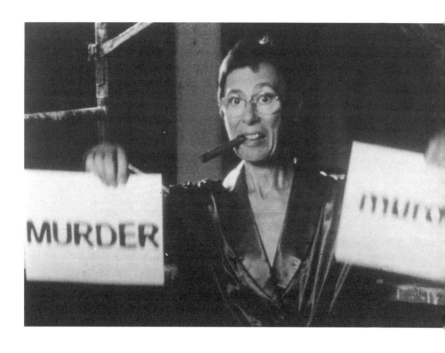

Yvonne Rainer, "the next contender," in *MURDER and murder.*

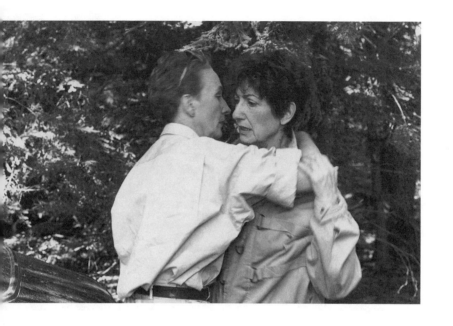

Kathleen Chalfant and Joanna Merlin go to the country in
MURDER and murder.

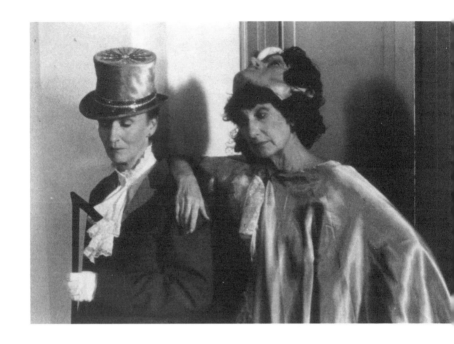

Kathleen Chalfant and Joanna Merlin at the masquerade in
MURDER and murder.

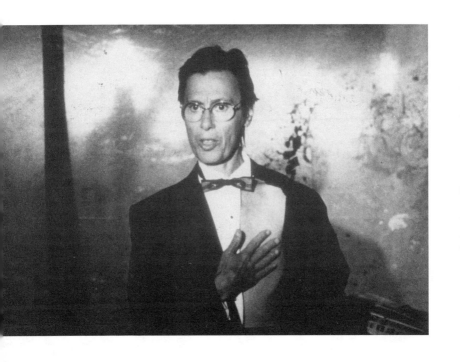

Yvonne Rainer, the "marked woman," in *MURDER and murder.*

III Film and Narrative

A Likely Story

This paper was delivered on a panel September 3, 1976, as part of the "International Forum on Avant-Garde Film" during the Edinburgh Film Festival. It was later published in *Idiolects,* no. 6 (June 1978). The panel of which I was a member—along with Peter Wollen, Manuel de Landa, and Simon Field—was on film and narrative. I recall Paul Sharits at some point asserting that everything was narrative, even his work, which of course derailed any possibility of subtle argumentation. It was at this conference that I first met Laura Mulvey and heard her speak about her now-famous essay "Visual Pleasure and Narrative Cinema." I gathered up my *chutzpah* to ask the poor woman "what about the female spectator?" as though she hadn't already been put through the wringer on this issue. She replied that she was going to be dealing with that in a later essay, which of course she proceeded to do in her usual breathtakingly thorough manner.

In a strict sense—and I always prefer narrow definitions because then we know where we stand—in a strict sense, a narrative state of affairs exists when at least one of certain conditions is met, such as indications of causality, or temporal or psychological coherence, or dramatic resolution dependent on a clear rendering of past and future time. Narrative demands that objects, events, and personages be connected, however marginally, by something other than fortuitous proximity in time and/or space or morphological and iconographic similarity.

Narrative produces an expectation and effect different from those produced by the distillations, transmutations, and perambulations between meaning and sound that characterize poetry. It also stands in opposition to the parataxic, a method of ordering that in its emphasis on the discreteness of things, presumes their *a priori* relatedness or equivalence, a relatedness that is not always immediately evident. Evidence and qualification are not as crucial to a parataxic method of ordering materials as to a narrative one. The latter continues to overwhelm and intimidate us with its hierarchies of contingent facts, its hordes of psychological priorities, circumstantial details, and extenuating circumstances; its excesses of circumspection—or irresponsibility, as the case may be—in revealing or concealing particularities of location and time; its potential to produce endless speculation, discourses on the real and the plausible, mistaken identities, and chronic complication, not to mention murder and mayhem. Is it any wonder that so many artists have given it a wide berth and a short shrift?

I suppose that there have always been those works that can rightfully be called neither narrative nor nonnarrative, works that share *both* narrative and nonnarrative characteristics. In such a work there may come a point where you realize that the point of departure, or center of gravity, or stylistic mode has drifted, forcing you to shift your attention and look or read with a new frame of reference. For example, a series of events containing answers to *when, where, why, whom*, gives way to a series of images, or maybe a single image, which, in its obsessive repetitiveness or prolonged duration or rhythmic predictability or even stillness, becomes disengaged from story and enters this other realm, call it catalogue, demonstration, lyricism, poetry, or pure research. The work now floats free of ultimate climax, pot of gold, pay-off, future truth, existing solely in the present.

Or perhaps a work that starts out being meditative, concerned with resonance, mood, or investigation of its own procedures and premises suddenly changes its density by appropriating elements of melodrama. And there may always be the possibility for a simultaneous fusion or coexistence of these modes rather than the succession I have described.

If I may shift to a more personal narrative for a moment, let me insert here that my own involvement with narrative forms has not always been either happy or wholehearted, rather more often a dalliance than a commitment. The reason lies partly in the nature of the predominating form of narrative film. The tyranny of a form that creates the expectation of a continuous answer to "what will happen next?" fanatically pursuing an inexorable resolution in which all things find their just or correct placement in space and time; such a tyranny, having already attained its epiphany in the movies (I think of *Gertrud, Senso, Balthazar, Contempt, Lulu*) such a form has inevitably seemed more ripe for resistance, or at least evasion, than for emulation.

My own forays into this territory border on a kind of banditry, the need for which has slowly evolved out of a dilemma imposed by subject matter. This dilemma has become more clarified for me on the completion of each of my three films, presenting itself in the form of basic, though variously oriented, questions asked—and not always answered—by each of these films and having, I would hope, wider application than my own work.

Can the presentation of sexual conflict in film or the presentation of the experience of love and jealousy be revitalized through a studied placement or dislocation of clichés borrowed from soap opera and melodrama? Can specific states of mind and emotion or subtleties of social interaction be conveyed in film without being attached or by being only provisionally attached to particularities of place, time, person, and relationship? And can such subject matter be presented without being "acted out"—in both the theatrical and psychoanalytic senses—via simulated dialogue and gesture? Are faces such as belong to Katharine Hepburn and Liv Ullman the only vehicles for grief and passion? Can a film achieve comparable impact through means other than these faces? And why in the world would one ever want to achieve an effect comparable to that wonder of art and nature, the smile fading from Hepburn's face?

Can an audience learn to abandon its narrative expectation once that expectation has been aroused by narrative elements in a work? Must modes of operation be consistent within a given work? Can subject matter dealing with perceptual and photographic phenomena be sequentially—rather than narratively—linked to material that has already been invested with "storyness"? When can one say—to quote from Annette Michelson's reading from Eisenstein's diary the other day—"Experiment external to the thesis is impossible"[1] and when is such experiment possible, or appropriate? Conversely, when is it inappropriate to use a narrative thesis? Why bother with it at all? What is the connection between lions and Jews? What is the relationship between a man stepping forward from a line of people and a distant car moving out from behind a foregrounded group of lions?[2] And does not a photograph of a forty-five-year-old peroxide blonde female lion-tamer tell us all we need to know about the "shit of the world?"[3]

What kinds of clues tell us, the audience, when to read an image—or series of images—narratively, when to read them parataxically, and when to read them iconographically? What constitutes continuity in the movies and what kind of clue tells us to "begin again"? Why this urgency in our acculturated and suppurating brain that propels us to find connections between what we simultaneously see and hear, between what we have just seen and what we are about to see? What constitutes unity in a film? Can the narrative and the other-than-narrative exist simultaneously in the same shot, creating a kind of strobe effect with regard to meaning?

Can something—say, a tiger—at a narrative level be at once illustrative of the heroine's vocation, symbolic of unknown danger, representative of endangered species—and at the same time function as an object of choreographic and cinematic pattern-making? Or does this something—say, a tiger—once having been assigned its narrative *raison d'etre,* refuse to be relegated to what may seem by comparison a limbo of purely formal filmic construction? Or, on the other hand, can this filmic construction infuse new life into an old story, create new meanings and levels of interpretation? (Witness *Critical Mass.*[4])

Is it entirely Quixotic to entertain notions of a work that might accommodate both a cone of light, and a wedge of pie being eaten by an escaped Brazilian political prisoner in the San Juan Hilton at 5:30 P.M. August 5th before meeting his brother-in-law, who has the keys to . . .

Will generational, or multifold techniques of reproduction of pictorial, kinesthetic, and behavioral material, or techniques for diffusing and fracturing the re-presentation of the real—will such techniques bring about a rapprochement between nonnarrative film and narrative and the irritation-cum-intellectual-deprivation that so often goes with film-as-pure-research? But now I had better stop asking questions. I've already started to rig the game. And besides, it isn't as if there aren't already lots of films that have achieved this—at least for moments on end.

Notes

1. See *October,* no. 2.

2. These references are to my film *Kristina Talking Pictures,* screened on the previous evening.

3. Reference to a paper delivered by Adrianna Apra on the first day, in which he said, "Structuralist films are not concerned with the shit of the world."

4. *Critical Mass,* a film by Hollis Frampton, 1971.

Interview

by the Camera Obscura Collective

The following interview appeared in *Camera Obscura, A Journal of Feminism and Film Theory/1* (1976). The first issue of this periodical was assembled by a passionate collective consisting of Janet Bergstrom, Sandy Flitterman, Elisabeth Hart Lyon, and Constance Penley. After reading the interview a friend described it as "the hare chasing the hounds." I had somehow found myself playing devil's advocate throughout, dragging my feet through their certainties and hell-for-leather faith in Brechtian correlations between form and social good. Now they are all dispersed in their widely divergent interests, from classic Hollywood to *Star Trek,* while I have stayed behind to struggle over and over with the same questions. It was fun while it lasted.

CAMERA OBSCURA: We're starting off with a very broad question to situate the general area we'd like to talk about. There is much in your radical formalism which has points of convergence with radical political concerns. (We are leaving these terms loosely defined for the moment.) Some of these shared concerns include a critique of illusionism of emotional identification, of the performer as "expressing self," and of the performance as virtuosic. Combined with these critiques is your assertion of dance or performance as work, as task, and of the dancer as "neutral doer"; moreover, each of these concerns is set within the context of social relations. Also there is your attempt at collective work, and the fact that, in all your writings, you are consciously involved with process and change.

Do you yourself see any connections, or analogues, between your radical formalism and radical political concerns, and secondly, do you see your work as making any kind of contribution to sociopolitical change?

YVONNE RAINER: The answer to the last question is an emphatic *no*. I see myself in the same predicament as many artists who identify themselves, or have been identified, with the so-called avant-garde. No matter how overtly politicized my work becomes with respect to subject matter, my thinking and making process will always result in a product that appeals to a very select audience, an audience already disposed to share my point of view and appreciate the manner in which it is conveyed. When I started making films I hoped otherwise, but now I know all that was wishful thinking, based partly on the notion that film—or video, for that matter—has a de facto appeal to the masses. 'Taint necessarily so. But it seems to me you're imposing certain questionable interpretations on my work. What do you mean, or where do you see, for instance, a "critique of the self"?

CO: We've gotten some of these ideas from your writings and previous interviews, as well as from your films. For example:

> w s/*Avalanche*: That attitude seems very similar to Nauman, who said in our 1970 interview, the work wasn't about himself, but about a person, any person. How did you come to that point? That's pivotal because it structures the whole relation of the audience to the performer.

> y r: That comes straight out of my awareness . . . of the way l phrased and delineated for myself the dilemma of dance as an art form. That more than anything accounts for where my work went from 1965 on. It was this trying to find an alternative to—I have consistently used these words—narcissism, virtuosity, and display. Coming to terms with my own exhibitionist nature. I mean people go into performing and dancing for this very reason. It has to do with the immediate confrontation with the adoring gaze of the spectator and living in that moment. . . . It led me more toward making dance that was involved with task, work, rather than with exhibition. . . . So being, I guess, a kind of renegade, or wanting to define for myself the battles that still remained, the arena seemed very much to lie with revealing to the audience some kind of "work" rather than "preening." Not showing off my skill but revealing my involvement. And the idea of task and a more concrete, autonomous-looking life on stage that was not constantly projected out at the audience seemed the way to handle this. (from the interview with Willoughby Sharp and Liza Bear printed in *Avalanche,* summer 1972)

Or, from your article "A Quasi Survey of Some 'Minimalist' Tendencies in the Quantitatively Minimal Dance Activity Midst the Plethora, Or an Analysis of Trio A" (in *Minimal Art,* Battcock, ed., 1968, and reprinted in your book *Work* 1961–73.):

In the early days of the Judson Dance Theater someone wrote an article and asked, 'Why are they so intent on just being themselves?'. . . Where the question applies, it might be answered on two levels: (1) The artifice of performance has been reevaluated in that action, or what one does, is more interesting and important than the exhibition of character and attitude, and that action can best be focused on through the submerging of the personality; so ideally one is not even oneself, one is a neutral "doer." (2) The display of technical virtuosity and the display of the dancer's specialized body no longer make any sense. Dancers have been driven to search for an alternative context that allows for a more matter-of-fact, more concrete, more banal quality of physical being in performance, a context wherein people are engaged in actions and movements making a less spectacular demand on the body and in which skill is hard to locate.

It is easy to see why the *grand jeté* (along with its ilk) had to be abandoned. One cannot "do" a *grand jeté*; one must "dance" it to get it done at all, i.e., invest it with all the necessary nuances of energy distribution that will produce the look of climax together with a still, suspended extension in the middle of the movement. Like a romantic overblown plot, this particular kind of display—with its emphasis on nuance and skilled accomplishment, its accessibility to comparison and interpretation, its involvement with connoisseurship, its introversion, narcissism, and self-congratulatoriness—has finally in this decade exhausted itself, closed back on itself, and perpetuates itself solely by consuming its own tail. The alternatives that were explored now are obvious: stand, walk, run, eat, carry bricks, show movies, or move or be moved by some *thing* rather than oneself.

In addition to statements of this kind, you describe in your book performances which you organized in opposition to the Vietnam War and political repression: *WAR* (1970); *M-Walk* (1969); the *Judson Flag Show* (1970).

You seem to give performance a social definition. We're really interested in the analogy we see between the analytical and distanciating form your work takes, the kind of audience involvement this form necessitates, and the implications, following that line, for social change.

YR: Some of those early writings had a decidedly idealistic bent. That kind of thinking caused me a great deal of difficulty when I tried applying it to my life as well as my art. Which now, of course, makes me very suspicious of the original impulse. It seems clear that I was trying to elevate my concerns as a dancer into a form that was more "serious" than the activity construed to be sophomoric then prevailing in the modern dance world. Utilizing references to the everyday, to athletics, to the bizarre, was our way of removing ourselves from the expressive artiness of modern dance. At that point it seemed that the original expressiveness of the pioneers—Duncan, Graham, Humphrey—had degenerated, all but disappeared, and was not available to us in an acceptable form. We had to start elsewhere. The problem is that in the attempt to justify and launch a movement as vital and audacious as that early '60s dance explosion, enthusiasm can easily become rhetoric. I won't say that I was the worst offender, but I was certainly one of them. For instance, the flaw in the ideal of the "neutral doer." I wrote that one can't "do" a *grand jeté,* one has to "dance" it. Well, neither can one "do" a walk without investing it with character. From the beginning, one of the reasons Steve Paxton's walking people were so effective was that the walk was so simply and astonishingly "expressive of self." But are you making a distinction between those who produce and those who express themselves?

CO: That doesn't seem possible. But we are interested in de-emphasizing the expressive and emphasizing the productive aspects of performance and of art-making, and of emphasizing a corresponding view of the audience—redefining the audience as participants in the production of meaning rather than as appreciators of artistic virtuosity. One of the projects that our journal is attempting is to talk about the politically progressive aspects of films which are reflexive in terms of the processes of signification and the production of meaning. That is not to say that avant-garde filmmakers necessarily consider themselves or their films to be political.

We find that there has been an arbitrary separation made between experimental, avant-garde filmmaking and so-called political films. We see one of our projects as an attempt to redefine political filmmaking to include the progressive aspects of formal innovation. It is not that specific formal strategies are progressive in themselves, but in a political context, they can be important tools. For this interview we don't want to draw a direct correlation between your work and socialist politics, but rather to evaluate some of the radical implications of your formal strategies.

YR: Are you trying to suggest a way in which social change occurs, and to underline how art is more effective than we know? One of the notions I acquired in the '60s—and I'm trying to change it—was about the uselessness of art, or its usefulness only to the people who are directly engaged in it. At the point where it's in museums and people go to see it, it really has not too much to do with their lives. And before that, it seems to be a pretty small part of the population, any population, that is immediately affected by art-making. Maybe you're trying to get at something else . . . and it's about the very nature of this work, and the decision-making process. Are you trying to find a correspondence between revolutionary art and social change?

CO: We think one of the ways this culture works to keep people separated is to encourage people to believe that they're autonomous, isolated individuals. By "critique of the self," we meant a critique of *that* notion of individualism, a critique which we would consider an absolutely necessary prerequisite to any kind of progressive social change.

YR: Here I would have to talk on a very personal level about my relationship to that concept and more about my social experience as an artist than about how my work reflects an attitude about this matter. What you will make of that in terms of your needs to theorize about the work, I'll leave that up to you for the time being. First off, with regard to the social framework within which I work, I don't collaborate, as I have said. It goes against the nature of my ambition. The way I arrived at a self-identity was through involvement with work on an individual level. It so happens that I was working in an area that was highly social; it involved people. It was not like being a painter with a canvas, or a writer. I went through various phases of acceptance of a directorial role in relation to the particular group I was working with in the late '60s. My needs for family became confused with ideas of equality, egalitarian cooperation towards a common goal. I imposed on this working situation a cooperative structure which the people in the group had very different degrees of ability to cope with, including myself. That was the beginning of the Grand Union. I found out only after that relationship was launched that it was not appropriate for me, for my ego needs, so to speak, my obsessions. My imagination and creative needs were not being satisfied by the way this group worked, and there seemed to be no way I could get these needs fulfilled through the particular structure of this group.

CO: Well, given the points of our interpretation that you do agree with, how would you situate your critique of illusionism? Most modernist artists undertake an examination of the dominant mode of representation, i.e., in film, a critique of illusionism and of a type of narrative cinema.

YR: The critique of illusionism is, by now, a firmly established tradition. In the theater it comes directly from Brecht. I myself discovered Brechtian justifications for my own anti-illusionism long after my initial involvement with it. His purpose ostensibly was to make the audience think about the ideas in a different or in a more vital way, remove themselves and come back so that they would not be passive recipients of entertainment. But for me, illusionist or rather, making illusionism apparent, or questioning it by all these devices, on one level very simply provides other material—not only the implied characters and the suggested plot and the fictions, but also the director and the camera and whatever; it's a way of incorporating as many parts of the total relationship between author, viewer and object as one can. The implication of this is to make the audience think about, and deal with, and share in the creative process in a different way than they do where the techniques or structure are totally invisible. So one justification of this approach is that it respects the intelligence of the audience.

CO: Yes, but you want them to think about something in particular.

YR: Well, I guess I should really be talking here about how I depart from Brecht even though I appear to be using similar techniques. I think *Lives of Performers* is much more Brechtian than *Film About a Woman Who . . .* Nothing in *Woman Who . . .* resembles the close-up of Shirley Soffer saying, "Which woman is the director most sympathetic to?" Nothing in *Woman Who . . .* steps out of the "picture" like that and confronts the audience. By the time I was assembling the script of *Woman Who . . .* I was interested in plain old Aristotelian catharsis. I wanted the audience to be swept away with pity and, if not terror, then a strong empathetic unease. The intertitle "She grieves for herself," stays on for a good fifteen seconds. I wanted to impregnate the audience with the depth of that grief. It is still a very uneasy moment for me to watch; it is too easy to see it as a kind of self-pitying indulgence.

CO: On the contrary, it appears to us that by having the intertitle on much longer than it takes to read it, the effect is one of calling attention to the intertitle itself rather than what the title says. To return to Brecht, his formal strategies were developed and used in order to foreground particular social/political situations. In your films, we see a virtual stacking up of situations which have their primary layer of meaning embedded in sexual politics, with, say, a man between two women, or a woman writing about her relationship with a man. The clichéd, fragmented, and often terse dialogue/intertitles go hand in hand with the formal strategies related to camera movement, point of view, repeated or disrupted action, lack of a frame, or devices which make you conscious of the frame. Those distancing devices make you examine what is going on, what is being said, and show you that those relationships are typical male/female sexual relationships.

YR: How does that differ from the way the man and two women are treated in a commercially distributed film like *The Mother and the Whore?*

CO: In *Lives of Performers* you question more of what you're seeing because you're constantly being led outside the film.

YR: Which you *might* look at as a kind of distraction from the sexual realities.

CO: Rather, it's a distraction from a particular character created as a fiction. You are able to place the sexual realities in a social context which is located outside the world of the film.

CO: One of these strategies is that of constantly breaking the narrative. It's inconsistent and fragmented, whereas *The Mother and the Whore* drags you into a monumentally involved deterministic kind of psychology which depends completely on the use of causal, linear narrative. It's a totally different way of approaching relationships. *The Mother and the Whore* is much less critical. We think your film, in the way it's structured, and in the kinds of things it makes the viewer do, critiques the relationships in a very concrete way.

YR: I wonder about that. The review in *Women and Film* (no. 5–6) of *Lives of Performers* suggested there was no commentary, and that is a very important question to me. Do the strategies provide the commen-

tary ? Do they put the demand for interpretation, and for forming conclusions, on to the audience, so they have to ask, "Well, what is really
going on here between this man and two women ?"

CO: Yes. We think that is definitely going on. One effective technique is
the way that the situational clichés are isolated. This makes you examine what you would not ordinarily pay attention to, making you look
at it in a fresh way. Take, for example, the conversation between Valda
and Shirley on the bed in *Lives of Performers.* If it were filmed in a naturalistic way, we would read it as an ordinary conversation. But here our
attention is drawn away from the content of their interaction by the
fact that it's done in long shot (rather than in close-ups, using shot/re-
verse shot), and by the fact that one of the stage lights on the set is included in the frame. So the architecture of the "conversation" is set up
and set apart as "a situation," a unit that prevents your participation in
the interaction and invites an analysis of it. We are forced to recognize
the idea of possible meanings, possible readings, which is very different
from the ordinary practice of instant identification and then on to the
next scene. Not only do we have to think about what this "situation"
means, but we realize that we have to think about it.

Also, the fact that the text is being quoted—we hear on the soundtrack the script of a conversation obviously being *read* by someone—
makes you pay more attention to the discourse, rather than to any individual's psychology. The long shot, the lighting, and the soundtrack
reinforce this distance, and make you pay attention both to the material construction of the shot and to the social construction of the situation.

YR: If you're going to talk about social change, and art being instrumental, or being one means toward a change in consciousness of more
people than the people who make it or write about it, then let's talk
about the audience watching these two films. Both are about a man
who can't make up his mind. Take an audience member—let's say a
woman who is in a similar situation—her lover is cheating on her with
another woman, and she has ambivalent feelings about it. How do you
suppose looking at *The Mother and the Whore* will affect her compared
to looking at *Lives of Performers*?

CO: That's a good question. You're right in tying up that discussion
with the audience and in trying to locate the analysis in the audi-

ence/film relationship. *The Mother and the Whore* can be seen as a paradigm of the type of illusionist, representational film in which one event follows directly from the preceding event, and which uses a kind of linear causality that seems natural to us. The chronological sequence is never called into question. We have a conditioned psychological reaction to this kind of narrative; it simply flows over us like water over sand. We're always told what's going on in a way that reinforces our dependence on psychological cause and effect, and is largely independent of social/historical forces.

You can't really remove sequences from the entire context of either film. By the time the scene with Leaud in bed with his two women comes up in *The Mother and the Whore* you've already identified with the characters, and have established a psychological bond between those figures on the screen and your own experience. But in *Lives of Performers* we constantly maintain a distance between ourselves and what is on the screen. You're constantly requiring the spectator to question this narrative, even in a very minimal way by making the viewer ask, "Now what's going on? Who's she? Who is *this* she? Who is he involved with? Who's #1 and who's #2?" You present it in a stylized and conceptual way, rather than through an emotional dialogue which works by making the viewer say, "Yes, I identify with that character; that's me up there." The traditional film works in such a way that people walk out of the theater feeling that they've seen the truth, that their life has been represented.

In the film *The Mother and the Whore* there's a similar situation, but you see the characters in an emotional trap. They're victimized by their psychological needs; they seem to have no real choices. In your films, on the other hand, compulsive sexual, and sex-role, behavior is also demonstrated, but the audience is forced to position itself at one or two removes from "reality" because of your conscious use of strategies which atomize the narrative. Situations in this film can be encapsulated, isolated, and made to appear banal in the same way that discourse, language, conversation are frequently lifted from a context and become trivialized—that is, made to seem commonplace. Or, conversely, situation and language may be intensified in their isolation, for example, the question, "Have you ever considered the possibility that if a man likes you he doesn't necessarily want to fuck you?" In contrast to Eustache, you deal with this kind of set-up situation as a problem, not as a predetermined phenomenon. And even if one comes away from your film with echoes of "I'm filled with self-loathing," pessimistic sentiments about women and possibilities for change, the fact is that by dealing with this complex of situations as an intellectual or analytical problem, rather than as an emotional problem, or by dealing with it in both ways, (YR agreeing) you provide the audience with a means of articulating it, of trying to resolve it, so one is not trapped by it in the same way.

YR: These are very impressive arguments, but I feel we're still not getting at . . . So you come away feeling the director's hand. I still don't see the relation of that to really thinking about the psychological situations in a different way, and learning.

CO: In *The Mother and the Whore* you *are* provided with situations that you can identify with, that you can see yourself in, but you're given no conceptual tools to analyze the situation. It has to do with questions of perception, with the way we see things. For example, when Vertov demystifies certain work processes in *Man with a Movie Camera* (working in a factory, working to make a film, working to make hydraulic energy, working to make public transportation, etc.), he's exposing the world in a new way, making new connections. Apart from the content of his films, the form really does something to change the way people perceive their role in the world and their relations with other people and their work. But it's at the perceptual level that a formalist strategy really works. It doesn't mean that you're untouched by films like *The Mother and the Whore,* but that these films provide you with a ready-made experience. Once you're inside that fictional world, you may see situations you can identify with, but when you come back out of that world, out of the theater, it's hard to transfer that filmed situation outside because it's so much tied to the characters and the emotional situations inside the film. When you watch a film that you have to think about in order to determine its coherence or relevance, you are engaging in an active process which is exactly the same inside and outside the film. You don't have to rethink the milieu of the film in order to examine the situation it presents.

YR: I couldn't agree more. However, I think one of the problems in talking about what films do is, you start talking about some kind of Everyperson. When you talk about people who might be affected by a different kind of film, you're talking about yourselves, still a very tiny segment of the larger population. And that's something I think I've had to come to terms with, that my films, my dances before that, have affected people who were ready in a certain sense, or already tuned in. At first I had some illusion that because I had started dealing with the areas of the emotions my films would be accessible to a lot more people than my dances. But I was underestimating, or overlooking, the difficulties and demands of the treatment.

Perhaps it is a mistake to compare narrative films from the standpoint of those which use distancing devices and those which do not. How can we say which type of film will make "people" think, or make them active, and which will not? A friend of mine thought that *The Mother and the Whore* summed up a particular male-female predicament in a nutshell. I got bogged down in the talkiness, the actors, my difficulty with Leaud, a thousand-and-one details. As she talked about it, I had to agree with her. What other film has so explicitly dealt with the child-man's expectations of women? She, my friend, came out of that movie critical and objective. I, poor soul, was adrift in that other tradition. It is very difficult to cross over to the other shore.

On the other hand, *Film About a Woman Who . . .* often elicits very strong empathetic responses, like "Did you intend for it to be about all of us?" I am not, however, convinced that my film gives people—no matter whether they empathize or are "distanced"—an understanding of the problems it reflects back to them. What is important is to get things out into the open, by whatever means. Eustache did it in his way. I did it in mine.

CO: Do you feel that your films are more accessible to women than to men?

YR: Sometimes. Men are more prone to dismiss them as soap opera. But I am continually pleased by how many men are deeply affected by the films, especially by the last one.

CO: Annette Michelsen in her article "Yvonne Rainer, Part One: The Dancer and the Dance" (*Artforum,* January 1974) wrote:

> New dance, like new film, inhabits and works largely out of Soho and those adjunct quarters which constitute the center of our commerce in the visual arts. They live and work, however, entirely on the periphery of their world's economy, stimulated by the labor and production of that economy, with no support, no place in the structure of its market. New dance and new film have been, in part and whole, unassimilable to the commodity value. Exist-

ing and developing within their habitat as if on a reservation, they are condemned to a strict reflexiveness.

This suggests to us that Michelson feels that because of this relative autonomy from the economics of the art world, this new art is also ideologically autonomous; that is, it doesn't participate in the ideology of, for example, the New York art scene. We wanted to know how you felt about Michelson's statement.

YR: The area where I started to work, and the composition of the audience, was in large part the art world rather than the dance world. It was largely artists and art-world people who were the supporters and fans of our work, as of the work of Merce Cunningham at a certain point. (It's not the case now so much.) My *economic* situation has been very dependent on the art world in that I am brought to colleges by art departments, and I have performed in museums a lot. Now that I am making films, and as film departments in universities increase in number, this is beginning to change. The economic support for my films has been from these fees, but also from grants received first as a choreographer, and now as a filmmaker. So my situation is getting more diffused in that it's the art world that continues to provide me with teaching situations, while I receive grants as a filmmaker.

Before now I never thought of my work as a commodity, as something that can be bought, sold and invested in. Being paid a fee for service rendered—performing, lecturing, etc.—feels different even though there are obvious similarities with art-object sales—fluctuating market price, for instance, and value based on reputation, notoriety, associations, previous sponsors (collectors), and media exposure. Now with the possibility of the sales of prints, I feel a need to define certain limitations with regard to the use of my work. Since I think of film in relation to an audience in the same way I thought of my dances, that is, as a public spectacle and not as something to be viewed by a few people in a living room, it follows, then, that I shouldn't sell prints to private collectors. (That there don't seem to be any collectors around buying up 3,700-foot films is beside the point.) And I don't like the idea that anyone is going to make a profit from *reselling* them. It's OK if they make a profit from screening them publicly, i.e., rendering service. As a consequence, museums, film archives, and educational institutions are the only prospective owners.

Even though a few art galleries have taken over film distribution, it is true that, for the moment at least, films are not being subjected to the speculative practices that characterize the marketing of art objects. The kind of film I make is also outside of the distribution system governing narrative films of mass appeal. This may constitute economic autonomy of sorts, but only if you ignore the fact that it is made possible largely through the current policies of subsidy by government cultural agencies. And to suggest that this has resulted in "ideological autonomy" is to ignore the extraordinary influence the art world—with its demand for novelty and innovation—has had on those outside as well as within the marketing system.

CO: It seems to be an ideological choice that you have in fact chosen not to make commodity art.

YR: I started to paint and draw at the age of sixteen. My father, a frustrated easel painter himself, discouraged me. That I was later able to immerse myself in dance as completely as I did can be attributed to an explanation somewhat more dynamic than "ideological choice." One attraction was that it was a profession in which competition with men was tolerated. Another factor was that by that time my father was dead. In the last several years it has sometimes occurred to me that the kinds of collages I pin up on my walls as "sketches" for books or films might be "hung" in a gallery, duplicated, and sold as quite respectable equivalents of a painter's drawings. If I haven't followed through on this idea it is because my heart isn't in it to the extent that my money-inspired motive is, or not enough to make me do the necessary work-plus-hustle the project would entail. Perhaps "ideological choice" is more applicable here, though I feel somewhat self-conscious about disguising both my venality *and* my sloth with such an encomiastic phrase.

CO: But you could make illusionist films, and you've chosen not to do that.

YR: I should say right here that there is a lot more illusion in my movies than any of us have admitted up to now. I mean, you wouldn't call silent movies anti-illusionist because they used intertitles.

CO: You would if someone made a silent film today with intertitles.

YR: Furthermore, I don't feel "modernist" techniques necessarily preclude illusionism. As for conventions of narrative time, my next film will probably deal with that in a more straightforward way. You will be able to distinguish chronological fictional time from edited time, which it is not possible to do, except sporadically, in the two previous films.

But I do know what you mean: a work in which the strategies are invisible to all but the trained eye. Whether or not I *could* make a film that used naturalistic acting and a causal narrative chronology (assuming I could obtain the requisite financial resources), this is not so important as the fact that I haven't, and most likely never will, make that attempt. My impulses remain very much what they were when I was a choreographer. I must call my own shots, create my own terms and definitions—I mean artistic terms—as I go along. You may call *this* an ideological choice, but I don't think it is as idealistic as you might wish. It is the result of coming in contact very early with the notion of innovation as a necessary component of work, a notion provided by contemporary art history. I inherited that; I swallowed it whole. I guess I am very American in that sense: refuse the past and embrace violent change. By now it is impossible to shake off this article of faith, but also, I am sure there is a large part of me that likes and needs the risk-taking that is involved. In that sense, I don't have much choice.

I had a discussion with Richard Foreman about the place at which a person gets tuned in to a certain kind of art, which may be crucial in determining the mode of expression you're going to choose. His first recognition of art as something current and vital was the New American Cinema in the late '50s—Anger, Brakhage, Smith, you know. I would say the first film that turned me on (and maybe it was one of my first art experiences) was Cocteau's *Orpheus*. And I sometimes wonder how that early infiltration of my senses has affected my work. Another early film experience occurred when I was ten years old. My father took me to the Palace of the Legion of Honor with him (where they continue to have Sunday movies). I saw *The Passion of Joan of Arc* there. And that I will never forget. When I went to New York I was barely twenty-one, and it was the Abstract Expressionist painters who were providing me with things to think about. I can't say I've ever been really at ease with painting. I'm stimulated intellectually, but it's not something that has, I would say, affected my gut, the way movies have. It was only when I took a dance class that I realized that this is what I would enjoy doing. It was about a basic kind of pleasure. And so I found my metier through my body, but I had already been turned on by certain film experiences and by the ideas generated in the art world.

I think that if at that age I had found that I had wanted to paint, I might not have had the independence or strength to pursue it. This was the late '50s. It was definitely a man's world. I would probably have had a very difficult time, being a woman. That's obvious. At that time there were four women painters who were accepted, who were given validation, so to speak. I would have had to struggle to establish myself as a painter, whereas I didn't as a choreographer.

I want to say some more about those poor misunderstood aesthetic strategies of mine. In the dances I made prior to 1972 I rarely entertained questions of a problematic nature about form and content. Once the nature of given materials was revealed to me, I simply went about devising a system to "explore possibilities" within predetermined limits, or devising a system that would give equal exposure to all the materials. Thus in a duet of 1963, variations on Kamakali sculptural positions were worked out while we spoke variations on "I love you," "Why don't you love me?," etc. The limits were stylistic: a flat monotonic delivery of the lines and a leisurely undramatic flow of movement. And in the 1965 *Parts of Some Sextets* and *Rose Fractions* of 1969, materials ranging from task through expressive dance through gymnastics to film were simply "distributed" over a period of time. Material with specifically emotional "content" was rarely differentiated in treatment from anything else. In this way I could presume to deal with all materials as equivalent, fully accepting the consequence that certain things would "pop out" of context in ways very unpredictable for an audience. One critic was moved to say, "She deals with everything as though it is equally unimportant." I, of course, would have said I was giving the multifarious items in my bag of tricks equal *importance*. As my concern with abstract dance and task activity began to wane, I was becoming more concerned with dramatic and psychological subject matter. This could not always be realized to my satisfaction by configurations of bodies in space. As a consequence, language—in speech and print—became a more insistent component. And simultaneously the ambiguities of the I-love-you, I've-never-loved-you approach, the pretense of an objective exploration of possibilities, no longer seemed adequate. I now found myself dealing with things that could not always be accommodated by inventories and lists, with their attendant ambiguities of meaning or point of view, which at times made irony appear to be the primary attitude investing the work. I guess I got tired of this "equivocating" and depersonalized voice. I was ready to make a commitment of greater depth to exploring the love conflict. This meant acknowledging at least a limited causality and finding ways to create more cohesion between isolated expressions of emotional states. You might say I moved from a kind of poetry toward narrative.

But not all the way. A novelist might well laugh at my makeshift dallying with storytelling. For me the story is an empty frame on which to hang images and thoughts which need support. I feel no obligation to flesh out this armature with credible details of location and time. *Lives of Performers* tried to do this to a greater extent than *Woman Who . . .* In *Woman Who . . .* I was much more concerned with interweaving psychological and formal content, i.e., with images being "filled up" or "emptied" by readings or their absence, with text and speech being "illustrated" to varying degrees by images. This made for a situation where the story came and went, sometimes disappearing altogether as in the extreme prolongation of certain soundless images.

It is necessary to go on about the relation of this work to narrative only because we are so conditioned by narrative films to pursuing a continuous thread of events to their ultimate correct placement in place and time, however disrupted the edited continuity in the given film may be. Those of my techniques that can be called "disjunctive" are not used with the intention of extending, obfuscating, or disrupting what might otherwise be a continuous narrative, which seems to be one aspect of many "new novels." Where narrative seems to break down in my films is simply where it has been subsumed by other concerns, such as the resonances created by repetition, stillness, allusion, prolonged duration, fragmented speech and framing, "self-conscious" camera movement, etc. Rather than being integrated *into* the story, these things at times *replace* the story. Because they are interesting or beautiful or funny, *not* because they alienate or "distance" the audience. That they may or may not do this to the audience is another story. In short, I am no more committed to narrative than to antinarrative.

CO: When you conceive a film, do you conceive it visually or verbally?

YR: Both. Sometimes a shot occurs to me independently of speech or text. I also accumulate stuff, from newspapers, my own writing, paragraphs, sentences, scraps of paper, photos, stills from previous films. Ultimately, the process of sorting it all out forces me to organize it and make the parts cohere in some fashion. Sometimes a given text suggests a visual treatment and I dispense with the text. There is always the question of to what extent I want to duplicate content in text and image.

Sometimes I feel I have to invent transitions as flimsy as "Meanwhile back at the ranch." In my notebook there is an entry that discusses the various merits of *meanwhile, in other words, but, as things stood,* and *in any case. In any case* won out. In the film I'm working on now (*Kristina Talking Pictures*) I hope to find more sound and camera-movement transitions, but only if they are needed. My method is that of a collagist as practiced by a would-not-be writer turned filmmaker.

I shouldn't talk about my next film. I know it will change drastically as I get into it. But I can talk about a combination of texts and photos called "Kristina (For a . . . Opera)" that was recently published in a German magazine called *Interfunktionen.* It is a very disjunctive story about a woman lion tamer.

I used found photos of a real Polish lion tamer named Kristina, and also Babette Mangolte made photos for it. The lion tamer is sometimes played by herself and sometimes by me in photos. I have her discuss questions of art and film, things like Godard, the acting in Godard's films, editing, etc., as though she is the author. Each page or double page has a different lay-out: photos with text in balloons, or columns of photos with adjacent text. Sometimes two or three pages of straight text with no photos at all. It was extremely interesting to do. After I'd finished the book *Work 1961–73* I thought, "Oh, I'd really love to work on another book now, using this kind of format." But a totally fictitious book. Make art for the book, rather than document already existing art. Rehearsals, discussions of dances that never existed. This thirty-page treatment has relieved me of wanting to do another book, for the time being at least. As for my next film—I'm still ruminating about how to do this in film . . . much more elaborately.

CO: For the sequence of stills in *Film About a Woman Who . . .* , why did you choose *Psycho?*

YR: I had been reading the Truffaut/Hitchcock book, and looking at the stills just as stills. I was thinking about using some of them (from a number of films) perhaps as an homage to Hitchcock. And then I decided I wanted something more coherent, and there is that double-page spread of the stills from the shower scene in the middle of the book. I think that's one of the most amazing jobs of editing that has ever been done.

As used in *Woman Who . . .* , the stills work on several levels. They serve as a cinematic reference to *Psycho.* And in a strange way, although presented in a totally different form, they recreate the feeling of the original. The fairly slow pace of the stills dissipates the shock of the original while intensifying the horror. Can I say that the horror has been "distilled" by the fact of each still "sitting still" for so long? The images depict a woman being murdered while the voice-over describes a woman being sick and lost. It works better than this description makes it sound because the sequence is tied in narratively to the voice-over, which begins, "She stumbles out of the theater. Her disgust with the film and actual nausea drive her body into the street." I wasn't trying to make any comment about Janet Leigh's predicament, although I knew that people would think I detested *Psycho* because my "she" is disgusted with it.

CO: In both your films you include long visual-quotation sequences from films which involve the victimization of women—namely, *Psycho* and Pabst's *Pandora's Box*; both the characters played by Janet Leigh and Louise Brooks are stabbed to death by psychopaths.

YR: Obviously I'm involved with victims and the female as victim. I think the choice of *Psycho* was unconscious, however, in that respect.

CO: There are scenes in the films where so much depends on the configuration made by bodies. Did you intend specific readings by deliberately posing the characters?

YR: Very often in *Lives of Performers* I left a lot up to the actors, much more so than in the second film. In that long shot where Shirley and Valda are moving, making small changes on the couch (with accompanying voice-over "What will Nina and Theresa think? . . .") I told them, "Well, just move one at a time; make small changes." And I didn't ask that they end up in that kind of conspiratorial relationship. It's almost like one is about to whisper something in the other's ear. The exact reading of each one of those positions was not so important to me. Whereas there is the sequence of three shots where first Fernando and John are on the bed, and then in the next shot, they have switched positions, and then Shirley and Valda appear in those same positions. Each shot is followed by a different intertitle. And that was an attempt to give totally different interpretations to each of three identical *tableaux*.

CO: We wanted to ask you about your use of a kind of "pseudostill." In the beginning of *Film About a Woman Who . . .* , the people on the beach assume a series of clichéd, stereotypical, snapshot poses. They pose, move, change positions, and then they pose again. What motivated that kind of strategy?

YR: I wanted to set up a familial relationship between John and Shirley and Sarah that later on would get complicated when we see Dempster and Shirley and Sarah together. It was also about family pictures and how often they can come out wrong. I told Babette to overexpose it; she could have done it even more. It glitters with amateurishness. From my dance days, I'm very involved with stillness and moving, so the reference to the still camera, through the lens of a movie camera, was a natural reflex.

CO: The word for photographic negative in French is *cliché*. So in a way, these snapshots are clichés about relationships and personal situations, and they're also symbolic gestures. The fight sequence in *Film About a Woman Who . . .* seemed to be, on one level, a demonstration of various permutations of movement—variations and combinations of stillness and motion—and frozen gestures.

YR: Also in the scene where Renfreu puts on her clothes, takes off her nightgown. She's moving as fast as she can, but the camera is going at forty-eight frames per second. Everything seems to float.

CO: That could be interpreted as a subjective device; it's like a nightmare when you want to run but can't. Another kind of motion takes place in the verbal content of the films. Things are transformed slightly, or have new meanings relative to their position in the text. In *Lives of Performers,* when someone says, "Oh God, you gave me so much room" the statement seemed to refer to *Grand Union Dreams,* where gods were designated, and to an epic space. And then it was reiterated in the context of the anecdote about Valda and Fernando passing each other on the stairs.

YR: Again I must say I am, or was, a dancer. I'm very involved with space and motion, so it's going to come out in a lot of different forms. The space of the frame, metaphors for relationships, the physical space of intimacy, of avoidance, attraction, flirtation, or hostility.

CO: In another sequence, the audience could read some of the words that surrounded the photo; for example, one of the lines that was going to be spoken later in the film: "Have you ever considered the possibility that if a man likes you he doesn't necessarily want to fuck you?" You make the assumption that this dialogue will concern a man and a woman. And then when you read the line later, the image is of two men sitting on the bed. In other words, we interpret this same line differently according to the image that accompanies it; the image of the two men is disorienting because it subverts our previous expectation. This form of retroactive dissociation occurs frequently in your films.

YR: I was concerned that that particular intertitle in *Lives of Performers* might subvert the appearances of heterosexual involvement. This also happens in *Film About a Woman Who . . .* The only scene in which you see the two men together in that whole film is during the trout sequence, where you see this hand come out and wipe the food from John's mouth and go down and get the cigarette. Then it turns out to be Dempster's hand. It was only afterwards that I realized the sexual implications. Sometimes it seems like negligence and sometimes I don't really care; then I run the risk of contradiction where certain technical maneuvers take priority over the significance or the psychological implications of gesture. I wanted a seamless movement, determined by very small events that were happening in the frame.

CO: Another example of meaning being determined retrospectively in *Lives of Performers* is the shot where Fernando is on the bed looking at something and the camera moves in a pan in close-up. It's impossible to determine what those textures that we are seeing are. The placement of the objects is completely indeterminate.

YR: Yes. I don't always use establishing shots.

CO: So you end up determining what the image is as it's unfolded, and you redefine the spatial relationships of the objects—the bed, the bedspread, and the floor. This is the same kind of retroactive dissociation that we just talked about in terms of the soundtrack. But here it is a spatial dislocation. A space is established in your mind through all the close-ups, but it's very confused. And then when you do get an establishing shot, you react, "Oh, but that spot was the *bed*; that's where it is." It really makes you conscious of the *imagined* space that you had established through close-ups when you got to the virtual, the "real" space.

There's a statement in *Lives of Performers*: "I'm simply doing another form of storytelling—more intimate, less epic." You were talking last night about your use of space, moving from performance space to more intimate space. The camera is able to pick up the small, intimate things, and the small modifications.

YR: One of the turning points in my move from performance to film was *Grand Union Dreams* of 1971, which was performed in a large gymnasium. I was struck with the absurdity of having a performer walk across the entire width of the place to tip his hat or shake a hand. It was an absurdity that worked once, twice, or even three times, but after that you knew the space was dominating the director rather than the other way around. That was the last gymnasium I performed in. The filmic frame is far more adaptable for my purposes. It can be intimate or heroic. It can press itself against your eyes or recede into infinity. I once said I didn't want to collaborate with a scenic designer or artist because I would be stuck with their decor for the duration of my dance. Now I don't even want to be stuck with that real space. Changes in lighting are not enough.

CO: How did you modify the fight scene from the performance piece *This is the Story of a Woman Who . . .* to the filmed version?

YR: In the performance piece *This is the Story of a Woman Who . . .* John and I did the fight. We screamed, squealed, and made sounds of pain or rage alternately. He did one and then I would do one. For the film, I taught the fight to the two women so that it could illustrate the narration at that point about her remembering the scene from the movie in which the two women tore each other's clothes off and she got so turned on by it. At the beginning of the voice-over you see the photo of the older woman in the field. This dissolves into the fight. I used a dissolve here (there are very few in the film) to make a stronger connection between the older woman and the younger ones. The end of the voice-over comes shortly after with, "She never told anyone, not even her mother." Halfway through the fight another voice-over (presented as half of a telephone conversation) describes a conflict of identity: Should she become a "big woman" or remain a "hunchtwat"? The fight ends abruptly as a whole new series of images starts—the girl in bed with subtitles describing seventeen abysmal self-evaluations. I describe all this because I think of it as having a unity. The mother, the rage against the mother transferred to the other woman, the soliloquy on maturation, and the matured woman's lapse into self-doubt superimposed on the terrors of (herself as) the child at night. I eliminated the screams from the fight in order to focus on what was happening visually. The camera speed changes four times during this shot.

In the show the telephone bit happened during the stylized conversation. We had studied our mannerisms during actual conversation, and later took turns trying to recreate gestures or facial expressions or nervous tappings. The idea of conversation was used totally differently in the film and in a different place. The slow pan back and forth over the three women's faces as the voice-over says that they're talking about sexual fantasies. The part in the film beginning with Sarah in bed was shown intact in the show. The subtitles were projected *beside* the film rather than over it. The difference in the way you associate image and text in these two instances eludes me, but I know there must be a difference.

CO: We're interested in your use of sound. In the films the sound is either spoken voice or sometimes music. Would you consider using other sounds, or live sound, for instance, traffic and other noises?

YR: In the trout scene you hear utensils . . . but that was very controlled.

CO: Yes, and controlled in the way that the lighting was controlled in that scene. Also it seems that in the film there are only a few images of "the world outside." The beach doesn't count because the beach is like a stage. But there are feet running in the rain; there's the subway. . . .

YR: Oh yes, I want to get out in the street more. As for sound, I was trying to make a silent film—with occasional sound.

CO: Are you thinking of incorporating noises as a component?

YR: I don't know how I'll do that. Certainly if I use sound, it will not be naturalistic, necessarily. In the next film I'll be playing around with lip sync and speech. The use of the utensils and chewing—I'm sure I'll do more of that kind of thing. I mean, so far my ideas about sound are pretty simple, when you think of what can be done. I still think of it as a very singular kind of event.

CO: Music in your films often plays a seductive role. For example, you show images without any sound, and they have a certain duration. As soon as the music comes in, the sense of time is radically different. You sense that the pacing of the image track will have a coherent relationship to the sound track. *You* (the audience) are no longer responsible (and feel relieved). The time passes faster, as it is marked and now quantifiable. So that you get a very sharp contrast when you are watching a silent image track, a silent screen in motion, and then suddenly emotive and rhythmic music is added. It's extremely effective in making the audience aware of the concepts of duration and expectation.

YR: I was also involved with pure hearing—the image just disappearing totally. I'm not that involved with opera, but this whole spectrum of seeing, hearing, seems really important. Or again, as a means of changing the context, like the aria in *Woman Who . . .* that comes on during the intertitle that stays on for a long time: "Oh Christ, now he'll never screw me again." First you read the whole thing; then you hear the music, which gives it a different flavor, and that goes on and on and then the title goes off and you're just listening to the music. And then you read, "Her mind drifts back," and it's about someone who is listening, and then the image comes on and there she is, sitting very still and "listening." So it was another way of providing a constant against which landscape, situation, and time could change.

CO: At what level do you think your films affect people?

YR: If my work stands a chance of helping anyone to change—although I certainly don't see that as an essential aim—it will not be because that work embodies an ideal of change, or even reflects my own growth. I want my films to reflect whatever complexities I feel about being alive, and the most I can ask of myself is that I create work that retains a powerful connection to my own experience, whatever distance from literal autobiography it traverses. Just as I can't manipulate my position in the scheme of things to match the ideal of the person I ought to be, neither can I bring myself to try creating an exemplary woman through my films. If anything can be said to be exemplary in this work, it is the idea that self-scrutiny can function as an active and positive principle.

Alongside of this, my women will probably continue to vacillate between being fools, heroines, and—yes—victims. Victims of their own expectations no less than those of the opposite sex, or of the prevailing social mores.

I find that it's a very important part of my process that I make new theories. I mean, I constantly change my theories, or justifications, as a result of working. I then have to find new justifications for the work, which may or may not hold up. But for the moment I have to use them and hold off calling them into question until after making the next work. I know that not all artists have this compulsion. I envy those who can exist in the world with more elegance and ease. But just as I make art to justify my existence, so I must sooner or later make words to justify my art. The latter offers the same powerful release as the former. Sometimes the words refuse to come for a long time after the art. Not until they do, however, can I breathe easily, "Now I can go on."

Afternote

From a letter to *Camera Obscura* written several days after the interview took place: "At the end we talked about whether I might work with a particular *image* of a woman in my next work. A triumphant heroine, a woman who 'wakes up' (A la Varda's Cleo). I said no, in effect. But my feelings about this are complicated. I cannot see narrowing down my concerns in any one work to a singular narrative line that would reveal a woman in that light. Aside from the fact that socialist realist art (which I naturally abhor) is based on this kind of transcendent simplicity, I have no more investment in triumphant woman than I have in sex-object woman. I can only reflect the reality of my own experience, which continues to be about loving, hating, acting stupid, 'waking up,' trying to 'sleep,' being in despair, being courageous, being terrified, getting excited, getting outraged, laughing. A story about a woman who is only courageous is not enough for me. Which gets back to the limitations of conventional narrative films: They cover a particular duration of time in which the protagonists transcend or are destroyed in the course of a single climax. Yes, it really is about bracketing time that I object to. I want everything I make to reflect my whole life. I think that is why those paragraphs floating in the frame fascinate me so: they have no time or space, they are pure events or states that the audience can very concretely apply to themselves, if they choose."

Beginning With Some Advertisements

For Criticisms Of Myself,

Or Drawing The Dog You May Want

To Use To Bite Me With,

And Then Going On To Other Matters.

Initially published in *Millennium Film Journal*, no. 6 (Spring 1980), this short essay includes excerpts from *Journeys from Berlin/1971*, my fourth feature (released in 1980), but also replicates the idiosyncratic style of parts of that script with its non sequiturs and ambivalences, in this instance, about the nature of film itself as a conveyor of truth. I have an affection for its throw-caution-to-the-winds play with syntax and barely successful resistance to the enticements of self-pity.

Is *Journeys from Berlin/1971* (16 mm, color/black and white, sound, 125 minutes, as they say in the filmographies) autobiography or fiction? Is it dadaist vaudeville or legitimate filmic research? Is its politics a set-up, a rigged game, mere window dressing thinly masking a formalist adventurism? Are its armchair terrorists and self-absorbed narcissists worthy of being made to voice serious moral-political concerns? Can I claim redeeming social value for this film? Is its emphasis on the individual act—the *attentat* or the act of suicide—in relation to totalitarian absolutism, is this emphasis an admission of the hopelessness of working for social change? Are its humanist yearnings and confessions a substitute for political practice?

Without delay a short grammatical intervention: Wasn't it Gertrude Stein who said the sentence is more important than the paragraph? Flitting and dipping are more to my liking than soaring and arcing. Stumbling over the hit-and-run of the quote and the snort is more habitual to my mode of thought than the intricacies of binary logic. The latter is my nemesis, I mean amanuensis. Inadvertent puns tripped over my mother's mouth where you would have expected malapropisms. A condition in itself not totally surprising, for, as one well-known critic once

said of her (mother), "She must suffer because she has no education."
(Mercy, pity, compassion: gimme, gimme.)

New paragraph. The function of the artist is to emerge periodically
from the (m)ire of her solipsisms. Yes, that's it. I think I've finally got it:
The function of . . . uh . . . memory is selective burial. Disinterment
being what it is, i.e., inevitable, seasonal, chronic, it behooves us to engage memory in the service of a perish-the-thought subjectivity mired
in (she was never very good at living with) contradictions. Hundreds
of seabirds rode the wind. She felt compromised at the drop of a hat:
by being asked a question she couldn't answer, by being held in high
esteem, by being in the company of two men, by being addressed by
one man, a younger woman, a younger man, a peer (To look for the
reasons one should not stomp on someone's face is to accept stomping
on it.), by her irresponsible memory which invariably copped out at the
punch line.

Know thyself, stay with your own class and sex. Only in dreams does
one sit at a long conference table with Ike and Mamie Eisenhower
laughing with them at a check for $148 made out to Shirley Eisenhower.
Why this—and the added necessity of ordering lunch—was funny I
don't know. "To declare that existence is absurd is to deny that it can
ever be given a meaning; to say that it is ambiguous is to assert that its
meaning is never fixed, that it must be constantly won." That's by Simone de Beauvoir in *The Ethics of Ambiguity.* Read it again?

Shall we proceed: The fatal glass of beer at this late in the day sees
print as harboring fact, and the filmic image as perpetuating representation (fiction?). And the voice? Well, the human voice is at once the
clinker and the crunch. It lies, sings, floats, or emerges from a mouth
from which it may or may not have originated. It speaks of things that
may or may not—usually not—have originated in the mind behind the
mouth in question. These three terms of possible dissociation—*word,
mouth, thought*—suggest a fourth: the thought as a cultural given rising
unbidden at a particular historical moment. And a fifth: the fourth in
relation to each of the first three. Where and when is whose voice uttering whose thought through whose mouth and what for? Film is the
place where the (extra)ordinary (im)balances between culture and expression can be most vividly demonstrated and enacted. Film is opaque
and convoluted and baffling, never doing what it seems to be doing,
never doing what one wants it to do. Today at the movies a woman sitting in front of me said, "I used to have a dress like that." She would remember the dress "up there," but not what the mouth on top of the

dress said. The movie of someone's Millennium will be total print or totally wordless, a sublime abstraction. No voices from the void, or from bodies gesturing helplessly, simulating approximations of desire and despair. Someone else's Millennium, not mine.

So when I finally put someone in front of the camera and had her open her mouth, whom did I have her represent and what did I have her say to whom? In *Journeys from Berlin/1971* she is a fifty-year-old patient in some sort of psychiatric situation talking at this point to a woman who has her back to the camera: "Here we are, locked in this hermetic, sclerotic embrace, beholden to no one. So what if we are the world? You owe me everything; I owe you nothing. Nothing but money. Paying you money gets me off the hook. What else do you want? Ha, funny thing for me to be asking *you*. But if equality between you and me is the issue, no one is measuring the virtues and achievements of one against those of the other . . . except maybe me. Oh Christ, why won't an asteroid land on us now? Why won't someone please get me off the cusp of this plague, this ellipsis, suspension, anticipation, this retraction, denial, digression, irony, this ravenous for admiration, this contemptuous of those who provide it. It's probably true that this contagion started spreading in the seventeenth century when they brought in silvered mirrors, self-portraits, chairs instead of benches, the self-contemplative self, the personal as a . . . slave? . . . the personal as a slave of autonomy and perfectibility. By now it's quite clear that where proleptic capitalism is concerned, both self-discovery and speaking past each other are express stops on the way to carpeting the ceiling. I asked them how to say *bow-wow* in German. His friend said to him, 'Why is she asking that?' The reply came back: 'Oh, you know these Americans, they're curious about everything.' Do you know that every time your pulse throbs, one more human being has come into the world?"

Cut to new shot. The only change is the therapist, who is now a nine-year-old boy. The therapist barks, "Wau-Wau!"

That's all for now, folks.

Postscript to a false ending, or another little trailer: The phone rings. The therapist answers it. A voice like Jimmy Durante's rasps: "My daddy called me Cookie. I'm really a good girl . . . I'm not one for fussing. Not like those movie women: Katy Hepburn facing the dawn in her posh pad with stiff upper chin. Merle Oberon facing the Nazi night with hair billowing in the electric breeze. Roz Russell sockin' the words 'n' the whiskey to the best of them. Rita Hayworth getting shot in the mirror and getting her man. Jane Wyman smiling through tears. I never faced the music, much less the dawn; I stayed in bed. I never socked anything to anybody; why rock the boat? I never set out to get my man, even in the mirror; they all got me. I never smiled through my tears; I choked down my terror. I never had to face the Nazis, much less their night. Not for me that succumbing in the great task because it must be done; not for me the heart beating in incomprehensible joy; not for me the vicissitudes of class struggle; not for me the uncertainties of political thought. . . ."

Enough vaudeville. Behind the teasing ambiguities lies an ominous reality that obtrudes intermittently in the form of expensive rolling titles, white-on-black, dealing with the post–World War II German State. I conclude this essay with the printed image that opens *Journeys from Berlin/1971:*

> Let's begin somewhere:
>   In 1950 a draft for a political criminal law in the Federal Republic of Germany contained the following sentence: "The danger to the community comes from organized people."

Noel Carroll

Interview with a Woman Who . . .

This interview was published in *Millennium Film Journal* (nos. 7, 8, 9, Fall 1980–Winter 1981). I am including Noel Carroll's introduction because it provides such an incisive and thorough philosophical contextualizing for *Journeys from Berlin/1971*.

The period in which Structural Film (as distinct from Structuralist-Materialist Film) dominated the American avant-garde scene appears past. Attacks by sentimental humanists, on the one hand, and professorial Marxists, on the other, are not causes of the decline of Structural Film but symptoms of what is already a fact. Structural Film is retiring from the field not because it lost the battle of ideas—if such a mishmash of amateur theorizing can be so called—but, more seriously, because it no longer crystallizes the attitudes, values, and fantasies of the avant-garde intelligentsia. The image of the filmmaker as part cognitive psychologist, part mathematician, part chess player—the epitome of rarefied intellect—is no longer compelling, perhaps because the qualities it mimes and projects—including professional coolness, expertise with systems and technologies, and controlled experimentalism—cannot, for all sorts of reasons, be regarded heroic in the way they were in the early '70s. The revived interest and attention given to documentaries and autobiographical film, as well as the appearance of the punk/no wave indicate the displacement of Structural Film from the center to a corner of the American avant-garde arena.

If the tempo of anticipation and discussion at major New York strongholds of avant-garde film bears any resemblance to reality—a proposition many non–New Yorkers may greet with a hearty harumph —then the tendency pretending to or contending for the throne is what we might call The New Talkie (All Talking, Some Singing, Some

Dancing). *Riddles of the Sphinx, Argument, Dora, Thriller, Our Hitler,* and *Journeys from Berlin/1971* are examples of this "direction" (rather than genre). As the title suggests, The New Talkie emphasizes language—specifically, in this sort of film, language is more important than image. Of course, Structural Film also often made language its topic—e.g., *Rameau's Nephew, Poetic Justice, Nostalgia,* etc. But Structural Filmmakers seem primarily interested in the possibilities of language (e.g., the polysemy of words) and its limitations, whereas practitioners of The New Talkie are preoccupied with this while at the same time with "saying something." Undoubtedly, it is the urge "to say something" that accounts for the rise of The New Talkie as well as for its energetic if not always admiring reception so far.

Though I am writing about the American scene, The New Talkie, as the preceding list evinces, is not essentially home-grown. Its origin is largely European, seasoned in some cases with devices garnered from American Structural Film. Nor is the grouping homogeneous. *Riddles of the Sphinx, Dora, Argument,* and *Thriller* go together as espousals of a cluster of interwoven ideas drawn from Marxism, feminism, psychoanalysis and semiology. *Our Hitler* is in a class unto itself; it is an eccentric working through of a poetic/imagistic idea about the rise of Nazism—that it was a case of art (bad art) becoming life—and about its significance—Nazism is a major moment in the Americanization of the twentieth century—that is utterly idiosyncratic. *Journeys from Berlin/1971* (henceforth *Journeys*) is closer to the other films cited—it shares related subjects and sources (Godard, Straub/Huillet)—but it is not of their ilk either. It does not so much allude to antecedent theories as represent, in the broadest sense of that concept, the contesting claims of politics, feminism, morality, psychoanalysis, and personal needs, desires, fears and myths, on an individual perplexed by urgent decisions about how to live and what to do. The film does not answer these questions nor does it recommend a theory with which to attempt to answer them. Rather, it is a highly stylized imitation of the tugs, conflicts and texture of the inner and outer debates such questions prompt.

Journeys is Yvonne Rainer's fourth feature-length film. The primacy of language has always been key to Rainer's cinema, but what can conveniently be called "content" has never before concerned her as forcefully as it does in *Journeys*. The major influences on Rainer's filmmaking are twofold, yet converging. Of prominent American avant-gardists, Rainer is the one whose work is most analogous to European film modernism of the Godardian variety. In the first half of the '70s, for instance, her use of quasi narratives (*cum* distantiating devices) distinguished her from most of her compatriots (though, of course, this is no longer quite the differentia it used to be). American avant-garde dance and performance of the '60s—of which Rainer herself was a pioneering figure—is another source of her film style. Both influences predispose Rainer to her favorite formal strategy—radical juxtaposition.

Juxtaposition defines both the gross and fine structures of *Journeys*. In terms of the gross structures, *Journeys* is a dialogue of dissonant and at times contradictory voices discoursing on topics like political and psychological domination (and oppression) and the interrelation of the two. There is no overt framework—like a narrative or an authorial commentary—that organizes the various debates. Rather the film is a species of free-floating forensics with voices antiphonally adding information and opinion to a breccia of neighboring issues. The voices include: an exposition of the Baader-Meinhof saga of German terrorism (mostly in printed titles); selections from Rainer's teenage diary concerning her emerging moral consciousness; a stylized psychoanalytic session in which a psychiatrist, played by three actors, listens to an attempted suicide, played by Annette Michelson and called "the patient," who grapples free-associatively with a skein of psychological "knots" involved with the nexus between self-loathing and relations with The Other; an offscreen exchange between two disembodied voices—a man and a woman—arguing about the propriety of personal (read psychologically compensatory) motives for political action, particularly about the relation of displaced vengeance and terrorism; memoirs by Russian anarchists; an interview with Rainer's nephew; and a videotaped "letter" of Rainer, as a character, addressing her fictionalized mother.

These voices follow and even interrupt each other in an apparently desultory manner but, in fact, they are not rambled together. Most often the speeches are linked by correspondences in subject matter or analogies between thematic issues from categorically different registers. For example, the man in the offscreen debate compares the Russian anarchists' cognizance of oppressed classes with the blindness of German radicals to the plight of foreign workers. Then suddenly we hear the young diarist discuss her moral unease when confronted by a tired saleswoman. Likewise the Russian anarchists' violence is explicitly compared to the Baader-Meinhof Gang's while the patient's attempted suicide implicitly stands as worth considering in relation to Meinhof's death. Along with these correspondences in subject matter, there are thematic correspondences such as the covert connection between the problem of equality and interpersonal acknowledgement in the analytic sessions and the revolutionists' concern with social equality.

But no sooner is a similarity bruited than it is dissected. Nineteenth century Russian terrorism and '70s German terrorism are not on a par —the Russians were more in tune with history. The two suicides are not the same; Meinhof's did have some political significance as an act against a patently repressive state whether or not her actions in general were somewhat compromised by her personal motivations. For every position in the film, its opposite appears. Though the patient derives benefit from psychoanalysis, Meinhof shows how it can be a harmful regime. When several characters realize the unreliability of trusting one's feelings—contra pop-psychology—and the imperfectibility of human nature, Jean-Jacques Rousseau chimes in with a contrary word or two. The spectator is turned into a dialectician, in the classical sense, weighing arguments and noting both shades of difference and telltale correlations in the evidence marshaled.

Journeys can be viewed as an inner dialogue, the various voices portraying radiations of a single consciousness at sea, pondering related questions from multiple, incongruous angles. Or, the controversies may be the product of several distinct disputants. In either case, the intellectual and emotional tensions are the same. And it is those tensions and their sources that Rainer aims to depict.

The bristling debates and the lacunae between different perspectives open onto deeper chasms. For at the heart of *Journeys* is the intimation that some of the debates are irresolvable, that certain fundamental perspectives about human life are irretrievably disjunct. For example, the contentious couple continually return to the issue of whether the possibly vindictive motives of terrorists should count in the evaluation of their acts. If personal motives are to be considered, the acts will be assessed more negatively than if they are not. That is, we can either judge the terrorists' actions (a form of deontic judgment) or their characters and motives (aretaic judgment), and the results from these two perspectives may not be the same, signaling an incommensurateness of the most rooted moral perspectives at the core of the concept of value. This, in turn, portends an inevitable discontinuity between the political realm and the personal (at the level of theory rather than practice, I hasten to add).

Rainer observes other, putative, profound disjunctions; she stresses a gap between what one feels to be right and what one knows to be right. She acknowledges the possible dissonance between the two while also sympathetically conveying the basic human intuition that things "ought" to be otherwise. The repeated shots of Stonehenge metaphorically bear testament to this "mystery." But unlike a philosopher, Rainer neither attempts to reconcile the preceding antinomies nor to prove that they are necessarily irreconcilable. Instead, she animates them, embodying and projecting the experience of fragmentation in an aesthetic form.

Politics and psychoanalysis are the ostensible subjects of *Journeys*. But I cannot help sensing that they are ultimately means for exercising an underlying preoccupation with moral questions. This is clearest in the political discussions where the political/historical consequences and effectiveness of the various assassinations and bombings itemized are less a matter of concern than their possible ethical impropriety. The analytic session is a way for exploring the fragmentation of the self, its multiplicity of contradictory motives and desires. But in Rainer's treatment, the analytic session takes on a strong normative dimension. It is a positive process of self-discovery and, I take it, of emancipation. It is a way of rectifying behavior if only by slackening the demands of absolute perfection enunciated by the super-ego. If *Journeys* is a journey through a mind, the mind is that of a moralist.

The fine structure of the film—its moment by moment articulations—is grounded in intricate word/image associations. Objects mentioned in the dialogues are arrayed along a recurring mantelpiece or in the background of shots of the analytic sessions; we see an image and recall an earlier word, or we hear the word and remember the earlier image. There are verbal images or literalizations. For example, when the therapist, played by an adult male who is taller than the patient, is presiding, the desk and chairs are mounted on a platform so that the camera "looks down" at the patient, but when the boy therapist appears the platform is reversed, emphasizing his "smallness" vis-à-vis the patient; and these features of the image refer to the power relations between the patient and the therapist. At times, the soundtrack literalizes what is said; the patient remarks that "some members of the family don't say anything," and then the audio goes dead; we watch her lips move, but we hear nothing. In other instances, the language/image relations are more attenuated. As the patient snaps at the therapist, "You always seem to be talking out of the other side of your mouth," there is a cut to a flipped image where what was previously on the left of the shot is stationed on the right.

These word/image associations abet a sort of cognitive and perceptual play; the mention of objects and their apparition is particularly important in this respect because of the way that it engages the spectator's memory. *Journeys,* in other words, is the kind of film that makes a space for audience "participation." At first glance, this type of "participation" seems merely equivalent to the implied invitation to participation found in many Structural Films (i.e., an invitation to participate in a formal game, e.g., recognizing the rubato schema of the "Interval" section of Joanna Kiernan's *Trilogy*). And yet, due to the context of *Journeys,* Rainer's avoval of participation accrues expressive overtones. This initially formal concept appears to take on moral significance, as it did, in different ways, for both Eisenstein and Bazin. That is, the participatory style itself operates as a metaphor of value, proposing the spectator as a "free" agent involved in the active application of "judgment" as he or she partakes in the "democratic" construction of the film. This theme of participation in the fine structures is, of course, strictly analogous to the position of the spectator in regard to the gross "dialectical" structures where the viewer (or perhaps more aptly, the listener) weighs countervailing arguments, judges them and above all *chooses*—not only what is relevant to what, but also a stand on the issues. "Choice" like "participation" is morally charged; the form of *Journeys,* in short, appropriates thematic connotations of vital importance to Rainer. As she has said of other matters, "Choice is something I believe must be consciously and repeatedly engaged in."

The following interview was taped during several meetings in February and March of 1980. Parts of it have appeared in my article "Mortal Questions," in *The Soho Weekly News,* vol. 7, no. 20 (Feb. 13, 1980), and in *Cover,* vol. 1, no. 3.

NOEL CARROLL: Let's begin somewhere. Perhaps you could give some production background?

YVONNE RAINER: Between 1976 and 1977 I had a fellowship from the German government, from the Deutscher Akademischer Austauschdienst, to live and work in West Berlin for a year. While there I shot three segments of the film. This was before I had a clue as to what my next film was going to be about. One section was the walking in front of the church. Another was the videotape of me composing a letter to my mother, and the third was the music lesson. We shot that in my Berlin apartment.

In the fall of 1977 I returned to New York and in the following spring shot a segment in Berkeley—those parts in which my nephew talks about the Berlin Wall and the homemade radio. Meanwhile I had been applying for grants and doing research on the Red Army Faction. By this time I had a general idea of the scope of the film. And then a British Film Institute grant came through which stipulated that I shoot the remainder of the film in London, which I did. Next I received a fellowship from the Center for Advanced Visual Studies at M.I.T. Last fall I moved up to Cambridge and edited *Journeys* in my apartment there. The sound mix was done at WGBH-TV in Boston, and the remaining lab work was done at Multicolor here in New York.

NC: What was your budget?

YR: It depends where you stop counting. At the first answer print the cost was just under $60,000.

NC: Did you have to dip into your own money?

YR: I probably put about $3,000 into it, but this too had come from the fellowships.

NC: Your films involve autobiography. Do you see your work against the background of autobiographical filmmaking as discussed by P. Adams Sitney?

YR: My work is somewhat different from what I think Sitney is concerned with. He uses the term in relation to personal vision. Sometimes I use autobiography simply as source material to create fiction. I use autobiographical writing, for example, as a convenient way to get at an authentic sound, for credibility. Like the readings from the adolescent diary.

NC: Is that your diary?

YR: Yes. It's a diary I kept when I was about fifteen or sixteen. It's a kind of writing I couldn't have invented now. I'm not a novelist. A good fiction writer might have achieved the effect of that diary. There's no doubt that when you hear those words you believe they originated in the mind of a very young person. I should point out that the diary itself preceded any notion of a *need* for it. I mean that the idea of disparate voices came partly from what I already had around. I'm surprised I didn't make use of it before now.

But *Journeys* is also autobiographical in the sense that I'm working out things that are close to me for one reason or another, like political violence, strangely enough.

NC: How is that close to you?

YR: That too comes from my past, from the literature I was exposed to during my adolescence, during the time I was keeping the diary. Living in West Germany brought back to me the kind of political option I had not really thought about since my adolescence, when I first read Emma Goldman and Alexander Berkman. Their books were in my parents' house. My father was an anarchist, part of a community of Italian anarchists, bohemians, and poets—including Kenneth Rexroth—that met every Friday night at the Workmen's Circle in San Francisco. Violence wasn't advocated there; the discussions were more philosophical than political. But people like Berkman, Sacco, and Vanzetti were household names when I was growing up.

So this film was an opportunity to bring together powerful themes from my youth with my later experience of psychotherapy, and thus establish a point of view—peculiarly but clearly American—from which to look at other—European—components of the film.

NC: How do you see *Journeys* in relation to your other films?

YR: My films have been expanding away from me in a certain way. I've always brought my own life into my work—at least before *Journeys,* I was central, in the sense I've described. I insisted on a forthright use of my own subjectivity, whether or not my presence as a performer was involved. But in *Journeys* I have dropped heavier rocks into the water so that the ripples form larger concentric circles, cover more area, away from that center. In a sense, the center has disappeared. This film certainly contained greater problems than I've ever had to deal with. I not only had to find ways to deal with personal life and emotion but also with emotion fairly close to, if not within, a moral and political context. I found myself confronted with things that were hard to reconcile or totally justify in terms of reasons for including them within a single film. There were problems at every turn that were different from the ones I had had to cope with previously. I think my previous films came much more simply and easily out of my performance background.

NC: How so?

YR: Previously I used whatever interested me. I was able to absorb and arrange most materials under some sliding rule of thumb governing formal juxtaposition. Everything was subsumed under the kinds of collage strategies that had characterized my dancing, and could even include a kind of mechanistic, or quasi-psychological narrative.

Journeys marks the first time that the content made it imperative that I examine my formal ideas much more carefully before incorporating them—like the language-image cross references—for the meanings and connections that particular themes had in relation to each other, like suicide and political violence. At every turn I was confronted with the possibility of making faulty or sinister connections. It wasn't as though I had started out with a thesis I was trying to prove or elaborate on. On the contrary, I had started out with two things that interested me, just as in *Lives of Performers* (*LOP*) I had started out with dance and emotional life. Previously it was a matter of getting the stuff organized and distributed and not worrying too much about psychological or narrative coherence. For example, in both *LOP* and *Film About a Woman Who . . .* (*FAAWW*) there is much playing around with stills and people posing for stills in order to contrast still and moving photography. The formal distinctions took precedence over the content. I wasn't overly concerned that I was dealing with quotes from films about women who had been stabbed by male psychopaths. In *FAAWW* I was interested in contrasting these stills with a story about a woman who was lost after seeing a movie in a strange town, in the *narrative* possibility that the woman on the soundtrack, who is talking about a movie she's seen, *might* be talking about *Psycho,* which is identifiable from the stills of the shower sequence. That narrative connection took precedence over making the point that both women could be seen as victims. It isn't that I made an effort to avoid or disclaim the second interpretation. It just seemed of somewhat lesser importance. Throughout *FAAWW* the viewer has the puzzling task of dealing with these discrepancies between what you see and what you hear. That task animates the film as much as the fact that it's about someone who is angry over a love affair. Or so I thought.

In *Journeys* I was using much more sensitive subject matter. And so I felt a greater responsibility for possible interpretations. It seemed important to start dealing with juxtapositions in such a way as to produce separation as well as incongruity. Thus the divisions into those clear-cut compartments: the intertitles, the voices, the analytic session.

NC: Speaking of *FAAWW,* there seems to be some tension about it in your interview with the Camera Obscura Collective.[1]

YR: Well, they tried to give the film a particular interpretation which I didn't feel was appropriate. They tried to interpret the formal strategies of *FAAWW* and *LOP* in terms of a critique of patriarchy. Their final analysis—which focused on the "Emotional Accretion in 48 Steps" from *FAAWW*—concluded that the woman had internalized the man's negative view of her. That conclusion cannot be drawn, at least in that section.

One of the reasons I chose to design that film in those very short segments was simply to thwart narrative expectation. At the time it seemed weird that anyone would come along and try to piece it all together to make a particular psychological reading. But it would be unfair to Camera Obscura if I failed to mention another area in which they were trying to work at that time, and that is the antinarrative impulse itself as demonstrated in the film. The fact that most of the situations in *FAAWW* concern a woman's rage at a man, or men, doesn't in itself make a political statement about patriarchy, but maybe the disjunctive text-image relations and the demand these make on the audience and their implicit critique of dominant cinema—maybe all this constitutes a political position. It sounds good until you try to make particular correlations—like disjunction equals alert viewer equals critique of patriarchy and narrative coherence equals passive viewer equals status quo—without also making a convincing ideological analysis of narrative in cinema. This they didn't do. I feel a little responsible for that. I think they may have been sidetracked by my focus on the response of the audience. The flaw here is that the audience is conditioned to collude with whatever narrative strategies they are observing, even "deconstructive" ones!

The Camera Obscura people have subsequently implied that I categorically deny that my films have any political significance. This is simply not the case. I would like very much to make the claims for those two films that they make, but I'm just not convinced by their particular argument. I'm aware that other theoretical work has been done on the ideology of narrative, or the novel, such as Barthes' and Jameson's. Until I read and digest the stuff, however, I can't use second-hand arguments to defend what I do. At this point my reading is sporadic and unsystematic. In fact, even after reading I may still not avail myself of relevant arguments. For the same reasons.

But I am grateful to Camera Obscura for helping to move things along. They gave me a particular set of tools for thinking about my work at a point at which I had all but used up the ones I had.

NC: The Camera Obscura incident raises some important questions about *Journeys.* Given the topicality of subjects like politics, psychoanalysis, and feminism in the avant-garde film world, I suspect that many people will approach *Journeys* with powerful preconceptions. I've already heard complaints that argue that (1) the film has no theoretical position on politics, psychoanalysis, and feminism, or (2) that it lacks a *clear* position on these issues, or (3) that it has the wrong position. In other words, people expect the film to be theoretical, whatever that means. Perhaps you would like to talk about the relation of the film to these issues.

YR: Number 1 is absolutely correct: the film has no theoretical position on politics, feminism, or psychoanalysis. Rather than theoretical exposition, *Journeys* offers contrast and contradiction. Therefore, in response to number 2, it follows that no "clear positions" are going to be delivered on a platter. I didn't make a filmic dissertation. Unlike certain works being made today by people trained and/or skilled in Marxist and semiological discourse, my work requires a certain amount of interpretation. The sequences do not illustrate or orchestrate a preconceived argument. In fact, I myself discovered what might be called "positions" in the process of, even after, making the film. I would hope that some aspect of that process might be duplicated in the process of watching it. I'll get into both these things later, perhaps.

Number 3 is the most serious charge: "wrong position." Yes, there are wrong positions in this film, but if one looks for them one can also find "correct" positions.

A confession may be in order here (by way of explanation and not disclaimer): I have—realistically, I think—little trust in myself as a political analyst. Like my fifteen-year-old counterpart in *Journeys,* I have more sympathy with victims than understanding of the uses of power.

Partly because of my particular psychological history, partly because of my socialization as a female. It is from the viewpoint of the victim that I became fascinated with the subjects of suicide and assassination, and with the condition of powerlessness—real and imagined—as something that has so much potential for erupting into violence. However, I don't think of violence as some kind of essence or force lurking in the human psyche, waiting to burst out, and I didn't want to make a film "about" political violence and suicide as if the one could be conflated with the other by ignoring particular cultural and historical conditions. I am aware that in a film about both personal and political matters the "correct" treatment might be to show how external social forces and ideology affect and distort personal relations. We are most familiar with the filmic solution that has a central character "swept up" by historical or social events while "acting out" his or her particular personal story.

In the preliminary stages of *Journeys* I found myself with a unique collection of "characters" (previously I might have called them "materials") that would have taxed the ingenuity of a far more experienced director in working out the above solution within the normal timespan. I found myself with Vera Zasulich and the "Russian Amazons" in nineteenth century Russia, with Ulrike Meinhof and the Red Army Faction in Germany around 1971, with the diary of an American female adolescent circa 1951, with a middle-aged therapy patient spilling her guts in the U.S.A., 1979, plus sundry supporting players like Emma Goldman and Alexander Berkman and an assortment of female Hollywood movie stars.

Had I followed in the footsteps of *Kristina Talking Pictures* (*KTP*), Meinhof would have run into Zasulich and Goldman in a Zurich coffee-bar and subsequently sailed for America to be psychoanalyzed by Rollo May, perhaps taking a stab at Hollywood stardom somewhere along the way. "Ulrike Talking Cure" might have been the outcome, and "Ulrike Talking Bore" might have headed the *New York Times* review of this picaresque vehicle.

Well, I made the decision to keep the characters' stories separate, to maintain autonomous channels of presentation and information, and to allow—as much as possible—the personal and political (p & p) to fall where they might, presenting them as clearly identified texts of distinctly different origins. In some cases I didn't have to worry about a "correct" proportion of p & p within a given channel: the texts themselves took care of this choice for me, e.g., the unedited adolescent diary and the Russian memoirs. The thornier problem was (1) how to handle political violence in Germany and (2) how to handle the patient's suicide attempt, in relation to p & p?

I was slow to come to the realization of the extent to which German state repression was the real star of the German drama (I've written about that elsewhere, in *October*, no. 10), and that any information about Meinhof's private life could easily be misinterpreted for use against her. I'm not saying I didn't have my own nagging questions—questions about rage and outrage and whether or not these clouded her judgment about, among other things, popular support. But under the circumstances—namely, my ultimate decision to focus on German state terrorism in a series of printed facts—it seemed important to isolate and bracket those questions in some way, if they were going to be expressed at all. This I did by assigning them to the voice-over conversation between the man and woman preparing dinner.

It is in this section that I am most vulnerable to the charge of "wrong position." These two characters, heard but never seen, obsessively run through a gamut of speculations and counter-speculations about political violence as endorsed and practiced by the pre-revolutionary Russians and contemporary Germans. The woman repeatedly contrasts Meinhof and the "Russian Amazons" in terms of their respective personal struggles, while the man repeatedly challenges her. The style of the exchanges has a casualness and sometimes distracted air that one recognizes as compatible with the task of preparing a meal and trying to attend to a serious conversation at the same time. Since she is the more voluble and persistent, and *he* is cooking the meal, her emphasis on personal morality seems to dominate the exchange. Wrong position.

I tried to cover as much ground as possible in constructing this scene: provide information and make valid comparisons between the Russians and Germans while pointing out the dangers attendant on such comparison. The "he" was used to put a skeptical damper on "her" more presumptive declarations. On the surface her criticism of Meinhof seems limited to discrediting her political acumen by pointing to her questionable motives, in this case personal vengeance. "He" calls this "gossip." Several people have pointed out the absence of the issue of political *efficacy* in the discussion, and I must admit that that did get lost in the shuffle. I went back to my notes and there it was: "political violence—effectiveness." The closest either of them comes to a criticism of the RAF from that point of view is "his" statement, "The biggest mistake of the RAF was their timing."

I can't get too excited over this lapse. For one thing, I think that what the criticisms of this section really reflect is a need for a definitive "voice." No matter what I might have had the "he" and "she" say, it would not change the fact that the film is constructed so that no one channel or mode of discourse can be received as the definitive one. Consequently, these two people cannot be construed as *the* authoritative voice of the film. In fact, nowhere in the film can such a voice be found. No one mode of address holds the key to all the others. Meaning must be wrested from the interrelationship of contrasting voices. For example, "her" questioning of Meinhof's politics by examining her motives may or may not be relevant, but it comes into focus in a different way when she reads from Vera Figner: "Social concerns had gained ascendance over personal ones for good."

There is yet another "voice" in this scene that provides a clue to its appropriate reading (should I say "hearing"?), and that is the sounds of the household in which the discussion takes place—a relentless cacophony of domestic clatter that at times all but drowns out their speech. Like the urban din of *Two or Three Things I Know About Her,* the sounds clearly point to a form of alienation. In this instance the hermetic activity—insulated from exterior life, echoed in the implied confinement of the images of views through windows and close-ups of personal artifacts on the mantelpiece—is analogous to the experiential distance between the couple and the events they are trying to understand.

Okay, I know I said earlier that *Journeys* has no theoretical position on feminism. I am now going to assay a feminist theory (with a little help from my friends) *about* the film that will be constructed *from* the film but which is not explicitly stated *in* the film. (I blew my chance to espouse theory *in* the film by deciding to make the woman on the other side of the desk a nut instead of a feminist mouthpiece.)

It is no accident that the most prominent voices and texts in *Journeys* belong to women—notwithstanding the single exception of Alexander Berkman, whose story is part of an extrathematic exercise. Neither is it an accident that the most serious parts of the patient's address are to a female analyst. A fair amount of discussion is given over to the subject of political violence. Although this subject does not appear specifically in the adolescent's reflections, her embryonic moral preoccupations might be regarded as a prologue to the adult concerns. And despite the primary focus—finally—of the patient on her suicide attempt, even she makes several references to violence of the kind that concerns the others. Fairly early she says to the woman analyst, "Forgive me, I have no right to blame you for my not being in a situation where I can say, 'We have begun a great thing. Two generations perhaps will succumb in the task, and yet it must be done.'" (The quote is from Sophie Perovskaya, who was executed for anti-czarist activity in the late 19th century.)

Why are these women so fascinated with people who have turned to assassination as a political expedient? And how is this fascination related to the suicide?

Hold onto your hat. At the beginning and end of the film the subject of melodrama is introduced, first by the adolescent, who is critical of the excessive and exaggerated feelings aroused in her by "intense drama," and later I myself describe—with what might be called "excessive feeling"—a filmed melodrama made in Berlin in 1933. The implicit attraction and revulsion to melodrama demonstrated here can be related to the hold it has on women and the oppressed in our society. I am thinking of women and soap opera, and of young blacks roaming the streets of New York carrying radios that blare out disco music. They shall have music wherever they go, a self-made cushion of melodrama against the racist culture that dogs their heels. The thrall of melodrama cannot be considered separately from the extremes of behavior intrinsic to the form. Suicide and murder are prime ingredients of melodramatic treatment, and, beyond that, embody the options that occur to desperate and oppressed people. In *Journeys* the photos of, and references to, Merle Oberon, Roz Russell, Rita Hayworth, et al., bear out and extend these implications. Female movie stars are—more often than not—victims, both within the melodramas in which they must be punished or otherwise deprived of personhood for their sexual threat to men, and outside, as part of the system that garners profit from sexual exploitation.

What I am suggesting is that a subtext of this film is that women constitute an oppressed class, to whom—as such, and under proper conditions—certain options present themselves more readily than others as a response to those conditions of oppression. Suicide in the personal sphere, assassination in the political. *Journeys* meets the requirement of violence in melodrama and also other requirements.

Ruby Rich has proposed a number of elements necessary to women's film melodramas, among them "the presence of a woman at the center of the film; a domestic setting; an ellipsis of time to allow for the development of emotion; extreme verbalization, which replaces physical action as the means of communication for the now interior movement; and finally, the woman's ultimate decision to release her emotions."[2]

Journeys meets these criteria with its central female protagonist (the adolescent, the patient, and "she" can be seen as one), the domestic setting, the extreme verbalization, and even the ellipsis of time.

Let's say the foregoing is a first draft for a feminist theory. The objection may be made that women as such do not constitute a "class" at all, and therefore it is not valid to compare their position to that of indisputable victims of class exploitation, such as blacks, especially in relation to the spokeswomen in my film, who—almost without exception—are upper middle class and have education, money, and time to sit around searching their souls. In the case of the patient it is not even clear to what extent her "oppression" is real and to what extent it exists solely in her mind. The comparison is to be taken seriously only at the level of a general outline—a point of departure for a more complex investigation—under the common ideological heading of "domination," an extreme outcome of which may ultimately be the same—say, suicide —but everyday reality produces totally different conditions: grinding poverty and other racist constrictions for minorities, and internalized "objecthood" for middle-class women. Diminished humanity for both.

I'll stick to my guns, however, in respect to psychoanalytic theory. I chose the psychiatric situation not to take a position on psychoanalysis but because it provided me with a theatrical format. The "presentation of self" in analysis has much in common with performance, and the theatrical space was one in which I could work out a number of performance ideas. These included the writing of a certain kind of text, and the transformation of that text into a monologue, into a manner of speech one would ordinarily never hear.

The analyst of someone I know came to see the film and remarked afterward that "that's not the way patients speak." I am the first to agree. In all my long history of going to shrinks I never said 85 percent of those things, and the other 15 percent were never said that smoothly or with that assurance. Another thing that puzzles people about my relation to the therapy session is the peculiar letter of Meinhof's at the end of the film. I discovered that letter rather late in the course of writing the script. It was written while she was in prison and deals with psychiatry and how the profession handles (brainwashes) political prisoners in Germany. I was struck by the passionate rhetoric of the letter, for one thing. Here was Meinhof villifying psychiatry, the ostensible basis for a very large segment of my film. Some people hold that since it comes at the end it constitutes my negative commentary on the profession. This is not so. I present it as a letter of Meinhof's. At the same

time I present myself as an American living in Berlin and I describe the
film I had just seen about a man getting out of prison. A contrast—and
consequent separation—is made between Meinhof and me, between
my emotionalism over a vicarious experience and Meinhof's over the
harsh reality of her own. Again the distance of the American "voyeur"
from the German events is stressed.

No, I don't think you can read *Journeys* as a rejection of psychoanalysis. It is critical of the ways in which analysis can be abused and
critical of the culture that places such inflated and false hopes in it. As
far as the patient is concerned, all of the insights that she has acquired
seem to have come out of the psychiatric situation, her relationship to
the shrink. She repeatedly refers to what the analyst has already said:
"I'm very impressed with something you said," or "You may be right
when you say . . . "

NC: Much of the formal organization of *Journeys* seems predicated on
precipitating a range of word/image associations. First, there are cross-
references. An image will remind the spectator of a previous word or a
word will recall a previous image. The mantelpiece is especially important in this regard; it's a stockpile of objects mentioned by the patient
and other characters. Often the relationship seems to be one of naming, albeit obliquely. For example, the woman (Amy Taubin) says,
"Ooh, strawberries" at the beginning of the film and later we see strawberries on the mantelpiece. But sometimes this cross-referencing is
looser. The woman reads from a text by Russian anarchist Angelica Ba-
labanoff, intoning, "Once when I saw some peasants on our estate . . ."
and then we see a loaf of black bread on the mantelpiece, a staple of
Russian peasants. Or, as the patient relives a childhood memory of the
beach, we notice a toy pail and shovel on the psychoanalyst's desk. And
along with cross-referencing, you rely on language often to mold the
way we see the images. Verbal reports of trips to Pittsburgh and Siberia
overlay images of train rides, so that the spectator associates the journey
seen with the one discussed on the soundtrack. Perhaps you could say
something about how you conceive of some of the language/image relations in the film.

YR: Okay. I'd like to talk with special reference to the *attentat* section of
Journeys—the one where the man (Antonio Skarmeta) and the woman
(Cynthia Beatt) walk in front of the church. This section seems to

throw a great many viewers off even when they've been absorbed in the rest of the film. I've decided that it's not useful to talk about the *attentat* section as if it embodies a set of problems distinct from those in other parts of the film. This section is more demanding because it lasts so long, about twelve minutes. But the strategy used here is not really that different from the strategy used, say, at the point at which you first hear disco music, which is initially explained in voice-over as coming from "the neighbors." In the next shot, with a change in volume and tone, it becomes the driving "melodrama music" that accompanies the crawling titles describing the escape of Andreas Baader from prison and now functions in the traditional genre of "movie music."

The relationship between these two shots can be described in terms of a shift in meaning of the sound brought about by substituting formal juxtaposition (meaning by association) for a more simple narrative attribution. In the *attentat* sequence shifts in meaning are also generated, only now it is the image-track that undergoes transformations in meaning rather than the soundtrack. The soundtrack consists of two successive accounts of attempts at political assassination, the first by Alexander Berkman and the second by Vera Zasulich. In the image you see a man and a woman walking, usually not at the same time; you see them in the vicinity of a portentous pagoda-like portico jutting over the entrance of a building. Although the people, place, and activity have been seen earlier, they have not been identified. The editing is crude and foregrounded, consisting mainly of match-cutting and jump-cutting, though there are a few cuts that refer to conventional narrative continuity, e.g., in camera setup A the woman walks away from the camera and rounds the corner, and in camera setup B, which is now "around the corner," she walks toward the camera. In a normal narrative context, such cuts would not draw attention. Statically framed in three different camera positions (the camera does not "follow" the action), the location operates as a stage with exits and entrances, a blank space waiting for incident. The goings and comings of the man and woman are purposeless. In fact so relentless is their repetitious traversing of the space that it is ludicrous even to attempt realistic explanation.

How then is one to reconcile this collision of depersonalized formal design and credible personal anecdote? By suspension of disbelief? Impossible. By an act of will?

The *attentat* section demonstrates to a greater degree than elsewhere in *Journeys* how the uneasy union between word and image produces that resistance to intelligibility that necessitates a wholehearted participation on the part of the spectator, a state of mind more active than the good will that comes into play in "suspension of disbelief" or the pleasureable scopophilia induced by the sensuality of images. Perhaps this is the appropriate moment to insert once again a note making a distinction between a personal history of aesthetic preference and the Brechtian "distanciation" effect, a term which is popularly applied to anything modern or in the least bit "difficult." My personal history evolved via Duchamp and Cage and is accountable for that sometimes fatal attraction to "the way things fall" with a minimum of conscious manipulation or to that oblique glancing—of both eyes and objects— that can produce unexpected collisions of meaning. However, the "distance-from-meaning" created between objects (images and sounds, words) by my sometimes allowing unpremeditated juxtapositions to take place is a far cry from Brecht's interruptions of diegetic flow (addressing the audience, slide projections, etc.) for purposes of critical assessment, especially when, as in so many modernist works, a diegetic context is never clearly established to begin with. And however salutary I may consider my revisionist aleatorical practices (and I wouldn't ask the audience to be more mentally active if I didn't; after all, wasn't I the one who titled that dance *The Mind is a Muscle*?) using the terms *Brechtian* and *distanciation* to describe them is really using Brecht's name in vain insofar as it suggests, at least at this particular moment when artists are getting high on Marxist theory, that the revolution may be nearly here. It's *not* here. It's nowhere near. And I doubt if making things tough for you in my work is going to bring it any nearer, because when it comes it will most likely be in a form that won't be recognizable as any revolution Marx ever dreamed of in his hydrogen-bomb-free nineteenth century.

But whether or not social change, i.e., revolution, is possible, *we must work as though it is.* And making things a little tough for you in my art is one small part of the work that must be done. A paradox? If so, a necessary one.

To resume: The experience of connecting word and picture in the *attentat* section is one of moment-by-moment synthesis, of finding instantaneous correlations within the frame between image and word in specific, though fleeting, grammatical equivalencies, e.g., movement to verb, space to preposition or noun, performer to pronoun, architecture to proper noun, cut-between-shots to noun or verb, etc. The very temporary nature of this grammatical parsing, while allowing the spectator the possibility of attaching a provisional identity to some element in the image, denies us that process of identification and/or repulsion that is so comforting and essential to our relief-craving psyches when we make our weekly escape to the "movies-are-more-dreadful-than-ever" flicks. But hold on: There is more here than meets de neye al. Once you get the hang of it, secret pleasures await you as unforeseen linkages suddenly emerge. Several of my favorites come to mind: in the distance Cynthia turns and leans against the column and faces Antonio in the foreground as we hear "conscious presence of death." And later just after hearing "You'll be damn lucky if you don't lose your head" Cynthia, having walked toward the camera (her head growing larger), leaves the frame and we become aware of Antonio's truncated figure at the top of the frame. But as I say, it takes a while before you get the hang of it. Then of course there is a whole other issue of the ghoulishness involved in applying playful formal means to the subject of political murder, but I just can't get into that right now. What I propose to do instead is point out the correspondences between the beginning of Vera Zasulich's story and descriptions of the accompanying image. Camera setups in the following arrangement are indicated by (A), (B), and (C).

SOUND	IMAGE
Then *I* lay down to *sleep.* It seemed to me that *I was calm* and totally unafraid of losing my free life. *I had finished* with that *a long time ago.* It was not even a life anymore, but some kind of *limbo,* which I wanted to *end* as soon as possible. I was oppressed by the thought of the *following morning,* that hour at *the governor's,* when he would suddenly *approach* in earnest . . . I was sure of *success—everything would take place without the slightest hitch*; it shouldn't be hard at all, and not at all frightening, but nevertheless *I felt mortally unhappy.*	(A) Cynthia walks in slow-motion away from camera. Cut to (C). Portico dominates frame. Cynthia walks toward camera, glances at Antonio, moves briskly past him. Antonio turns, looks up at architecture. She exits right. He follows her.
I had not expected this feeling. And at the same time, I was not excited, but tired—I even felt sleepy. But as soon as I fell asleep, I had a	Empty frame dominated by portico.

nightmare. It seemed that I was not sleeping, but lying on my back looking through the glass above the door, which was illuminated from the *corridor.* Suddenly I felt as if I was losing my mind. *Something was irresistibly forcing me to rise, to go out into the corridor* and there, to scream. I knew that this was mad, I tried to hold myself back with all my strength, and yet nevertheless I went into the corridor and screamed and *screamed. Masha,* who was lying next to me, woke me up. I was indeed screaming, but on my cot and not in the *corridor. Again I fell asleep* and *again I had the same dream*: against my will *I walked* out and screamed. I knew it was crazy but nevertheless I *screamed. So it went,* several times.

   Then it was time to get up: we had no watches, but the sky had begun to turn *gray*, and someone knocked at our landlady's door. We had to *hurry to Trepov's* before nine o'clock, before he began *to receive petitioners.*
   We rose silently in the cold *semidarkness. I put on a new dress*; my coat and hat were old. After dressing *I left the room*: a new cloak and hat lay in the traveling bag, and I would *change* into them at the *station.* This was necessary because the landlady would certainly want to say goodbye; she would praise the cloak and advise me not to wear it on the road. And tomorrow this cloak would be in all the *newspapers* and *might draw her attention. I had had time to think*

Shadowy figure emerges from behind pillar, moves toward door, beneath the portico.

Cut to (C), Cynthia walking up path toward portico, walks

beneath it, and out the far side.

Cut to (A): Cynthia walks right to left in slow motion.
Cut to (B): Cynthia walks toward camera along right edge of frame.

Match- and jump-cut: Cynthia walks away from camera
                                   toward portico.
(The frame and weather are "grayish.")
Cynthia's white scarf billows.

Cynthia exits right, re-enters.

Her gait changes as she walks back and forth in front of the portico, from slow-motion to normal speed and back.
She stands motionless at right, facing right.

Antonio walks down left side of frame, exits. Cynthia remains about everything, down to the most petty details.

It was already growing light on the street, but the half-dark *station was completely deserted.* I changed, exchanged kisses with Masha, and left. The streets looked cold and gloomy.

motionless (lost in thought?).

Flash frame. Cynthia exits right. The space is completely deserted.

NC: Could you talk about some of the considerations that went into writing *Journeys?*

YR: I've really forgotten some of the considerations in the writing as distinct from the directing, or even editing.

NC: What about the patient's monologue? What were you aiming for?

YR: I did, in a way, want to approximate one of the things that happens in analysis, where one gets involved in a kind of evasion that has to do with the fear of pain and the often painful work required in confronting the sludge of one's psychic maneuvers. You might say that the language I gave the patient—in its torrential verbosity—is a version of that evasion. There's something particularly shocking about her monologue if you think of a good part of it as a huge digression. At one point she even lists her own defenses (which come straight out of Lacan): "ellipsis, suspension, anticipation, retraction, denial . . . ," etc. Psychologically speaking, her monologue is permeated with defensive tactics.

As for the disjunctive nature of the monologue, I had accumulated a great quantity of material in a fairly haphazard way, ranging from short phrases from various sources, like your [NC's] own "genetic codes for opening refrigerator doors," to extended passages of my own writing. It didn't matter to me that, spoken end to end, most of the stuff would form non sequiturs; in fact the non sequitur is one of the guiding principles. What seemed to happen sort of naturally was that the shorter fragments fell into lists while the longer sentences were arranged with these grammatical and/or syntactical ruptures. For example, right at the beginning she says: "You know I've never threatened you with . . . I've never held the threat of [   ] over your head an average of five or six blacks executed by hanging every Monday morning for political terrorism at Pretoria's central prison, according to reliable reports, rejection and disappointment are two things I've always found impossible to take." This sentence is also a good example of the way in which I like to play the political off against the personal. The square brackets indicate an ellipsis, a ploy I first used to avoid showing my hand too early, i.e., revealing that I was going to be dealing with suicide. During the shoot Annette actually spoke the word "suicide" and later I cut it out of the soundtrack. Later on in the film the device is used for other effects, like humor, or covering up a couple of gaffes, or for ambiguity.

Then there is another sort of shift, where the patient not only changes the subject but changes her mode of address, lands and takes off on a dime, so to speak. But that has more to do with direction and performance than with writing. Let's see . . . the writing process did involve choosing the exact place for the change in analyst. There's that anecdote she tells about asking her friend how to say "bow-wow" in German, which ends with the non sequitur question addressed to the female therapist: "Do you know that every time your pulse throbs a new human being has come into the world?" At this point the female therapist is replaced by the young boy, who promptly barks, "Wau-wau!" in answer to the earlier question, but also in response to ". . . a new human being has come into the world." Yippee. A new human being has appeared in the frame.

NC: So the ruptures in the text are meant to promote the same kind of associative play within the language that the various word/image relations set in motion? That is, just as an object on the mantelpiece refers to an earlier speech, "Wau-wau" throws us back to an earlier question.

YR: Yes, only the word-object dislocations are less jarring than the change from one shrink to the other. It's like a jump-cut being "harder on the eyes" than "cutting away" to the mantelpiece. And the word/image dislocations are also less jarring than the ruptures within the monologue itself. These are particularly abrasive insofar as she not only "monologues," but is always addressing another person, ostensibly trying to communicate.

NC: *Journeys* is made up of fragments culled from many sources. When you use quotations, how do you use them?

YR: How do you mean?

NC: Some avant-gardists use quotations like flags, as a signal of their allegiance to the position or person being quoted.

YR: I'm thinking about Godard. Sometimes you can tell and sometimes you can't. Sometimes the quotation signals a different viewpoint from what went before, and it isn't appropriate to wonder if it's the filmmaker's opinion. I guess I use quotations in a similar way. I collect things that clarify, or provoke, or perturb. Not all the quotations in *Journeys* represent "my voice," just as in the crawling titles the interpolated "I" and "you" don't necessarily mean you and me. They designate a change in address, a going "against the grain" of the authority established by the context of crawling titles. *I* may believe the titles to be correct, but "I" also performed in Iran quite recently. "I" was wrong then; *you* had better check these facts.

NC: I get the feeling that what could be called the "naming" relationship between word and object is the fundamental formal obsession in *Journeys*. It is a major locus of aesthetic pleasure for the viewer who is preoccupied with connecting the words of the text to objects through the play of memory. But it also constitutes a veritable drive behind the structuring of the film. It's so excessive that it no longer seems merely a convenient formal device. It's as if you derive special pleasure from the process of naming, as if the operation of naming, of associating words with objects, meant something special to you.

YR: Like what?

NC: You want or need things to have names, perhaps?

YR: I'm not sure I understand what you're talking about. Is this an example? When the patient is first introduced in voice-over, she says, "First it was just a sense of the bed trembling." And then in the background of the next shot, a group of people lower a bed. But it isn't that the bed has been given a name; the name has been given a body. It's like the "strawberries" example that we already went over . . . Is this what you call "naming"?

NC: Yes. Correlating words and objects is what I'm naming "naming."

YR: I went through the whole script and extracted every "name" that might be embodied on the mantelpiece or in the gallery. There's also a kind of "embodying" that is imagistic and doesn't rely on the kind of separation between word and object that we've been talking about, for example, all those images revolving around death.

NC: I didn't mean that the only associative structures are concerned with naming. Some are synecdoches.

YR: Which ones?

NC: Well, I was thinking of the pail on the analyst's desk when the patient regresses to childhood. It doesn't so much name the event as represent the trip by offering an element of the event for the whole event.

YR: Yes, I guess the paving stone on the mantelpiece functions similarly. Suggests street barricades, revolutionary activity. I have to put all this in the context of finding alternatives to enacted representation. Like these views through the windows: It was a way of getting activity into the frame but also of bringing in the outside world in contrast to the internal worlds of the kitchen and of the mind of the patient.

Very often I first decide what I'm *not* going to do. I was damned if I was going to show those two people bustling around in that kitchen. Eliminating *their* image left me with the practical question of how to fill up all that time with *other* images. Eliminating the mimetic convention, however, rather than being a limiting factor, opened up the opportunity to use imagery that would have multiple relations to the soundtrack: to suggest the couple's environment, to complement or counterpoint their discussion, and to create cross-references with other parts of the film. The tracking shots of the mantelpiece could even be seen as a model of the editing process itself in the way that sight and sound "slide around." I didn't want moment-by-moment illustrations of the text. I had already headed off that possibility by arranging the mantelpiece paraphernalia in more or less random "pretty pictures" bearing very little correspondence to the order in which the objects appear in the script.

The mantelpiece works somewhat in the way the windows work. It is conceivable to think of that mantelpiece, at least at the beginning, as existing in the house, in the same interior space, occupied by the two offscreen voices. You can think of those objects as a world of memorabilia belonging to those two people. This type of associative play substitutes for visualized enactment.

NC: I think that you've just introduced yet another kind of image/text relation—one that we didn't discuss earlier, viz., leading the spectator to construct a narrative space. For example, tempting the viewer to see the otherwise unidentified image of a window as Meinhof's or as the couple's. This type of associative structure is particularly interesting. Most of the film works to destroy any notion of continuous space. But then, there are these correspondences which, so to speak, forge little islands of continuous space.

YR: I have to give the audience something more than dissociation. I'm not interested in maintaining a totally poetic or dissociated stream of imagery in relation to the language. It's these provisional meanings that I'm interested in. I have to give the audience anchors, if only for a moment. How many ways can I find to provide these anchors? When does it make sense to pull some of them up and substitute new ones, or say "anchors aweigh" for awhile?

NC: Do you really think that those suggestions of narrative space add up to "anchors"? I mean all those little islands of narrative space don't finally fit together. Take the window. At some points it's in Germany and at others it seems to be in New York.

YR: It is mostly in New York because I want to establish those two as American. But sometimes the view through the window stands for two contradictory things at once: the place they're talking *about* and the place we see (Hamburg and London). Obviously, you make a choice or accept the contradiction. And if you've already seen the film you may be able to take in the three or four possible meanings. Some of these "anchors" are no more than straws in the wind: one should be able to let them blow by. I think that probably this can be picked up on fairly early—once you realize that you're not going to see those two people preparing dinner.

NC: How do you identify with the contesting voices?

YR: You mean me personally? Ah, you're looking for "my voice" again, aren't you? I'd rather not say except with regard to the patient. The states of mind she plows up do in some cases come out of my own experience. I believe in confronting one's feelings of insufficiency and the things one is most afraid of in oneself. I think it is an important part of any good analytic or therapeutic process. The darker side of the self has to be acknowledged at some level, not once, but over and over again. "It [suicide] could happen again," she says. It perhaps marks a resolution, a coming to terms with the limits of therapy, that she finally buckles down to pursue the meaning of her "act." Earlier she had said, "You can tell me until you're blue in the face that you're not God . . . but I'm not going to believe you." She concludes that the feelings she had so longed to acquire—like compassion—would not be given to her as a reward for her personal struggles, but must be invented—and reinvented—by herself. And applied to herself. "I had no compassion for the life I wanted to end." Just before this the adolescent speaks for the last time: "I must learn to love myself and then I will love humanity." This line had always been somewhat embarrassing to me, giving rise to unsettling speculations as to how far I had actually come, baby, from the precocious, naive, isolated, romantic, confused, painfully shy sixteen-year-old who wrote it. The line finally found its home: It takes on a prophetic, terrifying dimension when one thinks about the possible consequence of a lack of compassion/love for oneself, as confessed by the patient immediately after.

NC: Is there a reason why the analyst is divided into adult/child counterparts? Is that an attack, an expression of anger and frustration that literalizes the idea that the analyst *is* a child?

YR: One way of looking at those transformations of the analyst is as a mockery of the patient's self-absorption. She's so involved with herself that she doesn't even notice that the person in front of her has changed identity. They could stand for her inability to see anyone else's situation, her inability to empathize. Hence, her inability to feel compassion. It's interesting, her very last words are "a world in which conscious choice and effort might produce mutual respect between you and me." It's as though she has "seen" the shrink for the first time. The transformations also function as comic relief from her obsessions.

NC: I've heard you speak disparagingly of some of the voices. There's Meinhof's letter. And you have dismissed the segment where you read that letter to your mother as sentimental and confused.

YR: I had, and have, rather complicated notions about that section in which my letter to my mother is intercut with Meinhof's letter from prison. It's one of the most loaded sections of the film for me, and that's one reason that I put myself there, in person. When I first considered using the Meinhof letter, I thought that its rhetoric would neutralize its denunciation of psychiatry in some way. It seems hysterical and so biased and colored by her situation and what she had gone through that I thought it couldn't be taken seriously. Well, of course, it was colored by what she had gone through: When I really began to think about her experiences—of being in that prison for three years, and of how she had been treated—I began to have much more sympathy for her. Her denunciation seemed more impassioned and justified than hysterical and rhetorical. At that point when our voices intersect one of the most powerful contrasts in the whole film emerges. They are voices at opposite sides of a culture—her rage and my cultivated sensitivity. The whole of Meinhof's letter is included. The problem about my part was how to edit it. To have left it intact and uninterrupted would have been a terrible mistake. It is extremely sentimental when you hear it in its entirety, much more so than in its present form. What landed on the cutting room floor are the parts with me drinking wine and getting progressively more drunk and maudlin.

NC: Your basic method seems to be radical juxtaposition. Do you see any limitations in this approach?

YR: Yes, I suppose what I've just described is a form of radical juxtaposition, although when *I* use the term I usually mean a less specific kind of contrast, something more akin to ambiguity. Like putting the box of frozen "Fish Fingers" (the English version of our "Fish Sticks") next to the photo of Meinhof. As for limitations . . . there's a risk that some of the things I most highly value and have worked out with the greatest effort will get embedded in the general accumulation of ambiguity—for example, the stuff in the patient's monologue about "egalitarian relations." Her power struggle with the woman analyst centers around this issue. In *her* mind one of them is always up and the other is always down. The risk is that this particular discussion—which she returns to several times—may be absorbed by the general clutter.

NC: You've mentioned Cage and Duchamp as sources for your use of radical juxtaposition. Do you see your work with The Grand Union as perhaps a more immediate influence?

YR: No. My concern with that goes back to my earliest dances, such as the "Solo Section" of *Terrain,* where I told a coherent story and simultaneously executed a series of short movement phrases which had been invented without reference to the story.

NC: How do you insure against losing things in the clutter?

YR: By bringing things back in another form. Repetition is a key strategy. Like cutting Amy's voice into the therapy session with the Emma Goldman story about inequality in the Russian factory after the revolution.

NC: Aside from repetition, are there other overarching, organizing principles in the film? Do you see it as having an overall direction or large-scale structure?

YR: I see the therapy session as one large structure set against or beside several others. Likewise, the readings from the anarchist memoirs.

NC: I mean—apart from there simply being large units—are those large units beside each other as the result of specific underlying principles? For example, does the film have a linear movement or, better, what are the considerations that lead you to follow a given scene with another? The film does seem to have a climax; it doesn't feel like things are being juxtaposed, come as they may; rather, there appear to be definite thematic movements.

YR: You might call those death images a kind of climax. But then there follows a hiatus of sorts during which the Berkman and Zasulich stories are told. It's more of a "choreographic" interlude than something that advances the drama. We get back on the track when the titles start rising again with more information about Germany, and then—after the deaths of Baader, Enselin, et al.—we return to the therapy session, where the patient will now get into the nitty-gritty of her suicide attempt. There are several clearly linear movements in the film: the titles with their chronological progression, and the monologue in the sense that it is "leading up to" something. And there is what might be called a conclusion when all the voices come together and deal with the same issues: egotism, feelings, self-improvement. I can't decide whether the videotape of me is an anticlimax or denouement. Maybe a postscript. Decisions about sequence varied according to whether I was dealing with large units—like the "kitchen scene" on the soundtrack—or shorter segments within the large unit. The sequence of images during the couple's discussion depended totally on what was being said or read. The placement of this large unit was determined by the decision to divide the patient's monologue into three distinct sections and these breaks occurred at places which didn't require the fancy cuts that make the boy shrink into the woman, etc. As I recall, sense, nonsense, and/or expediency dictated the sequence.

NC: Are there other large segments?

YR: Stonehenge is sometimes interchangeable with aerial video footage of the Berlin Wall. It is usually seen during readings from the diary, and the diary excerpts were often placed so as to elaborate recently introduced themes, like factories or "the ego." The mantelpiece in the way it refers to the past and future throughout the film is a unifying element.

NC: The mantelpiece, the analyst's desk, and the background of the shots of the analytic sessions seem to function in the same way—as repositories for objects.

YR: They are similar and different. The mantelpiece shots create their own visual logic. You see what the tracking camera shows you. The desk is different. You only see the objects if you yourself scan the image. The desk is a repository but also a barrier between two people. It establishes the professional ambience. Certain things fell into place once I had established the "household" and the "office." The two places could then share certain things, such as the telephone, the crank caller, the boat, the bed, the vials of pills, etc.

NC: The background of the analytic sessions at Whitechapel, then, is also different. It involves not only objects, but people. And the people are involved in performances, task performances, after the fashion of your dances like *Room Service* and *Parts of Some Sextets*. They bring in a boat and later a stairway.

YR: Instead of a mattress! The staircase harks right back to 1968 to the "Stairs" section of *The Mind is a Muscle*. It's obviously a favorite prop. In *Journeys* it initially appears in Zasulich's story: She says she woke up in her prison cell and remembered a staircase that went nowhere and that had strangely disappeared. (The staircase I used in *The Mind is a Muscle* was modeled after one that appeared in a dream: it had two tiny steps at the top and it "went nowhere.") Later the group in the background of Whitechapel struggles to bring in an enormous staircase, about nine feet high and twelve feet long. Annette at that point is rambling on with these variations on her possible parentage, another one of those lists. They make a terrific din as they struggle to get the thing through the swinging doors, making her raise her voice. Still later a woman ascends, then descends the staircase (the "higher" and "lower" motif again). We have already seen, in one of the tracking shots along the mantelpiece, a color photo of a very ornate stairway, which in turn links up with the patient's list of opulent architectural details

Let me say right here that the idea of shadowy figures in the background began to obsess me after I finished *Kristina Talking Pictures*. There is that single shot in *KTP* in which Ed sits in a chair musing about the "concerned liberal" while three women in black coats hover in the rear. They create a sinister ambiguous image. I never really spelled out for myself what they represented, but it's not too difficult to see them as hovering somewhere between the fates and moral arbiters of some sort.

In *Journeys* the people in the background bring things into the shots that will be, or have been, talked about. Or they do things that constitute metaphors. They sometimes merely wait around. Maybe they're custodians. Custodians of . . .

NC: Consciousness?

YR: Consciousness, oh shit. They make concrete, they act out, the things the patient doesn't. The patient is not allowed to "act out." In therapy this is a term for living a fantasy, not living in reality. I don't allow her to get up from her chair or allow her to be followed by the camera. She is allowed to express herself in words within the confines of the session. But I don't "represent" her going home, making love, doing her work, or doing *anything*. The background people perform activity that is denied to the patient. Sometimes they simply wait "to act." The activity with the rug constitutes a metaphor. They stand on it in a line, like an unemployment or immigration line. One by one each person is called out of the frame, and the rest of the line moves up. In the way that one feels on the spot in a government office, they're "on the carpet," just like the patient. The rug also allowed me to get some visual diversity in the background. The look of the carpet was substantial and interesting and when I later thought of "being on the carpet" that clinched it for me. Which goes to show that language doesn't always come *first* to me.

NC: On several occasions you've said that you see the interior shots in the film as emblems for the inside of the mind and that this raises the need for exterior shots—street scenes, etc.—to reintroduce "the external world."

YR: Yes. I've described the background of the Whitechapel Gallery as being a place midway between the patient's introspection and her public life. And it is literally so in the Whitechapel because you see the constant stream of traffic through those rear windows. The views through all the apartment windows also function as the "everyday life" in that Merleau-Ponty quote that Vito reads: "Principles and the inner life are alibis the moment they cease to animate external and everyday life."

NC: How did you cast the film?

YR: Before I began to write the patient's part, I asked Annette Michelson if she would be interested. I think I indicated to her that it would be long and arduous. She said she'd have to read it. As I wrote—over a two-month period—more and more I saw and heard Annette. I became quite attached to the idea of her doing it.

I might have done the woman of the soundtrack myself, but felt I wasn't experienced enough as an actress, which may or may not have been an accurate appraisal. I approached Amy Taubin because of her acting background in theater.

I chose Vito Acconci as the male voice because I was familiar with his work, especially his videotapes. I kept hearing his voice on the phone as the crank caller, as the heavy breather. He exactly matched my image of that voice. And then I thought—I bet he could do the man's part too. It didn't matter to me that both voices would be heard as the same person. That was a funny touch.

The trickiest job of casting was the young girl. I actually auditioned children and adolescents. I couldn't find a voice I could bear to listen to for an extended period of time. Lena Hyun, an adult with a young voice, solved the problem.

The group of people in the background at Whitechapel comprised pretty much whoever was available. They were paid very little and were whoever wanted to be around a shoot with me and could spare the time. It's surprising to read in the credits that so many people were involved; while watching the film you're not aware that many of those people were replaced by others in different shots.

NC: How do you see your work in relation to film history?

YR: *LOP* used the intertitles of silent film as an alternative to sync sound. When I first met with Babette Mangolte to work on *LOP* I said I wanted the look of it to be somewhere between Warhol and Bresson. That may have been to impress her with my seriousness as a filmmaker. You can see the Warhol connection in the use of static camera and long takes in *KTP*—the bedroom sequence—and of course in the analytic session in *Journeys*. Of course the life created in front of the camera is the other side of the earth from Warhol's world. With one exception: the film portrait of Henry Geldzahler, one of my favorite Warhol films. What kind of film historical connection do you see?

NC: What I had in mind was Eisenstein, his "collision of ideas."

YR: But not in terms of visual montage. The connection is more likely in his ideas about conflict and contradiction. I reread the chapter on dialectics in *Film Form* recently and was struck by his phrases "clash of opposing passions" and "Art is always conflict, according to its methodology." Right on. But that's probably what you meant.

If we're going to speak of collisions of ideas then we certainly must speak of Godard. I must say I'm somewhat abashed at doing so. I think of Godard as "worldly" in a way that makes my stuff seem like "miniature provincial." Much of this is by choice, insofar as I draw very little from Hollywood films. Whether or not their influence shows up in my films, when I think of FILM it is the work of Dreyer, Renoir, and Vigo that comes to mind, and all those Jean Gabin movies I saw in the late forties and early fifties. I shouldn't neglect Hollis Frampton's *Critical*

Mass, the perfect filmic treatment of domestic hell, and *Poetic Justice,* an archetypal film of some sort. To this day when I think of the title, I can't immediately remember what parts of the story I heard, read or saw.

I seem to be speaking of influences and resemblances interchangeably.

I like Marguerite Duras's *Le Camion* a great deal. At a certain point, while working on the *Journeys* script, I kept flashing on the similarity between the recurring scene of Duras and Depardieu on either side of the table and my patient and analyst on either side of the desk. I was struck by the utter simplicity of the structure of that film: from house to landscape, over and over. This may have strengthened my resolve to use the recurrent shots of Stonehenge and the Berlin Wall.

NC: *Journeys* is a stylistic departure from *KTP.* Except for the analyst, the characters aren't broken up the way they are in some of the earlier films. Each character is played by one actor/voice whereas previously some characters were represented by several different people.

YR: I suppose I opted for getting my feet wet in that area of acting nuances and values, making a more identificatory situation. But by playing around with the patient's speech—making it so disjointed—I undermined the possibility of psychological verisimilitude. The kinds of fracturing of persona that you see in *KTP* and *FAAWW* have been taken up by the dissociations of the patient's train of thought in *Journeys.* As for the voices on the soundtrack, I deprived them of bodily visibility *because* their speech was coherent enough to produce psychological credibility. Give with one hand, take with the other. Maybe someday I'll direct a totally naturalistic film. But I just know I'll then have to send a line of print charging across the frame every so often: "This is not reality this is not reality this is not reality."

At a screening in Hartford a young woman remarked afterwards that she wasn't convinced that the patient was the type of person who would attempt suicide. Of course all kinds of people commit suicide, often very unpredictably. That oversight on her part took me aback less than the fact that she was involved at that level with the characters. With all the fracturing going on in this film you would think that the desire to suspend disbelief would not swing into operation so readily.

I was also very surprised when you [NC] told me that you were repelled by the two people on the soundtrack preparing dinner. You said they were pretentious, pseudointellectuals who talk, almost playfully, about dire political things—who use politics as an arena to display their cleverness, you said—while making a gourmet meal. You named some academics and artists they reminded you of.

NC: Shhh.

YR: I guess I have to allow that that is going to be one of the possible responses to this film. Spectators will insist on identifying with or hating the characters in spite of the degree to which I have disembodied them or wreaked arty havoc in their environment.

NC: Ending with the recorder lesson suggested to me the idea that art could reconcile all the turmoil and confusion explored by the rest of the film. And this didn't just have to do with the fact that the scene was about learning a musical instrument but with the way that the scene was shot. It was very symmetrical, classic and the colors had an aura of serenity, peacefulness and friendliness. It seemed like a coda reassuring us that despite all the turbulence in the narrative (or narratives) there was still a realm of peace—Art.

YR: It's funny, the fact that it is art is quite secondary to me. The lesson is important to the film because of the way it brings the issue of equality/inequality into the picture again, and resolves it, in contrast to the torturous analytic session. Here we again have two women, but now in a relationship which—unlike that of the patient to the analyst—is direct, simple, and uncluttered with psychic debris. We see a situation in which the terms of inequality are both mutually accepted and real, where one person—from the superior vantage point of her skills—is imparting knowledge that the other lacks. It is indeed a coda. Remember, however, that it not the final shot; it is the penultimate shot. The last shot returns to a more sinister inequality with the quote from the head of the Federal Criminal Investigation Bureau in West Germany.

NC: You italicize the last part of that quote—"*the State's monopoly of force.*" I thought that was curious and that it revealed your anarchist background. I mean, since at least the time of Weber, the state—any state, whether capitalist, communist or fascist—has been defined as exactly that agency that in a given geographical region has a monopoly of force. Only anarchists find a state's simple assertion of this prerogative, in and of itself, a cause for raising moral eyebrows.

YR: Be that as it may, it seems to me that there is something very different about the use of language by public officials in Germany as compared with American officials. It is much more straightforward than anything we're accustomed to here. The definition of state power is constantly spelt out without any democratic, humanistic trappings. One's first reaction to this is horror; it is this language that leads one to believe that Germany represents an especially repressive situation. And yet, you're right. Possession of a monopoly of force is one definition of the state. But that's not the definition we're given in a so-called democratic society. For this reason I felt it needed special emphasis, so that it might be seen as other than unique to Germany.

NC: Have you been surprised by the misinterpretations of the film that you've encountered so far?

YR: Yes. I'm surprised that people are so confused by it. The very first question at the very first screening set the stage: "Are you for or against terrorism?" In an age of confusion people want simple, clear answers. I'm afraid I can't provide them. And from the left come those charges of INCORRECT that we've talked about: "How dare you psychologize the revolutionaries and foreground individual, personal experience over what they stood for." That's an incorrect reading of the film. Someone even called me a "combat liberal" à la Mao. And yet, in his essay "On Contradiction" Mao says: "The law of contradiction in things, that is, the law of the unity of opposites, is the most basic law in materialist dialectics. Lenin said: 'In its proper meaning, dialectics is the study of the contradiction within the very essence of things.'"

NC: I have one last question. How do you envision your ideal spectator? That is, how do you want people to follow your film?

YR: He is white, fairly well educated, perhaps at one time was familiar with the films of Brakhage and Frampton, but gave up on avant-garde everything quite some time ago. He most likely has a predilection for classical music and listens to Beethoven for relaxation. He has a very demanding job, perhaps in a publishing firm; maybe he's an editor.

He's between forty-two to fifty, twice married, twice divorced, has 2.5 almost grown children. He plays volleyball, is between five foot nine inches and six feet tall. He has time to kill after a doctor's appointment and wanders into the moviehouse to see *Rules of the Game*. He stays to see *Journeys from Berlin/1971*. He is bowled over. His telephone number is . . .

NC: Let me ask my question another way.

YR: I thought that was your last one.

NC: Well, you changed the terms a little. I was ambiguous about what I meant by "ideal spectator." Actually you've already answered this question in detail by giving lots of examples of the types of associative correspondences you plant for the viewer. But perhaps you would like to summarize the types of hermeneutic responses that are appropriate to the film? What would an instruction manual for viewing the film be like?

YR: If I could write or had to write an instruction manual for the film, I would've made a different kind of film. I haven't made a *Finnegans Wake.*

NC: I didn't mean that.

YR: Okay. Last shot. I have to admit to a secret evangelical impulse. I would like it to be more difficult for a viewer to sit through pap as a result of having seen *Journeys from Berlin*. I would like the outcome of having seen *Journeys* to be that this person might seek out and prefer to see this kind of film. There are people who you might say are on the edge of escapist cinema—going to the flicks but needing or desiring something else. I would like to swing that constituency toward more demanding and intelligent work. If *Journeys* contributes to that eventuality then I'll be satisfied. I'm talking as though there's some way to gauge that. There isn't. But that is what I would like.

Is that the answer you're looking for?

NC: Not exactly. It's better.

YR: Why does she refuse to understand the question?

Notes

1. Camera Obscura Collective, "Yvonne Rainer Interview," *Camera Obscura,* no. 1. (1976): 76–96.

2. B. Ruby Rich, "The Films of Yvonne Rainer," *Chrysalis,* no. 2 (1977): 115–27.

More Kicking and Screaming

from the Narrative Front/Backwater

This essay was originally presented during a panel on avant-garde cinema during a 1982 conference called *Cinema Histories, Cinema Practices* at the Center for Twentieth Century Studies, University of Wisconsin, Milwaukee. The panel was moderated by Stephen Heath and comprised of Annette Michelson, Scott MacDonald, and myself.

I remember Scott being somewhat outrageous by stating flat out to the assembled academics and intellectuals that he had no use for theory. I also remember someone in the audience asking me about the difference between film and theater. I was so taken aback by the magnitude of the question that I said something dismissive. Because my paper had nothing to do with theater (or so I thought!), I wasn't feeling very cooperative. From what perspective did the questioner want an answer: that of the director, the spectator, the actor, the lighting designer, the casting director, the art director/stage designer?? Now I deal with these differences in tiny increments when asked the oft-repeated question about my transition from dance to film, e.g., film offers more control of the spectatorial gaze, does not require suspension of disbelief, requires less external affect on the part of the actor, offered me a greater range of possibilities in the interweaving of sound and image. (This being but the tip of the iceberg, I would hope that in the aggregate the essays and interviews in this volume cover those differences in more depth.)

My paper was later published in *Wide Angle,* vol. 7, nos. 1–2, (Spring 1985). It pursues the investigation of cinematic narrative begun in "A Likely Story" and previews scenes from my next film, *The Man Who Envied Women,* which would throw down the gauntlet to psychoanalytic feminist film theory by removing the physical presence of the female protagonist from the picture. The fly in the ointment of this somewhat doctrinaire tactic, however, is the return of the repressed toward the end of the film in the form of a theory-spouting French femme fatale played by Jackie Raynal. (I've always taken pleasure in flouting edicts, self-imposed or otherwise.)

What with this annoyingly persistent involvement with psychology, I constantly run the risk of being nudged into an area in which I am neither interested nor especially competent to operate—I mean the area of narrative film in which characterization and plot predetermine such formal signifiers as lighting, mise-en-scène, camera movement, editing and speech itself. In the four films I have thus far completed, character and plot are almost an afterthought as they slide behind devices that foreground not only the production of narrative but its frustration and cancellation as well. Thus, in varying degrees, words are uttered but not possessed by my performers as they operate within the filmic frame but do not propel a filmic plot.

Part of this project combines the pleasurefulness of language with a removal or narrowing of the potential for emotional identification on the part of the spectator. A removal or narrowing of those operations that cause identification. Here may lie a key to my present narrative dilemma, a dilemma that seems to deepen with each passing year. From descriptions of individual feminine experience floating free of both social context and narrative hierarchy, to descriptions of individual feminine experience placed in radical juxtaposition against historical events, to explicitly feminist speculations about feminine experience, I have just formulated an evolution which in becoming more explicitly feminist seems to demand a more solid anchoring in narrative conventions. (I am not sure of the reasons, but I suspect the worst.)

Consider several examples. First, this female voice-over from *Film About a Woman Who . . .* (1974): "The man danced with the three-year-old child. It went on for a long time. He didn't take his eyes off of her. He manipulated her tiny soft limbs in time to the music. He bent down to her, lifted her up, turned her around under his hand, delicately balancing and maneuvering her body, which at times his two huge hands all but concealed from view. She could not stop looking at the two of them. The sensuality of the dance fascinated her, and then as time passed it became bizarre. She began to be uneasy in the realization that he knew that *she* in particular was watching."

And consider this from the mouth of the patient in *Journeys from Berlin/1971* (1980): "Once when we were making love the thought came to me—'what a waste that the flow of our pleasure should begin and

end with ourselves.' Just once. And once before that as I started to mas-
turbate, my mind was invaded by the image of American soldiers forcing a hand grenade into the vagina of a Vietnamese woman. Only once
such a thought."

And how about this: "I shall be bold. Sex for most heterosexual men
is by definition an enactment of power, the kind of power over a
woman that is intended to demean her whether or not she engages with
that aspect of it. Most women prefer not to acknowledge this intent of
their partners. Those of us who have lived with the same man over a
protracted period of time may recognize the relation between our eroticism and our desire to please, but must disavow the nastier implications
of our mates' complementary dominance, which exists irrespective of
the specific sexual practice, i.e., who is on top, sado-masochism, etc.
Maybe I am being brutal; 'demean' may be too strong a word. Okay,
'control,' 'keep her in her place' rather than 'demean.' In any case, the
sexual act can be described as the crucial site where a primary social
contract is enforced and the imbalance of dominance and compliance
is perpetuated. . . . Good grief, and here I've been thinking all these
years that sex was fun."

This last speech is excerpted from a script I'm still working on. It is
uttered in voice-over by a woman who is never seen but is identified at
the outset of the film as the estranged wife of the male protagonist
whose name is Jack Deller. What I'm getting around to observing by
way of these three quotations is that as my texts become more explicitly
theoretical or political, I feel a greater obligation to enclose them in a
more totalized narrative and assign their utterance to more unified
identities. Not that I intend to yield in every case to this obligation, I
tell myself. Just be aware of its siren song and deadly constraints. Thus
in the earlier film the voice describing the man dancing with the child
never reveals or identifies itself, never speaks in the first person, is never
synchronized with a physical presence, while the voice in the last example speaks entirely as a "first person." Although she too does not appear, her identity will evolve via her telling a great deal about herself
and also through her formal and emotional relationship to the pho-
tographed central character, Jack Deller. Whereas in *Film About a
Woman Who* . . . the voice-over in its impersonal role of narrator can be
interpreted as standing for the autobiography of the "author," this latest voice-over—for all its vying with the image as an arbiter of truth—
will constitute a fiction.

Am I now to conclude that the personal, i.e., descriptions of individual daily life, must be depersonalized in its transposition to film, while the political, i.e., generalizations about social organization, must be personalized? Maybe so.

The necessity for digressing from and undermining a coherent narrative line driven by characters, or simply refusing to comply with its demands for spatio-temporal homogeneity, uninterrupted flow of events, closure, etc., has always been a basic assumption in my scheme of things. The necessity for *inducing* identification has only recently become worrisome, because once it is hooked, how do you unhook this audience that dreams with all its eyes open? Destroying the coherence of this speaking moving fictional subjectivity within a single film is more difficult than one might think.

Allow me to invoke Godard. Although he has transgressed just about every narrative code in the book at some point or another, his films seem to fall roughly into two groups from the standpoint of character identification. The more discursive ones, for example, *Le Gai Savoir* (1969) and *Ici et Ailleurs* (1974), offer little or no possibility for psychological projection on the part of the spectator. However, in the more numerous—and more marketable—films the characters survive the director's incursions against their narrative integrity. For example, in *Two or Three Things I Know About Her* (1966) Juliette Jansen, in being revealed as Marina Vlady the movie star, becomes an even stronger object for voyeuristic identification. And in *Weekend* (1967), for all the digressions and fantasies that take over the story, the nasty bourgeois couple remains true from beginning to end. (Don't get me wrong; I love Godard.)

Sometimes I feel caught between a formalist and a realist approach. Am I a formalist on her way to being a realist? I doubt if I'll ever make the grade. Just when it seems to be shaping up, I must put my fist or foot through the picture of reality. Yet hold on and hello! Wasn't I just talking awhile back about an identity-ridden voice on my soundtrack relating to an identity-ridden performer in the frame? Yes, but . . . there is the usual collection of flies in the ointment. The estranged wife on the soundtrack will both address and periodically seem to observe Jack Deller from a physical vantage point similar to ours, and Jack Deller will be played by three different performers. One of the functions of the voice-over will be to arrest or short-circuit the seduction/repulsion syndrome I anticipate in the relationship of spectator to any one of three moving, speaking, visible Jack Dellers. No one is going to come out of *this* flick saying "I saw this movie about a guy who . . ."

A momentary retreat into memory: a section of a theater piece I made around 1970. Two people at a time, from a group of ten or more, having hung large signs around their necks, come to the foreground of the performing area to strike ordinary sitting and standing poses with gazes directed toward or away from one another. The signs read variously "sister," "brother," "mother," "other woman," "lover," "child," "son," "friend," "husband," etc. In sequential *tableaux vivants* "daughter" sits next to "lover" or "other woman" stands near "father," etc., until all of the possible combinations of relationship and intrigue are exhausted. This primitive exercise in attribution can hardly be construed as having created "characters," yet it remains for me an important point of reference, reminding me of how little it takes to indicate identity and relationship and point both in the direction of narrative. Introduce a prop or two and we have melodrama. Introduce language and it's time to clear the decks again. Buffeted by patriarchic metaphors: the siren call versus the sword of Damocles; narrative fullness versus '60s cleansing of the stables . . . start over. . . .

I fill in the gaping holes of a script while cautioning everyone within earshot to beware of underestimating the willful tenacity of that aforementioned sleeping-tiger audience. When faced with even vestigial evidence of narrative time and space, it suddenly becomes rampant and demands the whole *mishpucha*, i.e., total psychological coherence at the levels of role and image. The avant-garde audience is the worst of all in this respect. Brakhage and Breer are no preparation for adulterated and truncated narratives. Thus, after seeing *Dora* (1979) they say, "A mother wouldn't read postcards like that from her daughter so calmly." Or, after seeing *Lives of Performers* (1972) they say, "The women are OK but the men are all assholes." Or, after *Journeys from Berlin/1971* (1980) they say, "The patient is totally narcissistic." Or, after seeing *Jeanne Dielman* (1975) they say—and here I must confess to agreement—"That kind of woman wouldn't look as young and attractive as Delphine Seyrig; that kind of woman wouldn't look like a movie star."

Here we go again: ". . . it's about this guy who . . ." and "that kind of woman." It takes a stout heart and stern sense of purpose to sit properly in the audience-seat. Will anyone ever come out of the movie palace saying, "It's about this man you see and this woman you hear? He has been given a name, Jack Deller; she hasn't been given a name. When he speaks of her he calls her 'she' or 'my wife,' whereas she never refers to him as 'my husband.'" This proper spectator has given equal attention to the fictions and the production of those fictions, to the social relations and to the representation of those relations. Spectator-of-my-dreams, will my filmmaking pr . . . will my films ever produce *you*?!

But really now! Who are these people, this Jack Deller and this nameless woman-wife-not-wife; what do they do; where do they live? What? You don't like the way I'm putting these questions? You've learned my lesson too well. How's this: In what historical period has the director permitted them to live? What are the director's concerns other than making the audience sit on the edge of its seat in fear of pleasure? Where is the social reality in this film?

This man with the name is a professor of some sort. At some point he will deliver a lecture on . . . anti-trust violations under Reagan. The wife with no name is a choreographer. We learn that when the man-with-the-name talks about her to his shrink. We also see her dancing on the screen in the shrink's office. When her daughter from a previous marriage goes off to college, she moves out of the apartment she has shared with Deller into her studio from which she is being evicted. She fights against the eviction while also getting involved in a city-sponsored program that would enable artists to renovate abandoned buildings in poor urban neighborhoods. When the neighborhood protests, she finds herself on the wrong side of the fence politically. This film is about the housing shortage, changing family patterns, the poor pitted against the middle class, Hispanics against Jews, artists and politics, female menopause, abortion rights. There's even a dream sequence.

The scene is a kitchen. A woman moves about in slow motion. The voice of the woman without a name speaks: "I think I am dreaming. I must be dreaming because there's my mother and she's only forty-eight years old. Still in her apron." A man enters. Same voice: "My God, what's *Jack* doing in there? And there's the old dog and cat. Dreams mix everything up. Those animals had barely been born then. I should wake up from this. But who are all these people? Oh no, I can't believe it— my mother's telling that terrible joke from that movie about the guy with the duck sitting on his head who goes to the psychiatrist. The psychiatrist says, 'Well, what can I do for you?' And the duck says, 'Get this guy off my ass.'"

Cut to bedroom. Jack Deller and a woman in mask are in bed.

"What? What is going *on* here?! That's me in the bed. He and I shouldn't be making love. Jack and *Mama* are supposed to be married in this dream, not Jack and me. But there's my mother standing by the door. Mama, get out of there. What's he saying? 'I've always been *what?*' Now he's coming with a big long Oh. And no, I don't believe it. Mama is watching."

Cut to back stairs. "*Now* what is he saying. Something like 'I've always been . . . committed,' that's it 'committed to you.' LIAR. How odd that he should be expressing his love on the back stairs. I haven't been in a house with back stairs since I was a kid. And Mama's carrying *my* one-eyed cat. This is too much. Wake up, wake up. I don't want to hear her. Mama, shut up, shut up."

Medium shot of mother, who speaks in sync. "I don't mind one bit that you two are carrying on. Jack and I stopped having sex ten years ago."

Some Ruminations Around Cinematic

Antidotes to the Oedipal Net(tles) While

Playing With de Lauraedipus Mulvey, or,

He May Be Off-Screen, but . . .

This was written at the invitation of Martha Gever, editor of *The Independent* from 1984 to 1991, and published there (vol. 9, no. 3, April 1986). It was reprinted in *Psychoanalysis and Cinema,* edited by E. Ann Kaplan (New York: Routledge, 1990). Narrative and cinema spectatorship are still on my mind here thanks to my continued immersion in the writings of Laura Mulvey and Teresa de Lauretis. The title almost says it all.

The audience is once more perplexed after viewing my last film, *The Man Who Envied Women* (*TMWEW*).[1] Some of them are once again asking, "What does *she* believe? Where in this welter of ideas, aphorisms, opinions, quotations, ironies, rhetoric, collisions, is *her* voice? Are there really no arguments to follow, no resolutions or conclusions to be gleaned from this overload? Are the meanings so embedded in ambiguity that even the most assiduous concentration is unable to dredge them up, with the various discourses eventually neutralizing each other?" (The audience of my daydreams, like the voices of my films, is very gabby.)

I hope not. I am not an iconoclast bent on destroying all vestiges of "authorial discourse." (As a "lapsed" anarchist, I am only too aware that when it comes to authority our choices are merely better or worse compromises.) On the contrary, I would like to believe that I subject such discourses to pressures and tests, or dislocations, e.g., a removal from their ordinary contexts—the printed page, the classroom, or the formal lecture—to unexpected physical and psychic spaces. The space of real estate profiteering, for instance, or the space of seduction, or the space of sexual (mis)representation.

In many ways, *TMWEW* lies outside traditional narrative cinema.

There is no plot, for instance, and although the voice of the (absent) female protagonist can be construed as a narrator, this voice departs from convention by refusing to push a story forward or promote a singular thesis that would tie up the various strands. In the struggle for the film's truth this equivocal, invisible heroine is not always the victor. Consequently, in relation to the social issues broached within the film, the question of an externally imposed, predetermined and determining coherence looms very large for some. If the process of identification with the trajectory of fictional characters is thwarted, we look for opportunities to identify with an extra-diagetic author or ultimate voice "behind" the film, if not camera. We are still not fluent in reading films that, while seeming to proffer this identification process, undermine it at the same time by setting other processes in motion, processes that involve a more detached kind of recognition and engagement. Rather than repositioning ourselves as spectators in response to cues that indicate we are being multivocally *addressed* and not just worked on by the filmic text, we still attempt to locate a singular author or wait for a conclusive outcome. The Master's Voice Syndrome all over again. And why not? Why else do we go to see narrative cinema than to be confirmed and reinforced in our most atavistic and Oedipal mind-sets?

Well, now that I've so precipitously catapulted us into the psychoanalytic soup, I have to admit that I'm not entirely satisfied with the model of spectatorship so flippantly refashioned here. For one thing, who the hell is this "we"? Can this indolent pronoun possibly account for the people who like the movies I myself make? Let's say it includes some or all of us some of the time, or enough of us enough of the time for me to justify, within limits, my own cinematic practice.

But there is another reason for invoking this spectre/spectator, and that is to question its *sexual* homogeneity. Over a decade of feminist film theory has taught us the importance of splitting this undifferentiated pronominal mass into two, if not more, component parts. Let us now speak of male and female spectators. The "we" further unravels when "we" think about stories and storytelling. The stories we love the most are those that appeal to our deepest and earliest fears and desires that modulate and determine our placement in society as more, or less, successful adult men and women. The question has come to be asked (and must continue to be asked inasmuch as those with more power and privilege are always inclined to erase both question and answers): within these stories, quoting from Teresa de Lauretis's "Desire in Narrative,"

... whose desire is it that speaks, and whom does that desire address? The received interpretations of the Oedipus story, Freud's among others, leave no doubt. The desire is Oedipus's, and though its object may be woman (or Truth or knowledge or power), its term of reference and address is man: man as social being and mythical subject, founder of the social, and source of mimetic violence. . . .[2]

. . . [man as] hero, constructed as human . . . the active principle of culture, the establisher of distinction, the creator of differences. Female is what is not susceptible to transformation, to life or death; she (it) is an element of plot-space . . . a resistance, matrix, and matter.[3]

Monster and landscape, she adds elsewhere, Sphinx, Medusa, ovum, earth, nature, Sleeping Beauty, etc.

Given that Oedipus killed his father and married his mother, it can be said that

. . . the crime of Oedipus is the destruction of differences and that the combined work of myth and narrative is the production of Oedipus . . . a mapping of differences, and specifically, first and foremost, of sexual difference into each text . . .[4]

The consequence for the reader/spectator is that

each reader—male or female—is constrained and defined within the two positions of a sexual difference thus conceived: male-hero-human, on the side of the subject; and female-obstacle-boundary-space [on the side of the object].

She elaborates:

. . . in its "making sense" of the world, narrative endlessly reconstructs it as a two-character drama in which the human person creates and recreates *himself* out of an abstract or purely symbolic other—the womb, the earth, the grave, the woman. . . . The drama has the movement of a passage, a crossing, an actively experienced transformation of the human being into—man. This is the sense in which all change, all social and personal—even physical—transformation is finally understood.[5]

Another question that has subsequently arisen is, "What's in it for us ladies?" Do we (ladies) go to the movies to put our minds in the hands of our various Daddies—benign, malevolent, whatever? The oppressed often have a very curious relation to those in power, a perverse identification with the power they lack. Why else would a black taxi driver justify his voting for Reagan with "I want to be on the side that's going to win?" One of my earliest movie-going memories is recounted in *Film About a Woman Who . . .* :

> She catches herself snorting gleefully at the scene of the two women being totally bitchy to one another. She remembers a similar scene—was it Dorothy Lamour or Betty Grable?—in a movie she saw when she was no more than nine or ten. One woman had ripped another woman's dress off. She had stayed in the movie theater long after her friends had left until that scene came around again. And she must have felt guilty about it, because she never told anybody, not her mother, nor anybody.[6]

During this speech, which is uttered by a female voice-over, we are looking at a snapshot of an elderly woman sitting in a field. I have no idea what the original movie was other than its source, Hollywood, and the approximate year, 1944. I can account for my pleasure in watching that scene as vicarious satisfaction in the eruption of female anger on the screen, an anger that I was not permitted to express in my own family. Right now, however, I am more interested in looking at my response as an example of male sadistic identification. The spectacle of two women fighting over a man provoked in me the pleasure that was clearly intended for the male spectator who would "naturally" identify with the absent (from the scene) male character they were fighting over. I don't remember rooting for either woman, neither the one who would eventually "get her man" nor her rival. The perversity of the situation was that I took pleasure in the humiliation of *both* women. Like the taxi driver, I was identifying with the power of the actual "winner," the man, rather than with those with whom I shared the same psychosocial disfranchisement, the women.

How does this response, or my interpretation of it, mesh with de Lauretis's

> . . . If women spectators are to buy their tickets and their popcorn, the work of cinema, unlike "the aim of biology," may be said to require women's consent; and we may well suspect the narrative cinema in particular must be aimed, like desire, toward *seducing* women into femininity [emphasis added].[7]

Or With Laura Mulvey's citation of Freud's argument about female sexuality as "an oscillation between 'passive' femininity and regressive 'masculinity'" in her effort to account for

> . . . the female spectator's phantasy of masculinization [which] is always to some extent at cross purposes with itself, restless in its transvestite clothes.[8]

They are both pointing to a double identification. De Lauretis further specifies the figures of narrative (movement of the male subject) and image (narrative closure/the space and body of the female object) as exerting, in and of themselves, a dual hold on the female spectator.

I have no doubt that I dutifully identified with the more passive, feminine "desire to be desired," in de Lauretis's words, at other points in my 1940s oedipal drama. (And, as a story of one woman replacing another, it was quintessentially oedipal, a recapitulation of the classical Freudian account of male normative sexual development, with its demand for successful repression of infantile desire for the mother.) But those were not the scenes that kept me in that theater until they came around again. Auguring calamitous consequences in my adult life, it was the scene of the two women fighting each other that gripped me most, a scene that almost thirty years later would be transformed and played out as a real life melodrama of internalized misogyny in my private life. In patriarchal terms, I was a wash-out. It wasn't that I had refused to be seduced into dancing on the oedipal stage. I had simply gone to sleep and missed all my cues. Even the prince's kiss could not awaken me. I refused to wake up, and that is what nearly did me in. If the Medusa had not been sleeping in her cave, could Perseus have slain her? Must it always be either the prince or Perseus who gets you in the end? Here's another story:

On October 25, 1896, on the night after the funeral of his father Jakob, Sigmund Freud had a dream. "I found myself in a shop where there was a notice [*Tafel,* German for tablet (of the law) or table] saying 'You are requested to close the eyes.' . . ."[9] Using Marie Balmary's intricately fashioned key from her *Psychoanalyzing Psychoanalysis,* we can interpret this dream as an "injunction to 'close an eye' to the faults of the deceased." What might these faults have been?

Preceding his father's death, Freud was collecting indisputable evidence that pointed to the father as the cause of hysterical symptoms in the child. His theory of seduction was not well-received by the Viennese medical community. Within eleven months after his father's death, he emerged from depression and mourning only to "close an eye" to his accumulated evidence via the Oedipus complex, his new theory that repudiated his patients' stories by consigning them to the realm of repressed unconscious desire. With his father's death he laid to rest his own unconscious knowledge of his father's unacknowledged past. Rather than two marriages there had been three. The town records of

Freiburg reveal a second marriage to Rebecca, a mystery woman who is unrecognized in official Freud biographies. The fate of this wife and marriage remains undocumented. Balmary speculates that she committed suicide just before or just after Freud's birth.

Oedipus and Freud's theory conjoin as myth to conceal the "hidden fault of the father." Oedipus's father Laius had seduced his (Laius's) half-brother, Chrysippus, who later committed suicide "from shame." Freud's "closing his eyes" to Jakob's part in Rebecca's suicide (seducer and abandoner) is reenacted in his ignoring the part Laius played in the Oedipus myth (first as seducer of Chrysippus and later as violator of the gods' injunction against procreation), and is echoed yet again in the attitude psychoanalysis brings to the afflicted patient: "The fault is *your* desire rather than that of your father." And rather than that of The Fathers, or patriarchical society.

To varying degrees and from early on, all of us can characterize our lives as a struggle between closing and opening our eyes, sleeping and waking, knowing and refusing to know. If, as de Lauretis and Mulvey say, women oscillate between masculine and feminine positions of spectatorship and identification, then it must be said that we also oscillate between knowing and not knowing that this is what we do. It is not the first oscillation that is in itself dangerous, but rather a state of ignorance of that oscillation that will permit Oedipus (used here to stand for the *dominance* of men's faults, fears, and desires) in some form or another to do you in. My archetypal Hollywood Oedipus waited off-screen to claim his true love in what was for my nine-year-old spectator a no-win situation, a rigged game in which the precondition for participation as a female was the willingness to lose. My pleasure was that of a sleepwalker dreaming a dream of perennial tomboyhood. A more bitter reality lurked in the wings: the father I could neither have nor become, already prompting dialogue from the scenario governing the next phase of my feminine life. But this last was a story that no one was telling, therefore one which I could not know.

By now it must be more than clear that one does not have to probe very far into the psychoanalytic uses of Oedipus to find a phallocentric bias in both myth and theory. The terms of the oedipal formation of the human subject and its cultural expressions all seem to come down on one side, whether we're talking about women as signifiers of castration threat, voyeurism and the controlling gaze, identity and difference, scopic drives, visual pleasure, To Have and Have Not. The problem is that even as we employ these terms for describing and unveiling the workings of patriarchy, we implicate ourselves deeper into those very operations, as into a well-worn track in the forest. The very notion of lack, as proposed by Lacan, mirrors the prevailing cultural bias by privileging the symbolic threat of loss of the penis over the actual loss of the mother's body. Yes, I know that language is an all-important mediating factor and that loss of the breast predates the acquisition of language. Which then means, of course, that the breast is "less" than the penis. And how can this be otherwise when the clitoris is *nonexistent?* Psychoanalytic hierarchies of sexual synecdoche are mind-boggling and, for psychoanalysis, irrevocable. For women, however, psychoanalysis can only define a site of prolonged struggle.

All of this may seem far afield from my starting place, the authorial voice and fictional subject in cinematic practice, which we may now characterize as our (back to the undifferentiated pronominal mass!) desire for Oedipus in all or most of His manifestations. Although I may have to pay the consequences of breaking the Law of the Father in my daily life, there's no reason I can't give it (the Law) a run for its money as a filmmaker. If I'm going to make a movie about Oedipus, i.e., Eddy and Edy Pussy Foot, I'm going to have to subject him to some calculated narrative screw-ups. It's elementary, dear Eddy: play with signifiers of desire. Have two actors play Jack Deller, the male protagonist in *TMWEW.* Remove the physical presence of Trisha, the female protagonist, and reintroduce her as a voice. Create situations that can accommodate both ambiguity and contradiction without eliminating the possibility of taking specific political stands.

Shift de Lauretis's image/ground of narrative movement by frequent changes in the "production value" of the image, e.g., by utilizing refilming techniques, blown-up super 8, inferior quality video transfers shooting off of a TV set with bad reception, etc.—not in order to make the usual intranarrative tropes, however, such as the character's look at a TV show or a shift in meaning of the image to dream, flashback, or inner thoughts of a character. What I'm talking about is a disruption of the glossy, unified surface of professional cinematography by means of optically degenerated shots within an otherwise seamlessly edited narrative sequence.

Play off different, sometimes conflicting, authorial voices. And here I'm not talking about balance or both sides of a question like the nightly news, or about finding a "new language" for women. I'm talking about registers of complicity/protest/acquiescence within a single shot or scene that do not give a message of despair. I'm talking about bad guys making progressive political sense and good girls shooting off their big toe and mouth. I'm talking about uneven development and fit in the departments of consciousness, activism, articulation, and behavior that must be constantly reassessed by the spectator. I'm talking about incongruous juxtapositions of modes of address: recitation, reading, "real" or spontaneous speech, printed texts, quoted texts, et al., all in the same film. I'm talking about representations of divine couplings and (un)holy triads being rescreened only to be used for target practice. I'm talking about not pretending that a life lived in potholes taking potshots will be easy and without cost, on screen or off.

I'm talking about films where in every scene you have to decide anew the priorities of looking and listening. In *TMWEW* there's a scene in which Jack Deller delivers a rambling lecture to a group of students in what is eventually revealed to be a newly renovated loft-condominium. If one doesn't pay particular attention to the insistent, autonomous tracking of the camera around the space, but puts all of one's efforts into deciphering the spoken text with its ellipses, digressions, and dipping in and out of Foucault, Lacan, Chomsky, Piaget, et al., when Trisha's voice finally begins to talk about the disappeared in Central America and New York, you will have missed the meaning of that space, i.e., an expensive piece of real estate, as a crucial link between the lecture and instances of U.S. international and domestic imperialism. The visual track in this instance anticipates the sound track, but also supplies a subtext for the lecture with its retroactive associations of urban university landgrabbing.

Later in the film, texts are played off in a different way. In a scene in a narrow corridor between Jack Deller and his ex-lover, Jackie, the main thesis of Foucault's "power-is-everywhere" is intercut with documentary footage of demonstrations of power "somewhere" in particular, "on this side" and "on that side." Jack Deller's recitation of the Foucault material is further juxtaposed with Jackie's recitation of excerpts from an essay by Meaghan Morris in which she criticizes theory itself for having "no teeth."[10]

Other tensions abound here: the antimonolithic arguments of Foucault colliding with Trisha's invocation of military/police and medical fraternities, and the disparity between doing and speaking, or image and text, as demonstrated in the seductive moves of Jack and Jackie, a disparity that then collides with Foucault's "There is no opposition between what is said and what is done."[11] At another point Morris's description of Lacan's reign at the "costume ball" of feminine writing "not as lawgiver but as queen" is followed by a dream sequence in which a mother and daughter (played by one performer) play a queen of the kitchen who is alternately romanced by her son-in-law and watches him and her daughter in bed, in a short and shifty oedipal extravaganza caustically narrated by the irate daughter. If these scenes are about a conflict between theory and practice, or a contradiction between theory and everyday life, they can also be read in terms of a "return of the repressed" which, operating as more than cheap subversion, constantly pressures theory into re-examining systems of signification, reinventing its own constraints.

Finally, I'm talking about films that allow for periods of poetic ambiguity, only to unexpectedly erupt into rhetoric, outrage, direct political address or analysis, only to return to a new adventure of Eddy Foot or New Perils of Edy Foot. He may still shoot off his big toe while getting or not getting the girl, but he'll also ask a few questions or wait in the wings a little longer to see how the ladies work it out without him. And this time around she may start to rip off her rival's dress, but then stop to muse, "Hey, we're wearing the same dress aren't we? Why don't we pool our energies and try to figure out what a political myth for socialist feminism might look like?"

So they (she and she) make a movie together and . . .

Notes

1. 16 mm, color, 125 min., 1985; distributed by Zeitgeist Films, New York.

2. Teresa de Lauretis, *Alice Doesn't: Feminism, Semiotics, Cinema* (Bloomington: Indiana University Press, 1984), p. 112.

3. Ibid., p. 119.

4. Ibid., p. 120.

5. Ibid., p. 121.

6. Script of *Film About a Woman Who* . . . (16 mm, black and white, 105 min., 1974), published in *October*, no. 2 (Summer 1976), p. 61, and *The Films of Yvonne Rainer* (Bloomington: Indiana University Press, 1989).

7. De Lauretis, pp. 136–37.

8. Laura Mulvey, "Afterthoughts on 'Visual Pleasure and Narrative Cinema' Inspired by 'Duel in the Sun' (King Vidor, 1946)," *Framework*, no. 15/16/17 (1981), pp. 14–15.

9. From Sigmund Freud, the standard edition of *The Complete Psychological Works of Sigmund Freud*, 13:213, quoted in Marie Balmary, *Psychoanalyzing Psychoanalysis: Freud and the Hidden Fault of the Father* (Baltimore: Johns Hopkins University Press, 1982), p. 80.

10. Meaghan Morris, "The Pirate's Fiancee." In *Michel Foucault: Power, Truth, Strategy*. Edited by Meaghan Morris and Paul Patton (Sydney: Feral Publications, 1979), p. 159.

11. "Power and Norm: Notes" [taken at a lecture by Michel Foucault], ibid., p. 62.

Thoughts on Women's Cinema:

Eating Words, Voicing Struggles

Originally a paper delivered on a panel called "Making History: Revising and Representing" at *Viewpoints: A Conference on Women, Culture, and Public Media* sponsored by Women Make Movies at Hunter College, New York, in 1986. Margaret Randall and Lynne Tillman were on the same panel, as I recall. First published in *The Independent* 10, no. 3 (April 1987), it was reprinted in *Blasted Allegories, An Anthology of Writings by Contemporary Artists,* edited by Brian Wallis (New York: The New Museum of Contemporary Art and Cambridge, Mass: MIT Press, 1987). Oh for the good old days when one could immerse oneself at festivals in *feminist* films by women, or at least films that were not afraid to be called feminist. I was recently dismayed by an explication of Australian aboriginal artist Tracey Moffatt's *Night Cries.* The writer denied the political and feminist implications of that film in favor of a "generic" universal reading. As far as I'm concerned such a reading reduces the specifically ethnic and gendered anguish of that work to the universality of baby up-chuck. I can't say where Moffatt herself stands on this.

Polemics and manifestos having always served as spark plugs to my energies and imagination, I've been surprised when, following their publication, such statements were taken with what seemed to be excessive seriousness. Thus, in the mid-'60s, when I said "no" to this and "no" to that in dance and theater, I could not foresee that these words would dog my footsteps and beg me to eat them (or at least modify them) for the next twenty years. Such may be the case with my more recent stance toward/against/for narrative conventions in cinema. Raised, as I have been, with this century's western notions of adversarial aesthetics, I continue to have difficulty in accommodating my latest articulation of the narrative "problem"—i.e., according to Teresa de Lauretis's conflation of narrativity itself with the Oedipus complex, whereby woman's position is constantly reinstated for the consummation or frustration of male desire. The difficulty lies in accommodating this with a conviction that it is of the utmost urgency that women's voices, experience, and consciousness—at whatever stage—be expressed in all their multiplicity and heterogeneity, and in as many formats and styles—narrative or not—from here to queendom come and throughout the kingdom. In relation to the various notions of an avant garde, this latter view, in its emphasis on voicing what has previously gone unheard, gives priority to unmasking and reassessing social relations rather than overturning previously validated aesthetic positions. My personal accommodation becomes more feasible when it is cast in terms of difference rather than opposition and when the question is asked, "Which strategies bring women together in recognition of their common and different economic and sexual oppression, and which strategies do not?" The creation of oppositional categories of women's film or video, or, for starters, film *and* video, begs this question.

For what it's worth, here is a list of useless oppositions. Documentary versus fiction. Work in which the voices carry a unified truth versus work in which truth must be wrested from conflicting or conflicted voices. Work that adheres to traditional codes versus work in which the story is disrupted by stylistic incongruities or digressions (Helke Sanders' *Redupers,* Laura Mulvey and Peter Wollen's *Riddles of the Sphinx*). Work with a beginning, middle, and end versus work that has a beginning and then turns into something else (Marguerite Duras's *Nathalie Granger*). Work in which the characters run away with the movie versus work whose characters never get off the ground (Rabina Rose's *Nightshift*). Work in which women *tell* their herstories (Julia Reichert and Jim Klein's *Union Maids*) versus work in which they parody them (Ana Carolina's *Hearts and Guts*). Work that delivers information in a straightforward manner (Jackie Ochs's *Secret Agent*) versus work in which information accrues slowly, elliptically, or poetically (Trinh Minh-ha's *Naked Spaces*). Work in which the heroine acts versus work in which she does nothing but talk (my *Journeys from Berlin/1971*). Work in which she triumphs versus work in which she fails (Valie Export's *Invisible Adversaries*). Work in which she is a searcher or dominatrix (Bette Gordon's *Variety,* Monika Treut and Elfi Mikesch's *Seduction: The Cruel Woman*) versus work in which she is a victim (Lynne Tillman and Sheila McLaughlin's *Committed*). Work whose heroines you like

(Connie Field's *Rosie the Riveter,* Julie Dash's *Illusions*) versus work whose heroines repel you (Doris Dorrie's *Straight to the Heart,* Chantal Akerman's *je, tu, il, elle*). Work in which you nearly drown in exotic signifiers of femininity (Leslie Thornton's *Adynata*) versus work whose director can't figure out how to dress the heroine, so removes her altogether (my *The Man Who Envied Women*). *All* these films share a potential for political purpose and historical truth.

I could go on *ad infinitum* with these divide-and-conquer oppositions. There is one other example I'm not going to give equal footing with the others but will mention in passing only insofar as it bears a deceptive resemblance to the others: Films in which the heroine marries the man versus films in which she murders him. We have only to look in vain for recent films by women that end in marriage to realize what a long way we've come, give or take the baby. Marriage at the beginning maybe, but at the end, never. I challenge anyone to name one in recent memory. Murder, on the other hand, is a different story. As Joan Braderman pointed out last spring at the *Gender and Visual Representation* Conference at the University of Massachusetts, in the past ten years a substantial number of women's films have been produced that focus on a murder of a man by a woman or women. To name a few: Akerman's *Jeanne Dielman,* Marlene Gorris's *A Question of Silence,* Dorrie's *Straight to the Heart,* Sally Heckel's *A Juror of Her Peers,* Margaretha Von Trotta's *Sheer Madness.*

The phenomenon of man-murder in women's films points to the problematic of representing men. Do we wreak revenge on them (if for no other reason than the cinematic sway they have held over us for so long), turn the tables on them, turn them into celluloid wimps, give them ample screen time in which to speak self-evident macho bullshit, do away with them by murder within the story, or eliminate them *from* the story to begin with? Do we focus on exceptional men who escape the above stereotypes, or do we weave utopian scenarios in which men and women gambol in egalitarian bliss? Lynne Tillman and I pondered the question of whether it is politically useful to allow ourselves to be fascinated with men in our films even as we discussed the strange fascination with the 1986 World Series that had befallen the two of us along with every woman we know.

Following one screening of *The Man Who Envied Women,* a well-known feminist who subscribes to Lacanian psychoanalytic theory asked me why I hadn't made a film about a woman. I was flabbergasted, having been under the impression that I had done just that. But she, taking the title literally and taken in by the prevailing physical presence of the male character, had discounted the pursuing, nagging, questioning female voice on the soundtrack. By staying out of sight my heroine is never caught with her pants down. Does this mean the film is not *about* her?

It's also been noted that my female characters are not heroines. I would qualify that: My heroines are not heroic. They are deeply skeptical of easy solutions and very self-critical, constantly looking for their own complicity in patriarchal configurations. But neither are they cynical or pessimistic. The moments I like best in my films are those that produce—almost simultaneously—both assertion and question. Early on in *TMWEW* the assertion that women can't be committed feminists unless they give up men is uttered as part of a conversation, overheard by a man in the foreground, by a woman who is testing her female companion by quoting yet another woman whose relationship to the speaker is not identified and who never appears. The two speakers are also anonymous and are never seen again once this scene is over. I, the director, am not trying in this scene to persuade my audience of the rightness or wrongness of the statement. What is important is that it be given utterance, because in our culture, outside of a convent, giving up men freely and willingly—that is, without the social coercion of aging —is a highly stigmatized act or downright taboo. The linkage of giving up men, in this scene, with commitment as a feminist, however, is distanced and made arguable through the device of having the spectator become an eavesdropper on the conversation along with the foregrounded male character, then distanced once more through quotation. *"She told me,"* says this minor, will-o'-the-wisp heroine, "that I would never be a committed feminist until I give up men."

Whether an utterance comes across as feminist prescription, call-to-arms, or problem-articulated-ambiguously-to-be-dealt-with-or-not-later-in-the-film is always on my mind in the collecting and framing of texts. If the experience of watching certain kinds of social documentaries is like watching the bouncing ball come down at exactly the right moment on the syllables of the familiar song, watching a film of mine may be more akin to "now you see it, now you don't." You never know when you're going to be hit on the head with the ball, and you aren't always sure what to do when the ball disappears for long stretches of time.

Which brings me to what might be called a method of interrogating my characters and myself when I set out to make a film. Thinking about this has been facilitated by rereading Bill Nichols' essay, "The

Voice of Documentary," which poses certain questions that are relevant to both fiction and documentary. To what degree are we to believe a given speaker in a film? Do all the speakers convey a unified vision of a given history? Do the speakers emerge as autonomous shapers of a personal destiny or as subjects conditioned by the contradictions and pressures of a particular historical period? To what degree does a given film convey an independent consciousness, a voice of its own, probing, remembering, sustaining, doubting, functioning as a surrogate for our own consciousness? Do the questioning and believing of such a film question its own operations? Does the activity of fixing meaning in such a film refer to relations outside the film—"out there"—or does the film remain stalled in its own reflexivity? Is reflexivity the only alternative to films that simply suppose that things were as the participant-witnesses recall or state them, or as they appear to the spectator, in the case of fiction films?

Finally: Should a film whose main project is to restore the voice and subjectivity of a previously ignored or suppressed person or segment of the population, should such a film contain argument, contradiction, or express the director's ambivalence within the film either directly, through language, or indirectly, through stylistic intervention? Obviously, we can't afford to be prescriptive about any of this.

My own solution runs to keeping an extradiegetic voice, a voice separate from the characters and story, fairly active in every scene. It need not take the form of a narrating voice, although it often does. Sometimes it takes the form of a *Til Eulenspiegel*–like disruption, as when an anonymous woman enters the frame just before a troubling bit of sexual theory is enunciated, peers into the camera lens, and asks all the menstruating women to leave the theater. Sometimes it operates like a kind of seizure, producing odd behavior in a given character, as when the analysand in *Journeys from Berlin* speaks in baby-talk. Often it comes across in reading or recitation, which has the effect of separating the voice of the character from that of the author.

At this historical moment we still need to search out and be reminded of suppressed histories and struggles: prostitutes, housewives, women of color, lesbians, third-world people, the aging, working women. The method of representing these histories is a separate and equally important issue. I see no reason why a single film can't use many different methods, which is something I've been saying for years but didn't come close to realizing until *TMWEW*. In this film fictional and documentary modes come into play more fully than in any of my previous work, offsetting the calculation of my still-cherished recitations and readings with the immediacy of dramatic and documentary enactment. These last are, admittedly, the strategies that offer the spectator the most powerful sense of the real. But reality, as we so well know, always lies elsewhere, a fact that we nevertheless endlessly seek to disavow and from which we always retreat. I shall continue to remind us of that disavowal by challenging reality's representational proxies with assorted hanky-panky. I hope others continue to do likewise and otherwise.

Declaring Stakes:

Interview by Kurt Easterwood, Laura Poitras, and

Susanne Fairfax

The San Francisco Cinematheque published this interview to accompany its 1990 Rainer film retrospective. It was conducted by Kurt Easterwood, Susanne Fairfax, and Laura Poitras and revolved around my sixth feature, *Privilege.*

YVONNE RAINER: I started five years ago with a need to write a story. The story is a recollection of more or less something I was a participant in, in the early '60s, and this became the flashback in *Privilege.* So I simply wrote a synopsis of this story and began to assign names to characters, also thinking about ways that the story might be embellished, intervened with, challenged, and splayed out, so to speak. In part this was to avoid the closed-down potential that all story telling has, putting various elements and people into their respective places and social positions. I wanted to reveal contradictions and new meanings, including social meanings within the story, behind the story, underneath the story. Within *Privilege,* the story is both recounted and enacted by the character Jenny as a recollection of being a witness to an alleged black-on-white assault. I started with that, but there were also things left over from *The Man Who Envied Women* [1985], such as issues of menopause and aging, which were voiced at the beginning but never really gone into in depth. So here I had this story and a whole other area of investigation, and without knowing how they would fit together I pursued both independently. I started looking for texts for the participants in the story to speak, words that they would of course not normally speak, integrating these with so-called realistic plot elements that would get the story told. At the same time [1986–7], I was doing research into menopause and female aging. In 1987–88 I came out here [California] and started to interview, with my Sony-8 video camera, women whom

230

I've known for years, about things such as menopause, anarchism, et cetera. I kept on working on the script—nearly giving it up a couple times in despair over getting these different parts together in the same vehicle. I took one year off [1987–88] to work on a conference with Berenice Reynaud called *Sexism, Colonialism, Misrepresentation,* a film series with panel discussions that took place at the Collective for Living Cinema in New York. After that I began to get into the script some more and showed it to people who said, "You can't do this and you can't do that, why don't you do this and why don't you do that." After a certain point I said, "Enough is enough, it's got to go like this." By this time I had a couple of grants, and we went into production in June of '89, and after that it was like a snowball rolling downhill. Or like a rock.

KURT EASTERWOOD: You mentioned this conference. Did that find its way into the film, or did the script and story already have these issues of class and racism within it?

YR: It already did. I mean, some of the films by people of color we were going to show had already gotten me thinking about racial issues, in the way that years before, feminist writing had made me think about my life as a woman in relation to patriarchy. White middle-class feminism had been coming under attack for not taking into consideration differences in women's experience—racially and economically—and writing on race had been pushing at the limits of feminist film theory, so all of this was certainly affecting me. Five years ago Jenny's story was there but I had no idea how to deal with it, how to ask questions of it. Now with these new questions and challenges coming from black filmmakers—and I use "black" in the political sense—and from African/American and West Indian/Anglo cultural studies, I felt it was time to tackle it.

KE: This story, is it autobiographical?

YR: Yes, to a certain extent, but Jenny is also a composite of many different women.

LAURA POITRAS: The story, your story, which you referred to as black-on-white, seems to express something different than what the film ultimately puts forth. In other words, in *Privilege* you're attempting to break down the stereotype that violence is usually black against white and vice-versa. Were you trying to resolve the emotional impact of the experience?

YR: No. I wasn't interested in resolving it. I was interested in questioning the misperception and its misrepresentation. By asking how the story could be told, in a way that would make sense and be productive (which belongs in the area of my interest in narrative), and by challenging the stereotype: the bugaboo of the black rapist is still something that raises its head whenever there is some kind of interracial sexual violence. For instance, the gang rape in Central Park, which became a racial issue rather than a gender issue. Rather than questioning the social imperatives of masculine bonding, commentators repeatedly spoke of the incident in racial terms. I think this is a fallacious way to look at it. In other words, this story, my story, Jenny's story, could not be told in a simple fashion, but had to be turned over and looked at, sexually, racially, in terms of colonialism, in terms of social inequities and white domination. If I had been gearing this film to a mass audience, the story might have been told very differently: A young white aspiring dancer comes to New York City, lives on a street which is mostly black and Puerto Rican, is a witness to an assault of a downstairs neighbor, is subpoenaed by an assistant D.A., subsequently has an affair with him, and achieves fame and fortune as a successful dancer after the affair breaks up. End of story. Very neat. The other characters are all wallpaper, decorative elements in the narrative trajectory of this young woman. It would make a very entertaining story, like *Dirty Dancing* or that other dance story, what's it called . . . right, *Flashdance.* There could be a dance at the end where she wins a part in a Broadway musical. The perspective is all wrong; it is very one-sided. I did research to find language for the other participants, for Carlos, for Brenda, for Stew, characters whose prototypes I have little knowledge of. I went to various novels and histories of Puerto Ricans in New York City. I went to Frantz Fanon, Victorian medical practice, and archival footage. I sought out language which then could be assigned to the various characters. This is of course in keeping with my usual—what you might call—plagiarist practices, using literary and rhetorical material as speech.

SUSANNE FAIRFAX: The look of the flashback seems in some ways very glossy and Hollywood, and then this is juxtaposed with the video-8. What were you trying for with that?

YR: With the high-contrast black and white I was evoking *film noir* (my instructions to Mark Daniels, the cinematographer, were to make it look like the "dark night of the soul"). It's a very familiar look. I wanted it to have a different kind of seductiveness from the rest of the film, as well as to invoke those clichés of anxiety that that kind of lighting and mise-en-scène produce.

KE: You also see the crew in those black-and-white shots.

YR: Right. In some of the reverse shots, you see the loft/studio setting, equipment, people in the background. After being drawn into a scene, you then see some of the production elements of the scene. I find all that very pleasureful and interesting. I have in the past made a political justification for that, for instance, when people ask me, "Are you ever going to make a real film?," which means not having that kind of stuff, but I have to say that I'd be very bored making a "real" film. I like that edge of the illusion and the dropping away of the illusion. That is one of the things that keeps me interested in making moving pictures. Each production I do gets more complicated, and I want to get that into the film in as many ways as possible. I don't see why an audience can't take in two, three and four layers of reference at the same time.

KE: It is obviously not a conventional "narrative"; you have people directly addressing the camera reciting Eldridge Cleaver for instance. There is always some process of distancing that is operating. Do you think that these direct addresses need to be then subverted even more?

YR: My decisions for the presentation of those texts have very much to do with each particular text. The Cleaver "I became a rapist" speech is particularly problematic—that's the point where the black rapist is invoked in all his terror for the white world. How to distance that, to make it clear that this was not only performance and production, that this was a socially grounded text to be examined? The shot begins with the camera being literally distanced from the speakers—it's a crane shot—and I also put a white male actor in there to begin the speech, which is a reference to the way white male militants in the '60s defended that kind of rhetoric. The speech starts in the mouth of a white man, the camera is very far away, showing as much of the set and off-set as possible, and you see crew members, and we gradually move in to the Cleaver proxy, Stew. It is as though that speech had to be subjected to a whole range of visual mediations in order to be staged at all. Other recitations are not so problematic, such as Digna in Bellevue speaking Spanish and then English, or Carlos on the front steps. I thought of these as pedagogical kinds of speeches, which gave me opportunities to abandon the plot.

KE: But it's not so, pardon the phrase, black and white. During the Cleaver speech you hear Yvonne Washington say in voice-over, "Why are you telling me this, I don't need to hear how Eldridge Cleaver raped to save the black race. He made a much greater contribution than inflaming white paranoia."

YR: Right. That's another intervention. After each of the two Cleaver quotations by Stew, Yvonne Washington calls him on them. Following his rap on lesbians where he says their "ice has to be melted by his phallus," Yvonne W. says, "Are you going to let him get away with that?" And following that is a poem by the lesbian poet Judy Grahn about Venus having the ugliest mug in the world that has to be moved in on by men's imaginations, which is a kind of send-up of the notion of beauty as projected by men onto women—involving women's complicity, of course. All of the things which I have been describing are different kinds of interventions; the challenge is to keep these techniques, these devices, diversified, to keep the whole thing flowing, to keep things from getting bogged down. I avoided some of the pitfalls of *The Man Who Envied Women* which had these long monologues which were impossible to follow. They are very interesting to read, but they are over the edge when it comes to listening and concentrating. I paid more attention to attention span and duration of speeches in *Privilege,* with these counter-responses coming in at key moments. In many cases I identified my sources via titles, because I wanted people to know what they were listening to.

KE: What about the position of Yvonne Washington within the structure of the film? It appears that there is some sort of correlation to yourself, in that she has your first name. But Jenny's story is also, to some extent, your story, which creates an interesting division.

YR: There are a lot of dislocations. I play Helen Caldicott, some of my story is in Jenny's story, and there are two Yvonne's. I use my physical presence as a kind of hit-and-run driver and wild goose, as a diversion and diversionary tactic. I don't feel that Y.R. has to be foregrounded as the mover and shaker of the film. There is a real and fictional director, just as there are real and fictional interviewees. Yvonne is a common African-American name, and Washington is too. I liked the idea of the primal father-figure of our country transfigured as the mother of the film.

LP: The film begins with *Privilege* "by Yvonne Rainer and many others," and then begins again with *Privilege* "by Yvonne Washington and many others." What is the purpose of that?

YR: I've always liked the idea of beginning again. The first beginning has some loose ends that are never picked up. The Helen Caldicott speech introduces the sexuality motif with the lipstick. Then the black signer introduces the race, or racist, motif with the reversal of positions traditionally assigned to speaker and signer. In one-twenty-fourth of a second the speaker is "marginalized." The signer gives Yvonne Washington the opportunity to make a comparison of medical attitudes to deafness and menopause via their presumed status of "disease." And then we segue into the fictional documentary.

SF: I'm interested in the whole question of "actual" and "fake" documentary. It seems you're dealing a lot more in *Privilege* with questions of what reality is, and the way that documentary plays with narrative, and the fact that character is created in both. How does this differ from your use of documentary in *The Man Who Envied Women?*

YR: In *TMWEW,* the documentary segments were not contested as truth. *Privilege* plays around with documentary more. There are three kinds of documentary, three kinds of experience presented: the traditional professional talking head (the doctors who represent authoritative kinds of speech); the so-called "real" interviews—with their "spontaneous" speech—which have been highly selected from hours of material; and the "fake" documentary in which Yvonne interviews Jenny. I think all of these play on each other. I was in Australia recently, and in Melbourne one evening a dark-skinned woman asked me a question that made me realize certain assumptions I have about documentary that are not going to be necessarily shared. She asked me why I treated in documentary form women speaking about menopause whereas the material dealing with issues of race is only treated in this didactic fictional form. She felt that the speech of the women in the documentary sections is much more real or authentic than anything on race spoken by my fictional characters. Although I certainly make distinctions, I don't prioritize one kind of speech over another. I feel that documentary is as manipulated, selected, and molded, according to preconceived agendas as fiction is. Not that there aren't differences. Spontaneous speech, yes, has a different quality, it carries a different weight, it *suggests* a higher order of credibility. But I do not prioritize the truth value of so-called spontaneous speech over other kinds of speech. Obviously, the writing of Frantz Fanon is as "truthful" as what any of my ladies say about menopause. I saw no reason to cover every topic with a balance of representational formats. I find documentary is as up for grabs as a form as fiction is. What didn't happen—and here I'm offering a critique of my own film—is that I missed an opportunity to ask the women of color in the film how they felt race impinged on their aging and on their treatment by the medical establishment. I wasn't concerned with that because I was involved in the fictional conceit of the film that it was a documentary about menopause and not race. I don't know—if I'd thought about it more I might have tried to combine these two things in the interviews. But then I would have gone at these interviews with some preconceived agenda that they would have had to fall into. I didn't want to do that.

SF: Leaving it that way puts them on more of an equal footing.

YR: It does tend to universalize the issue of menopause, which is a dangerous thing to do. Poor women certainly have more problems vis-à-vis diet, access to doctors, and health care. They certainly have different problems from middle-class women. Although not all of my interviewees are equally well off, they are all better off than women on welfare, for instance. Which again refers back to the title of the film—that it is about privilege—both racially and economically.

SF: In *The Man Who Envied Women* you removed the image of the central female character from the film as a way of taking her out of the position of being objectified. Regarding people of color, their concerns with representation in cinema, or other media, has been almost the opposite. The question there is about *absence.* The last thing that one would think of would be to take someone of color *out.*

YR: Yes! It's a totally different matter when you've been under- or not represented. You want these exclusions to be redressed, not only by imaging blacks, but by making films that are extremely beautiful, lush, and as gorgeous as they can be photographically. Me, coming from the '60s white avant-garde, which is always talking about the degeneration, the degradation of images, I've always had this prejudice against the unified, glossy surface of mainstream cinema (not that I've done very much in the optical degradation department, not as much as other "avant-gardists"). But now I realize these are two very different aesthetic positions, very much connected to the social positions of the particular filmmakers.

SF: In *Privilege* there is a lot of talk about the similarities between women dealing with sexism and people of color dealing with racism, though at the same time you seem to be questioning these similarities. In terms of representation, how did you approach this? For instance, the characters of Carlos and Stew—how did you choose to represent them in the film; and how did that relate to those characters' concerns, which might be different?

YR: As I said before, I dealt with the stereotype of the black rapist by splitting him into three different men—Puerto Rican, black, and white—and lumping them all together as potential rapists, so that it became a gender issue. Regarding the question of how to portray Stew. Tyrone Wilson came up with this kind of jazzy, bouncy physicality, especially for the Cleaver/lesbian scene. It seemed important at that point in the film that he and Brenda laugh together, and it also seemed important that actual attraction be depicted in some way, so that it wouldn't be only about menace and threat. That speech is so ridiculous that I had them break up laughing. So the relationship of Brenda and Carlos/Stew is somewhat ambiguous. It gets played out in disconnected fragments, in which they are positioned in different ways in the room. At one point she lies down next to Stew, which is again about deconstructing that image of threat. She lies down next to him and says, "Your politics smacks of sadism like all the rest." She is accusing him, and at the same time is on a very comfortable physical footing with him.

LP: This question relates to what you just said about the sexual tension depicted. I am curious about how Brenda is referenced. At one point in the film Brenda says that women are trained to be victims. So it's ambiguous how her attraction within this confrontation is depicted. What kind of a role does she occupy? Is she playing the victim?

YR: I suppose I was looking toward a potential for comfort, or for racial and sexual rapprochement. The statement that women are trained to be rape victims is intercut with statistics showing that most rapes are white-on-white or black-on-black, which is something that most people don't know.

LP: But when Brenda makes that statement that "your politics smacks of sadism," is she by definition occupying a masochistic position?

YR: Well, how does one read these things? It's so un-naturalistic—at that point is it just argument, are they just mouth pieces? Or do you identify with them? I think it's on the edge there. At that point in the film, Stew is not the same man who entered her bedroom. It's very ambiguous how you read it in terms of identification, which is very deliberate. I wanted consistent characters to sustain a plot, but I also wanted to remove them somewhat from any fixed identity. I hadn't thought that Brenda might be read as the sexist stereotype of the woman who "wants to be raped." I didn't want to evoke that.

KE: Part of the problem of your flirtation with narrative is that one *does* start to identify. There are more things that are seductive in this film than compared with *Journeys from Berlin/1971* or *The Man Who Envied Women.* Five years ago you posited this progression that as your films became more explicitly feminist, you saw that you were having to work with narrative more and that you suspected the worst. . . .

YR: *Privilege* is certainly more into narrative then *TMWEW,* in which there is no plot, no climax, no closure—all of which is suggested in *Privilege* by this internal story. For reasons having to do with the ongoing debate about and around narrative as a form and a reinforcement of social positioning, I welcomed this story with all of its traditionally "hazardous" potential. Never before had I started with a story that had a beginning, middle, and end. And as soon as I had a story the gauntlet was down—I had to tell it and retell it, and de-tell it. I feel in a way my polemics have had some kind of fruition in this film, and have paid off in a certain way. The story, in being rooted in fact, offered me the opportunity to open it up with analysis and relooking, a very careful dissecting of it from many different angles. The fact that there is as much narrative as there is, and that there are sexual and violent elements in the film specifically recounted or enacted, will probably get *Privilege* more mileage than my previous films. Which in a way I'm glad about if it means more people will see it. But, by the same token, I don't feel I've made concessions that violate my ideas about filmmaking.

KE: This could almost be a bigger can of worms opening up.

YR: A bigger can of something.

KE: But also providing the audience with a space where they can be seduced, which could take precedence over the more distanced discourses that these characters or voices speak.

YR: I spoke to a black woman who said she was shocked at the assault in the film, that the alleged rapist was a Puerto Rican. She felt in her guts that even after all the turning over and re-turning, and voicing of social issues, she still felt kind of queasy about it. It *is* a queasy subject, and there is no getting around that.

SF: At one point a man accuses a woman of walking in front of the window with no clothes on. The potential is there to read some kind of seduction into that. It invokes the typical things that are said about women and rape. It seemed like there was a lot of room left for that interpretation.

YR: You mean to accuse her of "asking for it"?

SF: Right.

YR: The same ambiguity as before. In rethinking that, I might exclude that line. Its placement may be gratuitous.

SF: Everything's on these really fine lines, anytime you address anything that's difficult, or in a difficult manner. If people want to see something in a certain way, they're going to.

YR: People want to see themselves in positive images. We want not only fixed identities, but cultural experiences that will resolve our ambivalences, but I'm always putting these ambivalences back in. The fact that she walks around with no clothes on is no justification for rape. Right? OK. We can say that someone who does that is not discreet or cautious. I mean, women in big cities have to take precautions, she may not have been very cautious. Or maybe she was genuinely oblivious, or maybe it happened just once.

SF: Or maybe not at all.

YR: Or maybe not at all. Thank you very much. Carlos may have made it up. Right. He makes this observation at the end of a long slow zoom in to a close-up of his face. The close-up is an incredible device. Its effect must be like the experience of the baby suckling at its mother's breast—this big face looming up there. OK. Maybe I should have put that line somewhere else. Because that is where it got to you, where you really do believe what he's saying. Sound and image are totally glued, and he isn't even moving his mouth.

SF: In the videotaped interviews with women there seems to be more room left for chance or accident. Do you feel that the chance occurrences relate to performance that you were involved with earlier in your career?

YR: You never know what you're going to get in an interview. What I like about these interviews is the way little snippets of language can be pulled out and used in relation to other stuff. That happens in Minnette Lehmann's interview, where she contests the idea of the "real." I play that off of the doctor footage, which was not so much to contradict the doctors, but to convey a totally different quality of experience, and playfulness and vitality in contrast with the doctors' view of these depressed, hormonally deprived laboratory specimens. This comes across in a very economic way, with these women laughing and responding in spontaneous address. I find that very interesting about the possibilities of documentary—the way it can be played with and reshuffled. In *Lives of Performers* [1972], in the rehearsal sequences, which can be taken as chunks of spontaneous behavior, I was interested there in the way people stand around, look, enter into, practice, or drop out in contrast to the rest of the film, which is so controlled, framed, and ordered. I discovered the possibilities of documentary for play, which is another form of truth. Right? Another form of experience.

LP: Referring to the interview with Lehmann, where she contests the possibility of the interview being "real," we hear your voice off camera saying, "But there is something real I'm after."

YR: Her *experience* is real to her. Our experience is real to us. It's not an illusion, but through representation it has gone through a process. However we represent it, speak it, photograph it, throw it up in the air and put it back together, that is something else. Experience exists as subjectivity and representation. Not everything we experience is true either—we experience and internalize what we are told by the state, for instance. We are socially conditioned and placed in terms of our sex, race, age, etc. That is what this film is trying to get at: both that positioning and its representation, both social and narrative positioning. I think that is the best shorthand for accounting for all the devices, and my continuing interest in what I call "hanky-panky" with narrative.

SF: Is there a link between Jenny's story and the fact that she's telling it while going through menopause?

YR: The motivation for Jenny's story isn't only that she wants to talk about her youth. There is something bothering her, and one of the reasons she wants to confide this to Yvonne W. is that Yvonne is black. Call it guilt if you want to. There is that different tension that develops between them, and halfway through the story Jenny runs up against Yvonne's criticism about white women always universalizing victimization, and she realizes that she hasn't gotten it "right." Perhaps menopause has also made her feel "out of whack," or not "right." Perhaps "putting things right" is the common theme here: putting her menopause into a social, rather than medical, perspective; getting a handle on her white racism.

LP: Could you say something about the ending of the film, in particular the transition from Jenny's story to the wrap party, at that point where you insert the intertitle, "Utopia: the more impossible it seems, the more necessary it becomes."

YR: I liked the idea of showing all those people socializing with each other. So there is a utopian cast to it. Someone criticized it because it suggests the American melting pot fantasy, which of course lost its credibility long ago. I was aware of these connotations, so it had to be put into context as some kind of dream, or a utopian gesture, along the lines of all tensions and social conflicts momentarily forgotten or maybe at some time in the future, resolved, a coexistence with no racial conflicts. And that statement, "the more impossible it seems, the more necessary it becomes," suggests that we still have to work for utopia. It turns the tables: here is this somewhat sentimental intermixing belied by "the more impossible it seems." Here's a situation that might be construed as utopian, but we know utopia is impossible, it's always a dream, a doomed ideal. But then, on the other hand, it's necessary to work for it anyway. It's a variation on Alexander Kluge's, "Utopia: the farther away it gets, the more desirable it seems," or something like that.

KE: The Caldicott speech is something you had started and then dropped, and this relates to the idea of utopia because the speech seemed presented in a defeatist manner. I don't know if that is a correct characterization, but this whole thing about "we have no guts, and I'm one of you" . . .

YR: I think it's sort of funny. She's so full of these absolutist pronouncements—the end of the world, all this apocalypse and doom, as Jenny says. It *is* an indictment. I take that seriously, this indictment of the feminist movement, that it seems to have stopped short, so there *is* something there. But it's dropped. I didn't feel any obligation to pursue it. It's taken up in another form in Yvonne Washington's critique of white feminism. Not recognizing economic and racial differences among women is one of the failures of white feminism. Of course it's not one that Caldicott is admitting to.

KE: I'm interested in this notion of "getting off the hook," which is repeated by several "characters." One woman you interviewed says that menopause has gotten her off the hook, that it liberated her. And Stew says that Carlos thinks he's off the hook because he's Puerto Rican. Yvonne accuses Jenny of letting Brenda off the hook of being racist.

YR: And then there's that whole fish story. "Now that you've got me hooked," Yvonne W. says, "I want to see how your flashback turns out." And I'm always talking about the audience getting hooked on narrative. Isn't "getting off the hook" another way of saying, or declaring, what your stakes are or are not? For a white woman to make an alliance on the basis of gender with a black woman can be a way of not differentiating between stakes. Black women have a lot more at stake in claiming their rights than white women have, and they have to fight harder. The stakes are very different. The white woman [Helene Moglen] interviewed at the beginning feels off the hook, she can do what she wants, she doesn't have a stake in pleasing men anymore, right? She can please herself. And Carlos is trying to get out from having to declare himself black, and Stew is saying they have the same things at stake. And, although Brenda tries to establish a psychoanalytic connection with Carlos, it is pointed out that she doesn't have the same things at stake.

KE: But, regarding your own privilege as a white woman, one could say that you're letting yourself off the hook by creating this "alter ego" or whatever you want to call Yvonne Washington.

YR: It's true, the film has two directors, one white and one black. But the fact that Yvonne Washington and I appear in separate spheres—the fictional and the documentary—and the fact that my directorship is represented only in voice-over—don't these two tactics keep our identities distinct? We are not intercut in the same way I intercut Alice Spivak and Minnette Lehmann as Jenny and her double. In any case, my stakes are declared all through the film. I think my privilege is declared. I think you can see me, read me, in Jenny, and also in some of the intertitles. *Privilege* declares the stakes and the differences and the specifics of social positioning. I mean, it's all in the film. And after all, we've got to have something in common sometimes, don't we? Novella Nelson and I were in the same room making the same movie. And she had an input into the revision of some of her lines. But here I go confusing representation with the real, art with life. Have I gotten myself off the hook of your question? Or am I getting into hot water?

Interview by Scott MacDonald

The following interview, first published in MacDonald's *A Critical Cinema* 2 (Berkeley: University of California Press, 1992), is also about *Privilege.* It is here that I publicly "came out" as a lesbian.

SCOTT MACDONALD: In recent years every time there's a new Yvonne Rainer film, I read someplace, "This is new and accessible work from Yvonne Rainer. . . ."

YVONNE RAINER: Right. They said that about the last one, and I've heard it about *Privilege.*

SM: I didn't find *The Man Who Envied Women* [1985] more accessible than earlier work—though there were elements of it I liked—but I do find *Privilege* extremely accessible. I enjoyed it from beginning to end, and when I screened it as part of my film series in Utica I discovered it was accessible to a relatively general audience.

YR: This is a mainstream-geared audience?

SM: Pretty much. My series has a reputation, so the audience usually expects something unusual, but they're certainly not shy about leaving. At *Privilege,* I don't believe more than five people left, out of seventy-five or eighty. I've always assumed that your refusal to provide certain kinds of conventional pleasure was a defiance of what the audience has come to expect. But this film includes the audience in a new way.

YR: In Australia, someone asked me—after screening *Privilege*—"Why are you so committed to depriving the audience of pleasure?"

244

SM: They said that after *Privilege?*

YR: After *Privilege.*

SM: That surprises me.

YR: I was astounded because I have never thought of myself as depriving anyone of pleasure unless a shot or a sequence had a specific political agenda, like the tracking shot into the nude in *Film About a Woman Who . . . .* There was a specific mission there. It was an arduous experience for the audience to stay with that shot: *no* one could derive pleasure from *that* image of the woman's body. But in the general course of things, *I* always thought I was introducing *new* pleasures—the pleasure of the text, of reading.

SM: It's true; there are pleasures in many of the stories told in your films but not much *visual* pleasure, especially in the films after *Film About a Woman Who . . . :* that film and *Lives of Performers* [1972] have an unpretentious elegance and sensuality that's lacking in later films, especially *Journeys from Berlin/1971* [1980] and *The Man Who Envied Women.* So when *Privilege* struck me as thoroughly pleasurable, I thought that since, as Jenny says at the beginning of the film, the subject of menopause has come to *mean* unpleasure, you felt free to bring back other obvious kinds of cinematic pleasure as a defiance of the conventional attitude about menopause (and its implications for women), and as a way of modeling a new attitude about menopause (and about film).

YR: That may be a way of reading the progression of my films, but it was certainly not uppermost in my mind.

What *has* been on my mind is an ongoing relationship to narrative, be it about pleasure or nonpleasure. If narrative is a way of *engaging* the audience, I've gone further and further toward narrative conventions, such as *plot:* this is the first of my films that has a semblance of a plot; it's the first film to use so many professional actors. This is the first film that does not have some overly long passage that people just can't stay with—the theoretical lecture in *The Man Who Envied Women,* or the anecdotal, voice-over material in *Journeys from Berlin.* I have always thought of my films as containing dry moments, but compensating for those with offsetting moments—with animals or stories or irony, humor.

SM: This is also the first film where you use extensive interviewing, isn't it?

YR: Well, there's the housing hearing in *The Man Who Envied Women,* but I didn't interview those people. It's talking heads, people giving testimony.

SM: Women talking about their menopausal experiences is, actually, fascinating. Ironically, since it has been a taboo subject in movies, it has become as interesting as other taboo subjects that have to do with the body. The audience—at least the audience I saw the film with—seemed excited to hear these revelations.

YR: These are all young people?

SM: About half of them were college people; half were older people from the community.

YR: I often get the question from men, Who's your audience? At one point I was saying, "It's young women and men, because young women don't *want* to know about menopause, and men have no reason to, have nothing at stake."

SM: Unless a man is deeply involved with someone struggling with menopause.

Near the end, the Yvonne Washington character says,

> I try to monitor when my hot flashes occur. I'm watching a video cassette of "Sweet Sweetback's Baadaass Song." "Why does an embodiment of black protest have to be a stud?" flashes through my mind, and along comes a hot flash. I'm on the subway thinking about a friend. "Forget that family crap," I think. *Flash* . . . Ready to leave, I put on my coat in an overheated room. Instantly I am so hot, I must tear it off. . . . Reading about the Supreme Court's latest setback to civil rights. One of the justices is quoted as saying: "The fact that low-paying, unskilled jobs are overwhelmingly held by blacks is no proof of racism." *Flash* . . . Thinking about what I could have said, should have said: *Flash* . . .

The implication seems to be that you question whether at least some of the symptoms of menopause have anything to do with the physical changes occurring.

YR: That was physiological license; it was a way of bringing together the body and the external, social issues: race especially.

SM: I ask because during a particularly stressful period of my relationship with Pat [O'Connor, MacDonald's wife], she felt her hot flashes were pretty closely related to the psychic stress caused by outside circumstances.

YR: I've heard of only one corroboration of this. It certainly isn't my experience, but it sounds plausible. In *Privilege* it was a way of bringing together everything in the film, a kind of unresolved conclusion.

There are other wild goose chases: Jenny's remark that postmenopausal women don't have REM sleep, for instance. It doesn't seem to be many older people's experience that they don't dream anymore.

SM: How did you find your way to the people you interviewed?

YR: A number of them were old friends. Two of the women in California I've known since I was a teenager. Once I found one person, I found another.

SM: Were there people interviewed that you didn't use?

YR: Yes. And the original interviews are much, much longer. When I first started, I thought, "My god, this film's going to be ten hours long!" Then as I got the other parts of the film together, particular segments of the interviews began to pop out and be relevant.

SM: Have African Americans or Puerto Ricans played any role in your earlier films? I don't remember any.

YR: Yes. Roles, but not *as* ethnic Americans. Blondell Cummings was in *Kristina Talking Pictures* [1976]. David Diao, who's Chinese American, is also in that film. I was interested in an "interesting-looking" bunch of people. But I had no idea of dealing with racial or ethnic social difference.

SM: Was there a particular set of circumstances that led you to deal with race in *Privilege?*

YR: No single circumstance. It was a gradual awareness of, one, the limitations of feminist film theory as it has circulated around Lacanian, neo-Freudian ideas; and, two, this incident in my own past that constitutes the flashback in the film, which had been troubling to me. In the back of my mind, I always knew that I'd have to deal with it at some point. The so-called postcolonialist cultural writing of the last five years or so moved me toward thinking about a film around that incident.

SM: So Jenny's story is pretty close to yours?

YR: Jenny's *flashback,* yes.

SM: What in particular was it about the incident that made it stay with you so long?

YR: It had to do with a sense that in coming to New York I had been very oblivious to many things around me. Even though I had come from an anarchist background, when it came to self-development and realizing my own potential in the world, certain things got excluded: social inequities took a back seat, in terms of consciousness. Some of that had to do with my being in psychotherapy and coming out from under an oppressive marriage and having the chance to produce a lot of work. This incident occurred at the very beginning of this psychic and social advancement, and at first it had no effect on me. It was just something that happened and was very quickly forgotten. But twenty years later, it came back to haunt me with a lot of questions about the kind of life I led then.

SM: One standard thing to say about you, and maybe it's something that you've said about yourself, is that you relentlessly avoid the personal, the autobiographical, and yet looking back now, it strikes me that your films reveal more about you than many of the films of the '60s that are *called* personal actually reveal about their makers. It's because you deal with what you're *thinking about* at any given time, which is always a large part of "who we are."

YR: Yes.

SM: But I wonder, did you set out at the beginning with the idea of *not* making personal film?

YR: No. I certainly wasn't making "personal film" in the sense Brakhage does, in the way the New American Cinemists did—in terms of personal vision. I had no particular vision. And filmmakers complained about my films at the beginning because they weren't "visual"; they didn't play on the retina. My films weren't about making poetic or beautiful images. I got images where I could. And I didn't even do my own shooting! I didn't have a personal touch, in the sense of the painter's hand or a filmmaker's eye—although an eye was certainly there, in the way shots were framed. But my imagery was always at the service of a theatrical, emotional realm; *melodrama* was the perfect form for what I was after: the emotional life lived at an extreme of desperation and conflict. I wanted to explore the emotion of personal life, but it was equally important to me that the films be fictionalized in some way and that there would be no central person you identified with. There's always a lot of personal material in my films, but it's diffused, decentralized, contravened by antinarrative techniques.

SM: There's a healthy recognition that even if something *is* personal to oneself that one's personality shares concerns, ideas, feelings, whatever with lots of other people.

YR: Right.

SM: Your characteristic way of putting texts others have written into the mouths of your characters certainly diffuses—or makes more complex —our sense of their identity, *and* it provides the viewer with a précis of issues that you and many other people have been thinking about over a period of time. Did that technique come out of your performance work?

YR: It may be related to the separation of persona and speech in some of my early dances. A person would recite a story by someone else in the first person, but their body would not be expressing that story; the body would be involved in some other continuity. I was always working for disparities between sound and image. So yes, that carried over into the films. Also, quotation is an expedient way to produce characters: I don't have to worry about psychological credibility. And it gets certain texts out: *someone* has to speak these texts that I'm interested in. It's always a question in my films who's going to speak what, especially where the characters don't have a direct connection to what or the way in which they speak. In *Privilege* Carlos speaks a text that does reflect on his life, but a text that because of his class and education, he wouldn't normally speak. I've always used my actors as mouthpieces. It's a way of talking about the spoken and the speaker at the same time, and to alternate between them: when Carlos is speaking about color, sitting on the stoop, all of a sudden he says, "Hola! Brenda! Qué tal!" as she passes by, and there's a naturalistic scene where we see him as a street person making advances to his neighbor. It's not "realistic," but it can certainly be followed by the spectator. Everyone has that potential to "speak" themselves in some kind of detached way, and also to enact themselves.

SM: I think it's only *semi*-unrealistic because we're always mouthing ideas that we get from other people.

YR: Yes, absolutely.

SM: But mostly we disguise, or try to disguise, that we're doing it.

YR: Right. Right. It happens daily. You're impressed with something someone has said or that you've read and you incorporate it into your next conversation.

SM: I remember reading about a show at the Collective that you and Bérénice Reynaud curated [*Sexism, Colonialism, Misrepresentation,* the Collective for Living Cinema, April 25–May 8, 1988 (the program and related papers were published as the Summer/Autumn 1990 issue of *Motion Picture*)]. It was controversial.

YR: Because it covered feminist films and British black films and African films. It swept with a really wide brush. We were taken to task for that.

SM: Who took you to task?

YR: Coco Fusco, in *Screen* and in *Afterimage*.

SM: What was her take on the show?

YR: Well, the name of her piece was "Fantasies of Oppositionality" [*Afterimage* 16, no. 5 (December 1988), and *Screen* 29, no. 4 (Autumn 1988)]. The tack she took was that white experimental filmmakers and

psychoanalytic feminists are trying to make a bridge between themselves and black filmmakers or blacks in general, in terms of marginalization, and that by not examining our own "otherness"—in the panel
discussions—we "recentered" our whiteness. It was a hard lesson,
though I still feel Coco's overkill approach was not entirely justified.

SM: In *Privilege,* the Yvonne Washington character makes that argument.

YR: Yes, she's taken up a version of that criticism.

SM: Were you already at work on this project at that point?

YR: Yes. But the Yvonne Washington/Jenny face-off hadn't been written.

SM: How much response to the film by African Americans have you
seen? In Utica the audience was about twenty percent African American. It was pretty much the same audience that had, earlier in the fall,
seen *Sidewalk Stories* [1990]. At that earlier screening, I was shocked to
realize that some young African Americans in the audience had a hard
time watching the couple in *Sidewalk Stories* kiss, apparently because
they weren't young and attractive enough for the movies. So I won-
dered how middle-aged women discussing menopause would affect a
similar student clientele. As it turned out, there seemed to be an appreciation for the kinds of African American women who show up in the
film and the way in which they're presented, and present themselves.

YR: I've had very little response from nonwhites so far. I took the film to
the Frederick Douglass Institute of African American Studies at the University of Rochester. I expected at least a fifty-fifty balance of races in the
audience, but it was an almost totally white crowd. Karen Fields, who
is the head of that institute, was very appreciative of the film. In fact, I
remember she said, "How did you come to deal with something as ex-
plosive as a black on white rape with such restraint?" When I go out
with the film, it's pretty much white audiences. After this year is over,
when I stop taking care of my official bookings, I'm going to do an out-
reach and try to bring the film to community groups. I have to find the
black audience. The discussions have been really interesting, and there's
no reason they wouldn't be equally interesting with black audiences.

SM: You mentioned to Lynn Tillman in the *Voice* interview ["A Woman Called Yvonne," Jan. 15, 1991, p. 56] that Novella Nelson had an input into the film.

YR: I was giving Lynn an example of why the opening title credit says *Privilege,* a film by Yvonne Rainer *and many others.* I've never submitted a film to so many people or asked for so much criticism. So there was a contribution there. In rehearsal, Novella corrected my vernacular. She substituted "dude" for "guy"—things like that. And there were a couple of key moments like the one I mentioned to Lynn: Novella's response to Eldridge Cleaver, for example. She was very involved and made comments along the way.

SM: At one point late in the film, there's a tussle where Jenny and Yvonne Washington laugh and wrestle about being in front of the camera. Jenny feels she's been in the hot seat long enough and that it's Yvonne's turn. Yvonne Washington ends up being in front of the camera and talking about her menopause. This raises the issue of the filmmaker exposing herself to the eye of the camera to the degree her interviewees are exposed. You are in front of the camera in the Helen Caldicott reading, but you're not identified. You never do talk openly about *your* menopause. There seems an implicit irony here.

YR: Well, the film is very artificial. It continually plays with the so-called truth value of documentary, and with the authenticity of identity. I'm split across any number of people in this film. You might say the whole film goes on in my own head. Anyone who knows anything about my life will recognize little bits and pieces here and there. But it's not a roman à clef, where you figure out, Oh that's this one and that's that one. It's just a way of using material that has an authentic ring to it. Jenny's menopausal story comes from a particular source but not from me. And it parallels the story of the Cuban woman at the end, who is a real interviewee. My menopausal story is there, here and there, but it's not identified. Is this an issue for you?

SM: Well, only on the level that the real filmmaker isn't revealed as clearly as the "filmmaker" in the film.

YR: I play Helen Caldicott because it was convenient, and I enjoy making these Hitchcock-like appearances. I also pop up later, making the comment about Brenda not being desired by men.

There *is* an irony in my flu-ravished face. I'm sick every time I shoot a film. Here, I pop up with this smeared lipstick and drawn, pallid face and talk about desirability to men! The same kind of irony comes with putting "My Funny Valentine" over my middle-aged face. Of course, it prefigures what is going to be discussed at much greater length in the film. When Novella came in, she actually thought she was going to be handling the camera and be filmed as she was shooting. I wasn't about to go that far in developing her as a literal alter ego. It suffices for me to say in the credits that she is the filmmaker and to have said she's making a documentary film. You either take it or leave it.

I deliberately put Yvonne Washington on the edge of the frame until that key Marxist speech when the camera comes around the couch and finally frames her in close-up. That has a very specific metaphorical meaning about marginalization as does the shot of the black signer, center screen, signing for the white speaker in the oval on the side.

SM: It had never occurred to me how ludicrous the normal way of including a signer on the TV screen is: the person *signing* is in the small hard-to-see space at the corner of the image and the person *talking,* whom we can hear without any image at all, in the big space.

YR: When it's important to *see* the signer!

SM: It's like the moment in *The Man Who Envied Women* where you reposition the slicing of the eyeball from *Un Chien Andalou* so that we realize its violence against *women.* After decades of teaching that film, the gender implications of that shot had never occurred to me!

YR: Really! Wow. It's always been thought of as the "eye" of the camera, hasn't it?

SM: I'm a little puzzled about the dream where there are two black men looking at the *New York Times* want ads and two black women in the bed underneath them.

YR: Well, Jenny and Yvonne Washington have just been talking about REM sleep. Jenny mentions that she's heard that older people don't have REM sleep anymore, and Yvonne Washington protests: "I don't believe that, I still dream. Just the other night I had the weirdest dream . . ." and we're into the dream—or actually it's preceded by another dream image, of Jenny running in terror from something *off*screen. Then we see the two black men looking at the *Times* help-wanted ads. The camera pulls away and there's a sign beneath the *Times* that you really can't read: it says, "Lost: memories, muscles, husbands, friends"— all the things that are lost in the aging process or *look* like possible losses. And then you see these two women entwined in bed. It happens too fast (and there's also a voice-over that doesn't quite jibe with what you see), but the two *women* in bed are a reference to lesbians not *needing* men: the men are looking for work!

SM: [Laughter] Hmmm. I missed it.

YR: I don't think it's that obvious. But *then,* there's a reverse shot of Jenny looking down, suggesting a racial thing, the threat of the white woman coming between the black women. It's a dream within a dream.

SM: The title *Privilege* was used by Peter Watkins in a 1967 film about rock musicians receiving privilege as a means of siphoning off the political energy of young people into the rock concert phenomenon.

YR: I don't remember that film.

SM: How did you decide to use that title?

YR: It had to do with Jenny's status in the flashback event. She had privilege and didn't know it, and was also lacking privilege and didn't know it. To her neighbors the Jenny character represents a white norm and a privileged lifestyle. The aging process has put her in a different relationship to privilege.

Every character in the film can be seen as either having or not having privilege, depending on race, sex, class, age. If they didn't have it, I gave it *to* them. I privileged Digna to be the commentator, to be more omniscient than Jenny, and to be able to follow Jenny around without being seen. *Privilege* is a crucial term in the film, a kind of prism through which all these issues—and techniques—can be observed.

SM: At the end, you do an interesting thing with the credits, particularly given the line we see during the credits: "UTOPIA: the more impossible it seems, the more necessary it becomes." You intercut between the textual credits and what I assume is the wrap party for the film (you also include additional interview information). Do you see the party as a kind of momentary utopia?

YR: Yeah.

SM: Is the process of making a film your attempt to model utopian interaction?

YR: Originally, the ending was going to be a dozen postmenopausal women in bright red lipstick and black leather jackets, pouring out of a bar, trying to zip up their jackets [laughter]. It was going to be some climactic moment attacking stereotypes: these raunchy, spunky women. And then I kind of abandoned that and thought, "Oh, well maybe there'll be a dance." I thought I'd show all these women dancing to "Sounds of Soweto" or something, and then that seemed too corny. And finally, I decided, why not document what was already going to happen. I invited all the interviewees to the party. Only a few could come. Actually, Shirley Triest, the tall thin woman, flew from California: it was the first time in her life she's been out of California. I was very touched by that.

SM: At the end of the film, just before we see the wrap party, Yvonne asks Jenny, "So, did you ever make it with Brenda?" and Jenny says, "Hell, no! I was terrified of women." That, the two women in bed in the one dream, and a textual statement (it's quoted in one of the stills you made for *Privilege*)—"The most remarkable thing was the silence that emanated from friends and family regarding details of my single middle age. When I was younger, my sex life had been the object of all kinds of questioning, from prurient curiosity to solicitous concern. Now that I did not appear to be looking for a man, the state of my desires seemed of no interest to anyone"—leads to my last question: What *is* the state of your desires?

YR: I've become a lesbian.

SM: Ah.

YR: I mean I can only say that now because I'm deeply involved with someone. But for the last five years it's been on my mind. I've gone through these backbends to find some way of describing a state of non-active, unrealized sexual identity. I did a lecture in Australia where I called myself "a lapsed heterosexual" and an "a-woman" and "a political lesbian." At the level of politics, and emotion, my empathy was with lesbians. But I was settling into a celibate life. I didn't know how to proceed.

That's something I want to learn more about in my next film. I want to interview lesbians who *became* lesbians in middle age. That's the stereotype: a woman is not wanted by men anymore; therefore, she turns to women.

SM: That's a stereotype I've not heard, actually.

YR: Oh? It's in the culture. I don't think I invented it, and I really want to investigate it: *Is* it a stereotype? *Privilege* does raise all the stereotypes about desirability and women getting "old" before men get "old," and the old maid stereotype.

SM: I guess the stereotype I've heard is that old maids are lesbians whether they know it or not—though I'm certainly not in touch with the conventional stereotyping of lesbians.

YR: What's very interesting to me is that the instant you get involved with someone of your own sex, it's like crossing the Rubicon! I mean, suddenly, I'm not a "political lesbian" (well, I *am* a political lesbian), I'm a lesbian. I felt I couldn't *say* that before, which was odd, because years ago, there was a time I couldn't say I was a feminist because I thought, "Oh a feminist is a political *activist,* not just someone who makes art." I got past that, and have been an avowed feminist for years.

You know, this is the first time I've uttered all this. No one has asked me directly.

SM: *Privilege* gave me the sense you wanted to be asked, but I wasn't sure I'd have the nerve to ask you.

YR: I'm glad you did. It's the beginning—for me—of talking about it. Which means the beginning of fomenting a film.

Rainer Talking Pictures:

Interview by Thyrza Nichols Goodeve

Conducted by Thyrza Nichols Goodeve, this interview was published in *Art in America* (July 1997) following the release of *MURDER and murder*.

THYRZA NICHOLS GOODEVE: You have been a working artist now for three-and-a-half decades, and you are finishing *MURDER and murder,* your seventh film. History and memory seem appropriate devices for framing this interview. I'm interested in the way your personal and formal concerns dovetail with each decade's *zeitgeist.* Let's go back in time. It's 1952, who are you?

YVONNE RAINER: I'm a depressed adolescent. I graduated from high school in 1952 and went to San Francisco City College. The Beats were about to explode in San Francisco—poetry and jazz—following on the heels of the older bohemian generation consisting of anarchists, World War II conscientious objectors, poets and painters. In 1956 I attended Allen Ginsberg's first reading of *Howl* at the Six Gallery. All through my adolescence I had been going to the Workman's Circle, where people like Kenneth Rexroth and Kenneth Patchen gave readings, and attending anarchist picnics. In my early teens I was exposed to a heady mix of poets and painters intermingled with older-generation Italian anarchists, also Jewish anarchists from New York who'd come out to San Francisco after the war.

TNG: Were anarchists drawn to San Francisco more than to other parts of the country?

YR: It was a gathering place for Italian anarchists like my father around the time of the First World War. Alexander Berkman and Emma Goldman probably passed through. My father came from Italy about 1912.

TNG: And your mother?

YR: My mother's parents emigrated to New York from Warsaw in the 1880s. My mother was born in Brooklyn in 1896. I incorporate some of her stories in *MURDER and murder*. Like the time she went to Coney Island with her girlfriends and ended up alone in a rowboat with a man who told her women with thick ankles are very sensual. My mother went into this man's tent—they were sleeping in adjacent tents—and, as she recounted, they "had a sexual relation."

TNG: Why did she tell you this?

YR: She told me that story when I was eleven years old as a cautionary tale against sleeping with men before I got married. So then her periods stopped and she thought she might be pregnant. She couldn't tell her mother, and it was unthinkable to move out of the house and get her own apartment. She had girlfriends—one named Alice who had eight sisters. About three or four of these sisters had hitchhiked across the country and ended up in California with these Italian anarchists. They wrote to my mother and said, "Why don't you come out here! The sun is always shining and we're meeting all these great men." So my mother took the train (with a trunk full of very nifty clothes, I was told many years later by Ida, one of the sisters). Another bit of family lore is that she met my father in a "raw food dining room" and they had an immediate bond because he, too, was a vegetarian as well as an anarchist. It feels odd to tell these stories. They became frozen in my ten- or eleven-year-old imagination. My father died when I was twenty-one, and my mother almost immediately began to go down the tubes with an Alzheimer's-like brain deterioration. So I never got a chance to clarify these knots of information that cling to my memory like carbuncles.

TNG: Let's jump forward. It's 1962: who are you?

YR: That was the year of the first Judson Church dance concert.

TNG: You'd been dancing for how long at that point?

YR: Off and on since 1957, a year after I moved to New York, but seriously from 1960. I was choreographing from 1961. I was very ambitious, worked all the time. I was also dancing with Jimmy Waring and his company.

TNG: What was New York like then?

YR: At that point 10th Street was still full of galleries. At the Green Gallery on 57th Street, Richard Bellamy started showing Oldenburg and Rosenquist and the Minimalists. There were loft bashes every week. Every weekend you'd go to an opening or a series of openings and the grapevine would tell you whose loft was having a bash. You'd go there and dance your brains out. I was also going to lots of theater, dance concerts at the 92nd Street Y and, of course, Happenings.

TNG: Now it's 1972 . . .

YR: 1972 was the year of my first feature film, *Lives of Performers,* but I was still dancing.

TNG: Was it difficult to start making films?

YR: It came out of the autobiographical mode that I'd been exploring in performance work. My access to film was through rationalizing my autobiography. *Lives of Performers* was the result of that.

TNG: And that was radically different from dance?

YR: Right. There was no narrative in dance. Well, sometimes I incorporated story-fragments from various sources, some of which were autobiographical.

TNG: Did the autobiographical material develop in response to the formalism of dance?

YR: Not exactly. Formalism had always run neck and neck with dramatic elements in my work, which is what distinguished me from the Minimalists, I suppose. I never wanted to be restricted to Minimalism's antimetaphorical strategies. In fact, as a dancer I knew it was impossible: the body speaks no matter how you try to suppress it. So when I strung disjunctive pieces of movement together in the solo *Ordinary Dance,* in 1962, I also recited an autobiographical litany of street names and grade school teachers. Or when I staged a running dance, I accompanied it with a grandiose section from Berlioz's *Requiem.*

TNG: Exactly how did the transition from dance to film take place?

YR: The first three films [*Lives of Performers, Film About a Woman Who . . . , Kristina Talking Pictures*] grew out of earlier versions combining live performance with slide and film projections, and I always thought of those versions as an interim project on the way to making the finished film. I can't quite account for that; I just knew I was going to make films. Fortunately Babette Mangolte, who became my cinematographer, had just come to the States. Annette Michelson introduced me to her, and she was very interested in working with me. I learned about filmmaking from her. I was also going to Anthology Film Archives, seeing their cycle of avant-garde films. I had been following avant-garde cinema since the early '60s, when I had seen Maya Deren's work at the Living Theater on 14th Street and Sixth Avenue.

TNG: Were Deren's films an influence for you? It seems an obvious connection—a woman dancer who becomes a filmmaker—but I've never heard you talk about it.

YR: The influence was quite conscious on my part. If you look at some of the editing in *Kristina Talking Pictures,* it's right out of Deren's *At Land.* Like the scene where she is running on the beach, and her movements seem to be continuous but the landscape changes from shot to shot.

TNG: *Lives of Performers* is also a commentary on Minimalism—one easier to see now than before. For example, when we see Shirley and Fernando hugging and the camera tilts up their legs—he is in white pants, she in black pants—the relationship is transformed into a Minimalist image of black and white forms. The film seems to point to the constraints of Minimalism as an esthetic form, and the way it couldn't contain the ferment of personal relationships. You do have all of the characters bursting out of a Minimalist-style box at the end.

YR: Minimalism had its excesses, and I didn't escape them. There were formal concerns in performance and experimental cinema at that time, like extended duration and repetition, that are very trying for audiences today and may seem dated. In fact I am relieved there aren't many documentations of my dance work. I think a lot of it would seem insufferable now.

TNG: How did people react when you started using autobiographical material in your films? At that time it must have seemed a lot more shocking than it would now.

YR: By the early '70s the stage had already been set with Carolee Schneemann's *Fuses,* Jack Smith's *Flaming Creatures,* and Warhol's films. Still, there was a bit of the sensational in *Lives of Performers.* People either took it as a roman à clef or thought my performers—since I used their actual names—were the real subjects of the film. And I also included a long letter, read by Valda Setterfield, that had actually been sent to me by the "other woman" in my life. I always thought of my autobiography as source material, as something that could bring a note of authenticity to an otherwise flat, uninflected mise-en-scène and performance mode.

TNG: Did you ask the woman who sent the letter to you for permission to use it in the film?

YR: No.

TNG: How did she react?

YR: I don't know. I never saw her after that. To be honest, there was a kind of secret satisfaction on my part, a vindictiveness that was operating because it had been a very hurtful episode.

TNG: Set in the Minimalist performance context of the '60s, *Lives of Performers* must have felt like watching voyeuristic glimpses of someone else's private life.

YR: There were people who knew me and therefore knew the whole *Sturm und Drang* of my life and those involved in it. But even for those who didn't know me, it may have been a bit shocking. The stylizations of Happenings and experimental theater didn't prepare people for the kind of emotional candor or specificity they encountered in my work.

TNG: When you first made *Film about a Woman Who . . .*, were you thinking about melodrama as a *woman's* genre?

YR: I wasn't thinking of emulating Hollywood melodrama in a generic sense. If I had, l would have made a very different kind of film. But remember, the subtitle of *Lives of Performers* is *a melodrama.* I was using the term partly for its resonance, at the same time beginning to investigate my emotional experience as a woman and contrast that with classic melodramas such as Pabst's *Pandora's Box.* Even as a dancer I had a heightened awareness of myself as an "object of the gaze," an awareness of my own narcissism and exhibitionism as possible objects for investigation. I didn't differentiate between the male and female gaze as feminist theorists did later, but some of my early dance work had been about the audience "looking" and looking at me, a female self-dramatized performer. By the early '70s, reading *Sisterhood is Powerful* and all those outpourings of rage and outrage, I began to think of myself as a feminist. But it took a while. I was resistant. l thought feminists were people who went around in knee breeches. Yet *Film about a Woman Who . . .* reflects that kind of female anger. Some people called it "pre-political."

TNG: The art-historical scenario of those years stresses the way that the high male drama of Abstract Expressionism is followed by the distancing from emotion that occurs in Minimalism. Then artists like you come in, combining the formal and the autobiographical in volatile ways, exposing the power dynamics that go on "between the sheets" of people's personal lives. At this point you are preparing the ground for the kind of theoretical and analytical work that took place in the 1980s. When I was watching *Kristina Talking Pictures* again recently I was surprised to see how prescient it was of your later film *The Man Who Envied Women* [1985].

YR: How?

TNG: *Kristina* is a film about gender and subjectivity. There's a scene where you and your brother Ivan are sitting upright in bed together. He's reciting a text about a ship while you recite one about the mating habits of animals. It shows the way that two people in a relationship share a common experience but their inner lives are so different. There was also the critique of the white liberal male.

YR: "Do you believe in Chairman Mao and refuse to curb your dog?" Some of that was tongue-in-cheek.

TNG: Sure, but it shows how private actions are imbricated with larger social issues.

YR: The contradictions between public and private. In *The Man Who Envied Women* there's the Marxist, progressive academic who is a philanderer. Yet, there's no contradiction there; I mean it's such a commonplace that we don't think of it as a contradiction. But I guess I've always had a puritanical streak or a kind of utopian strain that wants to integrate the public citizen with the private person. But in our society, as the Jack Deller character says, "I'm a mass of contradictions—what else can you expect under capitalism?"

TNG: But there are some contradictions that one has to live with and others that one can choose to not participate in or exacerbate. But we've gotten ahead of ourselves. Who are you in 1982?

YR: We're really leapfrogging through the decades. I seem to chart my life by these films. In 1982 I had *Journeys from Berlin* [1980] behind me.

TNG: How long had it taken you to pull yourself out of being a dancer and choreographer and just be a filmmaker?

YR: *Journeys* came out at a time when film nomenclature was shifting from "avant-garde" to "independent." Younger filmmakers were beginning to have a different attitude to Hollywood, less adversarial, more yearning. The high camp of '60s and '70s avant-garde, as exemplified by Jack Smith and the Kuchar brothers, was being challenged by both feminist theory and the beginning of the "crossover" phenomenon, à la Lizzie Borden's *Working Girls*. I had officially stopped dancing in 1975, and by the '80s I was known as a filmmaker, though still "avant-garde," and had a body of work to prove it.

TNG: Your work produced in the '60s is influenced by the context of high art—Minimalism, but also the rebelliousness of that decade—and in the '70s you make films about relationships . . .

YR: . . . where there's a very reduced social life. The social space of my films in the '70s is quite cloistered. This expanded after I returned to New York from Germany in 1977. Indeed, it was to be a long journey from my year in Berlin (thanks to a grant from the DAAD) to thinking about political violence (the Baader/Meinhof group and Russian nihilist women), feminist film theory, New York real-estate depredations, and the activism of the left against U.S. imperialism in Central America.

TNG: Let's reflect on the continuities and discontinuities between your past work and present work.

YR: I suppose we can list them in terms of subject matter. Heterosexuality has shifted to homosexuality. Domestic and sexual conflict is still a concern. Specific social issues keep overlapping from one film to the other: political violence, U.S. imperialism, social privilege, gender inequality, notions of disease, aging. Autobiography and quotidian activity are constants. Narrative is also a constant, though my use of narrative conventions has totally changed since 1972. Each film has worked out a lexicon of narrative strategies, moving from the static, disjunctive tableaux of *Lives of Performers* to the full-blown characterizations and enactments of *MURDER and murder.*

Finding Topics on the Doorstep

TNG: To what extent did the recent critical discourse on identity and sexual identity help to open up the possibility of a relationship with a woman for you?

YR: Certainly being around dykes opened up that possibility. Also, in a funny way, receiving a MacArthur Fellowship. It made me relax in some fundamental way, enabled me to enact some deep-rooted component of my fantasy life—being protective, being able to take care of someone. I was thinking today about what makes people change. Yes, environment and economics change people, and ideas change people. The *New York Times* ran a series about corporate downsizing. Are these upper-middle-class people going to undergo a change in consciousness about free enterprise? I'm probably being overly optimistic, but let's hope the labor movement is finally going to be revitalized.

TNG: You're like a sponge in regard to your historical moment. The interaction between you, your cultural surroundings and your geographic location becomes material for you to work into a film.

YR: Or certain moments in cultural history give me permission to deal with specific incidents in my life. It is funny how my life parallels certain theoretical moments—most recently becoming involved with a woman coinciding with all the writing on sexual identity as a political issue. I always felt I couldn't handle topics until they fell on my doorstep. Even though I was calling myself a political lesbian for ten years before I became sexually active, I didn't feel I could make anything of that until I had the experience. So once my life takes a certain shape or direction I can start collecting material and start thinking of a larger social picture.

For instance, I wouldn't have dealt with women's health before I got cancer, although some people do, young people do. I had the title—*MURDER and murder*—before I had a mastectomy and was looking around for an appropriate social or institutional murder to go with the domestic strife and fantasies of murder that the film deals with. Then I was diagnosed—and there it was on my doorstep again. It's a weird way of working. In my more self-effacing moments I see it as a failure of imagination, or as the legacy of literal-minded Minimalism.

TNG: It becomes almost like a pun: for you the work has to be embodied quite literally.

YR: Yes, maybe that's my dancer's legacy. But it enables me to deal with things in complex ways. How the intimate is experienced alongside political and economic stresses.

TNG: That idea brings me back to your earlier films, where you take the very intimate—the scandalously intimate—and combine it with critical analysis and polities. As a result, the viewer is drawn back and forth between these two spaces and a complex experience—part emotion, part critique—emerges. Both the highly personal and the blunt analytical material become easier to absorb because of the relation you set up.

YR: The difference in *MURDER and murder* is that my main characters are not the mouthpieces of the political and social texts.

TNG: They're actually characters. When one compares the script for *MURDER and murder* with your earlier scripts, one now finds dialogue. Whereas in *Journeys from Berlin* or *Kristina Talking Pictures* your scripts are composed of lengthy monologues. What allowed you to feel comfortable with the characters being just characters?

YR: It came out of the writing. I found I was less involved in monologue than dialogue.

TNG: Why is that?

YR: Well, this film is about two women in an equilateral relationship, something I had never developed before. There was the character played by Annette Michelson in *Journeys from Berlin*. She has a relationship with the shrink, but the shrink is very recessive; it's still pretty much a long monologue. In *The Man Who Envied Women* the main character, Jack Deller, is mostly alone. There I chose to take the narrator—Trisha, his estranged lover—out of the picture. So he's doing these endless lectures, or talking to an off-screen shrink, or walking in the street overhearing things, while she carries on by herself on the sound track. There's no interaction. Relationship is indicated, but not enacted. Even the encounter between Jack Deller and Jackie, the femme fatale, is short-circuited by the nature of their language, a theoretical "speaking past" each other. But in *MURDER and murder* the relationship between Mildred and Doris had to be played out.

TNG: Your other films involved heterosexual relationships, but you didn't use dialogue. So what shifts in *MURDER and murder*? In the least traditional relationship you use the most traditional cinematic codes.

YR: This is such a rarely represented kind of relationship—older women *and* lesbians. I can't think of a single film dealing narratively with older lesbians, and by "older" I mean in their fifties and sixties. It seemed necessary to make the relationship more "credible," at least more recognizable, via the conventions of shot/reverse shot and extended scenes with almost classical structure in terms of development and climax.

TNG: It is radical to make the spectator identify with two older women in love.

YR: I think I've made a situation where young and old, male and female, gay and heterosexual audiences can identify with this couple. I'm a little amazed, but I'm quite sure there's that possibility here. Already someone has used that squishy word "universal."

TNG: It's a film which successfully treats older women *and* a lesbian relationship as part of everyday life. It's just about that, and it isn't corned up. Well, there are moments when you do corn it up.

YR: Where?

TNG: The scene in bed when Mildred says to Doris, "Well, *your* credentials as a bona fide lesbian have never been in question."

YR: Do you mean it's sentimental? Fuzzy?

TNG: Sentimentality is fine, but I tend to recoil when gay work has to announce the difference between lesbian and hetero sexuality. I want to see a film—a lesbian film—that isn't preoccupied with that opposition. When Mildred said that line in *MURDER and murder,* I thought, why does it have to be about marking the lesbian authenticity, or lack thereof, of the once-straight lover?

YR: That scene echoes what I encountered when I first got involved with Martha. It is what I found young lesbians talking about a lot: what does it mean to be a lesbian? What is a *real* lesbian? It goes on all the time. "How do you know?" "Who is and who isn't?" I actually ran into the attitude that you're not a *real* lesbian until you've been on "the barricades."

TNG: And what do you think about that?

YR: It's a discussion that disappeared between me and Martha within six months. I think it's a kind of game-playing necessitated by marginalization. One becomes part of a secret club with all that that entails and this in spite of all the gains in visibility. Because of the novelty of this relationship to me and, at the time, Martha (who hadn't been involved seriously with someone for a while), I think it just had to be played out. But it seems in our culture and climate that the specialness of being a woman with a woman has to be articulated by the subjects themselves.

Murders Large and Small

TNG: The title *MURDER and murder* isn't completely clear to me. You have *murder* in both upper-case and lower-case letters.

YR: *MURDER* in capital letters refers to actual death, by homophobic assault or by industrial toxins. Lower-case *murder* is fantasized murder in domestic or familial situations. "When I was growing up I fantasized poisoning my older sister."

TNG: What's the point of the comparison?

YR: As I say in the film, "Fantasies don't kill. Thoughts can be murderous, but thoughts don't kill." These other things kill: DDT, PCBs, dioxin in breast milk, blood, and semen; nuclear tests, electromagnetic fields, 177 organo-chlorines stored in our fat.

TNG: But you are making connections between the murderous aspects of homophobia and breast cancer.

YR: Right, homophobia can kill.

TNG: But homophobia is a thought—a thought-toxin.

YR: Not when it's acted out.

TNG: I understand. But what are the "lower case" murders?

YR: Getting enraged at the person you are living with.

TNG: How has your use of cinematic framing changed from your earlier films to *MURDER and murder*? For instance, the camera in *Kristina Talking Pictures* or *Lives of Performers* seems to have its own life; it's very much an independent character as it moves about. Whereas in *MURDER and murder* . . .

YR: In *MURDER and murder* the camera's presence is rarely foregrounded. There's a scene where the camera tracks and pans repeatedly over Mildred and Doris as they lie at opposite ends of the bed. This is the scene in which lesbian identity is being discussed (starting with

Doris's "Your credentials as a bona fide lesbian have never been in question"). In this case the spectator engages with the two characters rather than, as in *Kristina Talking Pictures,* with shots of furniture and a printed text on the floor.

TNG: Although *MURDER and murder* is more traditionally shot, you do choose to collapse various narrative spaces into one another as in your other films. For instance, the scene when you enter in your tux as a character.

YR: Well, at this moment the frame is packed with personalities—Jenny, Young Mildred and myself—and consequently with diverse time zones. Jenny is Doris's deceased mother stuck in 1918, Young Mildred is Mildred's eighteen-year-old incarnation, just graduated from high school, and "I yam who I yam," to quote Popeye or somebody. It was important to establish that the three of us are invisible to Doris and Mildred throughout the scene. So when Mildred puts down her bag of groceries almost in Jenny's lap, Jenny has to scoot out and reposition herself. Scenes like this make one long for 35 mm or Cinemascope!

TNG: So you're still wrestling with narrative but not via seamless editing and identification. You're making the space on-screen a tableau that contains different narrative trajectories.

YR: I do tend to think of things as flat—squared away. My director of photography, Steve Kazmierski, was always thinking of angles and motion. Space was much more malleable and sculptural for him. Even in my early work like *Kristina* I often wanted a person's face to be bifurcated by the frame or to see just parts of a body or an elbow. I have worked with tableaux or tended to have people just sit looking at the camera straight on, while in *MURDER and murder* Steve went for oblique angles. I accepted most of his ideas.

TNG: In what way is narrative still an issue for you in the '90s? What has changed about how we perceive difference, not just male/female difference but racial, sexual and class difference, and therefore how we represent these narratively?

YR: I still, and always did, see narrative as a political issue, but for different reasons at different times. Up through the early '80s, narrative—

in cinema, at any rate—was "bad" because it was seen as something that enthralled the spectator in vicarious experience and wiped out his/her critical faculties. Hollywood was the arch-demon; it "sent the mind away." Narrative sold the consumer a bill of goods. After theorists like Hayden White and Teresa de Lauretis got done with it, narrative could be dismissed as a tool of imperialism and patriarchy. But then in the early '80s pressure was put on the prestigious cultural institutions by all these previously disenfranchised folk who wanted *their* stories to be heard—African Americans, Asian Americans, Chicanos, gays and lesbians, women, Jewish and African diaspora people. And all of a sudden we (whites) realized that it was all very well to criticize narrative as an injustice-producing structure in the hands of the dominant class, race, and gender, but what about all those stories that had not been allowed in the door? Did *their* structures contain the same inequities? Was the subtext of *all* narratives about power? I can't answer that, and I don't know that the theorists have either.

My own relation to narrative has become increasingly complicated. It is the most effective "gripping device" or means of engaging an audience, and as such must be considered and mastered. This means that situations and characters must have varying degrees of credibility. Time and space, however, can and must be played with—for comic relief, for disruption, for foregrounding the "apparatus," for allowing analysis and commentary.

TNG: Reading Sally Banes's book *Greenwich Village 1963,* I was struck by your situation in terms of public funding. Your career developed during the years that the National Endowment for the Arts, which was started in 1965, grew up. The NEA has gone through the late-'80s attacks and the Gingrich era. Is funding more difficult for you to find now?

YR: Each time I make a film I think I won't be able to get this much money again. And now I think I *have* gotten to the end of it because I have received everything there is to get: a once-in-a-lifetime MacArthur, two Guggenheims, a once-in-a-lifetime Wexner Prize. The NEA is now a shambles, the New York State Council for the Arts is drastically cut, and the American Film Institute no longer awards production grants. Since 1972 each of my films has cost almost twice as much as its predecessor. *Lives of Performers* cost $6,500, and *MURDER and murder* will come in at around $225,000. The point is that in today's economic climate—and especially if you're past sixty years of age and persist in writing commercially unviable scripts—you can't make a feature film with a couple of $10,000 grants. So you see, at this point it's hard for me to conceive of making another film.

Self-Exposure and Slapstick Modernism

TNG: Last fall, when you took the students in the Whitney Independent Study Program on a journey through your work, you started with a film of your dance performance, *Trio A*. What is it like to watch yourself dancing decades later, when dance is so removed from your current life?

YR: Oh, I wish I'd danced it better; that's always my first thought when I watch that film. It was made in 1978, when I had not performed for a few years. I was also having some health problems.

TNG: Watching you watching yourself dance, I couldn't help but think of the other subject of *MURDER and murder*: breast cancer. You expose yourself in all your work—from the "scandalously intimate" moments of *Lives of the Performers* to the moment in *MURDER and murder* where you appear with part of your shirt cut out, revealing your scarred, breastless chest. Was the exposure of your scarred chest any more difficult than previous exposures?

YR: "Exposure" in most of my previous work was indirect and fictionalized, even when I myself performed. I knew that *M and m*, however, was going to involve literal exposure. The first time I had to go on set in the costume, I was pretty self-conscious and threw a towel over my left shoulder. But then when I saw that the cast and crew were as cool as cucumbers, I threw modesty to the winds. Of course I knew everyone had to get a good look, but they didn't do it when *I* was looking at them! I had a lengthy discussion with Linda Gui, the costume designer, about the extent of the opening in the tux. First she just made a little hole in the shirt and jacket, which only revealed the scar, but it didn't read. You had to see the whole side of the chest to get the kind of impact I was after.

TNG: This is an abrupt shift, but one hopefully in keeping with the sensibility of your work: your vaudevillian humor has become much more prominent as you've progressed as a filmmaker. One doesn't exactly associate gales of laughter with your early works like *Lives of Performers* or

Film About a Woman Who . . . . Yet by now you've developed quite a repertoire of slapstick. In *MURDER and murder,* for instance, you have a masquerade party that has a real Keystone Cops feeling to it.

YR: *MURDER and murder* has farcical moments. During the masquerade revel I'm on camera, talking about the corporation that manufactures both chlorine and tamoxifen. That's why I put the Cop-Docs in there.

TNG: The Cop-Docs are the ones running about in the white coats with the police batons?

YR: Yes. They are talking about early detection of cancer, not only about saving lives but making bigger profits. There is a company in the U.K., Imperial Chemical Industries, which has a subsidiary in the U.S. that runs campaigns for early cancer detection. At the same time they produce all these chemicals that cause cancer.

TNG: It's like Philip Morris manufacturing nicotine patches in order to recoup the profits they are losing to the antismoking campaign. But what is it about that kind of slapstick, one-liner humor that appeals to you? Is it because it's almost Brechtian in its way of intervening in narrative flow?

YR: I love the irreverence of such humor, the more wicked the better—flying in the face of good taste.

TNG: Like the moment when Young Mildred asks what's the difference between a lesbian and a tumor?

YR: The answer to that riddle is: "One ages well and the other doesn't." Or, "What did the lesbian say to her breast?" Jenny responds, "Ugh, I don't want to know." "That's it! That's what she said." Then they start whacking each other with rubber clubs.

TNG: Masquerade and performance are clearly important in *MURDER and murder.* Talk about your use of these, especially in relation to such scenes as when you have Mildred, as a university lecturer, citing part of Joan Rivière's essay "Femininity as Masquerade."

YR: I used the Rivière essay after a scene where Mildred says to Doris, "You are a bitch, you know; you still haven't thanked me for the gloves," and Doris backs away and says, "You want more than gratitude." Then we see Mildred delivering a lecture and quoting Rivière.

The essay was published in 1929 when the "aggressive" professional woman was still an object for psychoanalytic pathologizing. Rivière describes the efforts of her female patient, a professional academic, to take on "womanly" attributes after demonstrating her competence and knowledge on a par with that of her male colleagues. In other words, she tries to disarm herself, but gets enraged at not getting the recognition she feels she deserves for "having the phallus." The essay is retrogressive insofar as Rivière continues to pathologize her patient—not for "masquerading" as a man, however, but for her rage at having to masquerade as a woman. Along the way, Rivière brilliantly analyzes the female stratagem for being unthreatening to men. I needed a lecture for Mildred, and this one is so interesting in relation to sexuality and gender roles.

TNG: In other words, Rivière's female intellectual suffers not from penis envy but from a lack of "phallic" recognition for achievements, which, according to the ethos of the period, were masculine.

YR: People might be confused at how I take this essay, and of course I certainly don't want to dismiss it. Society dictates that even the butchiest of us masquerade as women sometimes. And some of us even enjoy it!

TNG: Why, in the performance number that the character Doris does in *MURDER and murder,* do you give her some of Kathy Bates's lines from Rob Reiner's recent film *Misery?*

YR: I simply love it. I thought it was perfect for Doris, this kooky performance artist who combines all sorts of weird things, like a collagist. So why wouldn't she use a speech from a Hollywood movie? Joanna Merlin, who plays Doris, had been teaching an acting workshop in Berlin, and she brought back Xeroxes of photos of expressionist dance poses from a book about Valeska Gert, a 1920s German modern dancer. It was Joanna's idea to do something with them. And I said, "Great." So we have the Madonna-like costume: sexy fishnet stockings, leather miniskirt, smeared lipstick, a breast-plate made of gold coils. We have the Kathy Bates speech from *Misery* about going to the movie serials every week and feeling betrayed when Rocketman doesn't go over the cliff the way he was supposed to. "That isn't what happened last week. He didn't get out of the cockadoody car!" And we have these German Expressionist poses. And that was the performance. Totally uninterpretable. Although in the film Mildred tries her damnedest to make something of it when put on the spot by Doris.

TNG: The ending of *MURDER and murder* is a kind of culmination of the interest in everyday life that began in your performance and dance work. It's a lovely, simple scene between these two women—they're eating chicken soup for dinner. To be honest, I didn't like the ending when I first read it in the script. It seemed clichéd in the wrong sense. I said to myself, "So they're eating a meal together and that's how this is going to end?!" But in the film it actually works beautifully. And it made me think of the endings of your other films. I've always loved the end of *Film About a Woman Who . . .* , with the words "You could always have an ocean ending" superimposed over an image of the ocean.

YR: It ends with text rather than image. The actual image of the ocean fades out before the printed text fades out.

TNG: That's an example of your slapstick modernism—calling attention to the conventions of film endings, but with a vaudeville wit.
   You're a gifted writer. In fact, I think of the script of *Journeys from Berlin* as a great piece of modernist writing. Do you think you might ever write a book?

YR: I keep toying with the idea of a memoir, but my memory's so selective and lousy. I don't remember enough.

TNG: But that's the point about memory and autobiography: they *are* selective. A past is only what and how you remember.

YR: But as someone reminded me recently, I've already written my autobiography in my films. I have to give the idea of a written memoir more thought, if for no other reason than that I don't want my films to be seen as autobiography.

TNG: I'd like to end by asking you not about history or recollection but about emotion. If you were going to attach an emotion to each of your films what would it be? For instance, *Lives of Performers*: what's the emotion?

YR: This is hard. OK, *Lives of Performers* is about infatuation.

TNG: *Film About a Women Who . . . ?*

YR: Rage.

TNG: *Kristina Talking Pictures?*

YR: Mourning.

TNG: *Journeys from Berlin?*

YR: That one's also about rage. Rage projected outward *and* internalized.

TNG: *The Man Who Envied Women?*

YR: Outrage.

TNG: (laughter) We're getting a theme here.

YR: I mean literally "out"—rage out.

TNG: *Privilege?*

YR: Ambivalence.

TNG: *MURDER and murder?*

YR: Love.

Odds and Ends

The following are excerpts from far-flung interviews not in-cluded in this collection, which, at the risk of redundancy, may cast more light on some prickly representational issues, such as "suspicion of narrative," "the gaze," and "the other." Although there are contra-dictions—for instance around the necessity (my own) for disrupting narrative—these particular bits reveal an evolution of sorts, if only through changes of emphasis and focus.

Quoted in a review of *Film About a Woman Who . . .* by Carol Wikarska in *Women & Film* 2, no. 7 (Summer 1975), p. 86

"I wanted to reveal some very painful realities which I had suffered through or had observed others suffering through; and I could not think of any presentation of these realities that surpasses the impact of the written form. I had experimented with language in dance. Now, in this film, I was faced with the problem of creating a continuity through image and text without encouraging the anticipation of a con-tinuous story, and yet not subverting the content of such a story which I wanted to reveal with as much clarity and nakedness as possible."

From an interview with Mitchell Rosenbaum, in *Persistence of Vision* no. 6 (summer 1988)

MR: Can you talk about what you do with the gaze in [*The Man Who Envied Women*]? You seem to have taken care of the male gaze in a twist on Buñuel's dual actresses in *That Obscure Object of Desire*.

YR: In the Buñuel the female characters become objects insofar as they are interchangeable for the male protagonist, who can't tell them apart.

In *The Man Who Envied Women* the male characters are interchangeable, thus becoming objects for the gaze of the audience but not for an
embodied female character. This seemed to me taking quite literally the
problematic of the image of the woman as the object of the controlling
male gaze [as elaborated by feminist film theorists]. Here, I removed
her physical presence totally while having two men play the same role.
But it then becomes unclear how the gaze operates. The strategy removes it from filmic narrative convention, and there's something going
on here that disproves a lot of this gaze stuff. The overheard heroine,
because she is unseen, cannot be said to be the object of a controlling
gaze internal to the film, but then neither is Jack Deller, though both
of them are objects of identification for the audience. This is a case
where the traditional axes of gaze, power, identification have been
skewed somewhat, allowing the female spectator a less ambivalent access to the image through the voice of the heroine. The male protagonist is not, however, objectified through a simple reversal of codes. His
"imaging" is constantly tempered by his powerful "discourses" and by
his monitoring and mastering behavior, in the metaphor of the head-
phones, for instance. He becomes an emblem and agent of patriarchal
abuse. His case, from a narrative standpoint, remains unresolved. He is
never brought "under control" as his cinematic "wild-woman" counterpart has traditionally been. That would have been too simplistic.

From an interview with David Laderman, *Art Papers* 13, no. 3
(May/June 1989), pp. 18–24

DL: I'm interested in what kind of role you see men playing in the feminist struggle in general or perhaps even in how they can be represented
in films.

YR: I think I'm facing the same problem in dealing with issues of
racism, as a white middle-class avatar, you might say, of cultural supremacy. You have to acknowledge your position of advantage, certainly. You can't, as Trinh Minh-ha says, speak for the other. You have
to speak "beside" the other . . . and you don't want a balancing act. After three years of struggling with a new script [*Privilege*], I realize that
it's a matter of foreground and background. Even where you have the
voice of the [female or nonwhite] "other"—from the point of view of a
man, a woman's voice; from my point of view, a black voice—that voice
can still be coopted or undermined by the position of the author, who
in my case is a white woman. At this point I see it as partly a topologi-

cal problem. What ends up being the predominant or uppermost voice? I think men have something to contribute to feminism in addition to lending support to women's efforts. I would be interested in men talking about their sexism. But it's tricky: does it end up being "poor me" or "us fellow victims"? [The Sunday *New York Times* column] "About Men" should be more about sexism.... There was one that fascinated me, about a man who went on a deep sea diving trip. When he was on the bottom he got a signal that he must come up immediately because something was wrong with the generator on the deck, and he had very little air left. Later, when he realized how close a call he'd had, he felt the most extreme contempt for his wife and children and his role as a father and husband. He couldn't understand it. Somehow the exhilaration of that brush with oblivion made him feel total contempt for his life as a man with obligations to women and children (that's the way I interpret it; he didn't put it that way). I thought that was an amazing confession and explains a lot about men's projects in the world, from war to various kinds of aggrandizement, from going to sea to going into space—a flight from women, even at the cost of their lives. He had no idea or theory about what had happened. When he told the story to friends, they said, "Oh, it was just an emotional reaction." The event was left up in the air. It was one of the most interesting and suggestive revelations in that column. Men's contributions to feminism might be anecdotes or analyses of experiences like that.

From an interview with Gabrielle Finane—after a screening of *Privilege*—Melbourne, September 1990

GF: I was struck by a question asked at the screening of the film, "Why do you always concern yourself with exposing the conditions of production of filmmaking and do you see yourself as progressing beyond it?"

YR: Right, "beyond" it as though it's a failing you have to overcome.

GF: And also the question suggests that you're doing it for simply antagonistic or contestational reasons. I'm interested in the positive conception of formal playfulness as opposed to the "negative" connotations of the deconstructive position, or are the two bound up together?

YR: It *is* fun; I find it pleasurable. That's my new tack. [laughs] And I would hope that it's also fun to watch. But there is, of course, a more serious justification that has to do with the fluidity of signifiers and disruption of fixed social positions. If narrative structure is an analogue for social hierarchy—and there has been much theorizing about this—then the disruption or messing around with narrative coherence has a positive function in pointing toward possibilities for a more fluid and open organization of social relations. This is, of course, an ongoing project, not at all subject to aesthetic fashion, not something you "get beyond," or "cross over" from, or rise above. You find ways to keep up the good fight, because it *is* a good fight, and continues to be worthwhile.

From an interview with Christianne Mennecke in Berlin during the Berlin Film Festival, January 1997

CM: Could you explain why you are suspicious of the narrative—or where the dangers are?

YR: Teresa de Lauretis and others have written definitively about this from a feminist perspective. For awhile I followed the arguments closely and was influenced by the critiques—particularly Laura Mulvey's "Visual Pleasure and Narrative Cinema"—which construed mainstream cinema as a vehicle for men to overcome female obstacles to their self-discovery, fear of castration, and attainment of manhood. These writings described the deployment of female figures in the noir and western genres as the creation of enigmas to be deciphered and controlled or of threatening landscapes to be traversed and possessed. And narrative structure, with its development, climax, and denouement, was in and of itself implicated. But subsequently I realized that there are all kinds of narratives, histories of marginalized or "disappeared" people who have not had a fair shot at being represented, and it seemed obvious that narrative structures can be used for both progressive and oppressive ends. Consequently, it is difficult, for me at least, to sustain a political critique of narrativity. Let me just say that I am interested in creating situations for different kinds of spectator engagement within a given film. And narrative is only one of these.

I find it odd that people who are otherwise sympathetic to avant-garde theater and film complain about my disruptions of narrative flow, especially in this last film [*MURDER and murder*]. It appears that the more I move toward fulfilling the spectator's desire for narrative by narratively expanding and developing the illusion of desire, the more disappointed some cinephiles will be when the character-driven story is replaced by print, commentary, or other nonnarrative modes of ad-

dress. As I attend more screenings of *MURDER and murder,* I'm finding at least one response of this sort in every audience. All I can say is
that if coherent and seamless narrative is the measure of a "real" or
"good" movie, then I don't, and never will, make real movies. "Good"
is another matter altogether.

. . . .

YR: Yes, individual consciousness is informed, produced by social institutions, but is also the instrument of both perpetuation of and challenge to institutions. Some of us manage to break out now and then
from the determinations of biology, gender, race, and class. The old na-
ture/nurture debate. We are not born conscious . . . and yet . . . and yet,
the infant seems to "know" an awful lot, and our endocrine systems
dictate some of our development into subjects and citizens.

A metaphor for this debate occurs at the beginning of *MURDER
and murder* when I first appear and say directly to the camera, "I'm the
director, Yvonne Rainer." If you have never seen me or a photo of me,
how do you know that that's Y.R.? It could be an impersonation. It so
happens that I, Yvonne Rainer, play this character called Yvonne
Rainer. And although it is almost incontrovertible that the mastectomy
scar revealed later on is "real," is it really Yvonne Rainer's? In a manner
of speaking, that is not me (like my girlfriend who denies that the Mildred character is "she." In fact, some of my monologues contain un-
truths, e.g., the reference to a sister: I don't have a sister.) I am playing
a part. That statement "I am . . ." is an act of performance; it's a kind
of trickery or play; there is a kind of parody of the notion of the truth
of film, at the same time establishing a credibility and an illusion of authenticity.

Why is it so important for me constantly to remind the audience—
via all kinds of strategies—that these apparitions on the screen are fab-
rications? Around 1985 I wrote, "Words are uttered but not possessed
by my performers." When I first started using more than one performer to play a given character—in *Film About a Woman Who* . . . two
women stand in for the "she"—it was more an aesthetic or formal
rather than political choice; mixing up the referents simply made things
more interesting and lively. Later I could say that detaching meaning
from the speaking subject was one way of forcing the spectator to deal
with issues in a broader social field rather than being vicariously swept
away on a tide of simulated individual experience. The visual decentering of the subject has a philosophical and historical origin in
poststructuralist writing, like Barthes's "Death of the Author," Fou-

cault's "What Is an Author?" and Julia Kristeva's work, which I was reading around 1980. The romantic notions of unified personhood and stable identity were under attack for the next decade. Kristeva's "subject-in-process" was especially appealing to feminists who were struggling to get out from under the tyranny of gender masquerade. With the advent of postcolonial writing, however, the focus of discussions shifted from gender to race, and there were wonderful films made about black experience, particularly those of Charles Burnett, Julie Dash, and Isaac Julien and the English black film cooperatives. . . .

An afterthought: From my earliest choreography, I never thought of my chosen medium as a vehicle for "self-expression." This was partly John Cage's influence; somewhere in my head I hear either him or Merce Cunningham saying, "If you want to express yourself, take up basket-weaving." Which subsequently made little sense, given Native American traditions and the cultural and social functions of basket weaving. But at the time I interpreted it to mean that of all the things in the world available to the artist, the self is only one inconsequential element. Of course, in terms of Cage's ethos, disposing of self-expression was key to the elimination of personal choice in art-making via aleatory methods of composition.

IV   The Horse's Mouth

Privilege

This script from the film (16 mm, color and black and white, 103 minutes, released in 1990) was previously published in *Screen Writings: Scripts and Texts by Independent Filmmakers,* edited by Scott Mac-Donald (Berkeley: University of California Press, 1995).

The following is a list of abbreviations used in this film script:

CU—close-up

LS—long shot

MCU—medium close-up

MOS—without sound

MS—medium shot

POV—point of view

sync—the visual image is synchronized with the soundtrack

v-o—voice-over

WS—wide shot

MCU, interview with FAITH RINGGOLD, *an African American woman in her late fifties.*

FAITH: The attitude is wrong . . . I mean, getting older . . . getting older is a bitch! *(She laughs uproariously.)*

MS, interview with SHIRLEY TRIEST, *a seventy-four-year-old white woman. She is seated at a diningroom table. Yvonne Rainer questions her from off-screen.*

285

YVONNE RAINER *(v-o):* Did you have any symptoms, like hot flashes?

SHIRLEY: No, nothing at all.

YVONNE R.: Then we have no story here.

SHIRLEY *(laughing):* Yes, we have no story here. I told you . . . the parts of me that work, work *very* well!

MS, interview with HELENE MOGLEN, *a white woman in her late fifties. She is seated in front of windows which look out on trees and distant hills.*

HELENE: Yes, I realize that one of the things that has made it so much of a positive experience for me is that my life is so very comfortable. So I have genuine alternatives now that I can take advantage of. And I think it would be very different if I didn't.

Film clip from TV movie Between Friends. *Elizabeth Taylor and Carol Burnett are drinking white wine in a fire-lit, well-furnished room.*

TAYLOR: Well, it's no big deal. It's no big deal for him. He doesn't have a uterus. Anyway, I don't want to go around uterusless.

BURNETT: Y'know, when you're over forty the whole apparatus seems to reorganize. Wouldn't y'know, after all these years I finally got my head together and my ass falls apart. *(They both laugh.)* Oh god, I'm going to *will* menopause away!

Cut to black velvet drapes. Audience applause is heard as YVONNE RAINER *enters and sits down in CU. She is a white woman in her mid-fifties. She removes her glasses and earrings, and then looks directly at the camera.*

Music begins: Chet Baker playing "My Funny Valentine" on the trumpet.

Intertitles appear on a word-processor screen.

PRIVILEGE

A Film by
Yvonne Rainer
and Many Others

with

ALICE SPIVAK
BLAIRE BARON
RICO ELIAS
GABRIELLA FARRAR
DAN BERKEY
and
special guest appearance by
NOVELLA NELSON

Cut to YVONNE R. *in front of black drapes. She picks up a large bottle of moisturizing lotion and holds it next to her face. Camera pulls back to Medium.*

Footage from an educational film on menopause: A white, middle-aged male DOCTOR, *sitting in a garden, addresses the camera.*

DOCTOR: In our counseling we emphasize the fact that even though the role of motherhood is over, the menopausal patient can now enter a new role as a wife and a woman, a role which needs redirection and reevaluation.

Footage from same film: Another white, middle-aged male DOCTOR *addresses the camera, from behind a desk.*

DOCTOR: I think we should not forget that our ultimate objective is to improve the relationship of the couple. Tragic though it may be, this is often the only chance that this couple will have to talk to a sympathetic and understanding third party. And the doctor may have a golden opportunity to improve the well-being of the couple as well as of the wife.

Intertitle:

Related materials on menopause are available from Ayerst Laboratories.

A series of titles follows in quick succession, delineating warnings, precautions, and possible adverse reactions as a consequence of undergoing estrogen replacement therapy.

YVONNE R. *reappears in front of black drapes.*

Music fades out.

She smears flaming red lipstick over her lips without regard for accuracy, then begins to read aloud:

YVONNE R. *(sync):* It's sort of appropriate that this is my last major, I think, public address here to talk to women, because I do believe that the future lies with us—in a very deep way. And one of the reasons I'm stopping is that I have to go away and work out how we do it, because *we've done nothing yet.* And, uh,

MS of CLAUDIA GREGORY, *an African-American woman signing in American Sign Language (ASL). She stands center-frame in front of the black drapes.* YVONNE R. *(still speaking in sync) appears in a small oval in the lower right corner.*

we talk all this equal rights, and we beg men for equal rights and we've achieved nothing. Like—I could say a rude word, I'm an Australian, but I won't say it. Fifty-two percent of us are women. And where is the proportional representation in the Congress? Like, *nowhere!* And it's not right. And you know whose fault it is? It's ours, because we are pathetic. We haven't got any guts. And I say this advisedly and with deep sorrow, and I'm one of you. And I haven't got any guts either. And do you know why I'm retiring? Because the men did me in. . . .

Intertitle:

PRIVILEGE

A Film by
Yvonne Washington
and Many Others

YVONNE WASHINGTON *(v-o):* I was bone tired. I had been careening around the country at a break-neck pace

Again cut to SIGNER *in front of black velours, signing the v-o.*

for too long. Even to *my* ears my lectures were beginning to sound like ranting and raving. I had been threatening to retire, so why didn't I stop beating my head against those would-be benefactors, those smug English-speakers charged by the nation with improving the plight of the deaf, while turning a deaf ear to the history of struggle by the community of signers.

YVONNE R. *reappears in lower right corner. ASL* SIGNER *continues to interpret center-frame.*

YVONNE R. *(sync):* OK, nuclear war. Every single town and city in your country is targeted with at least one bomb. All the nuclear power plants are targeted. If you drop a big bomb on a reactor, you can terminate permanently an area the size of West Germany. All military facilities are targeted; all universities participating in nuclear and military research, which is this one; all corporations making weapons, which is almost all the corporations now in the United States of America. So everything's targeted. Nuclear war will take about one hour to complete bilaterally. . . .

Intertitle:

Helen Caldicott, 1986

ASL SIGNER *reappears, still center-frame.* YVONNE R. *is gone.*

YVONNE W. *(v-o):* The deaf community has historically spurned the pathological model of its situation, favoring instead a social model: deaf signers have seen themselves not as deficient but as different, and what makes the difference is not their hearing loss but their ostracized language of signing, a language that has been actively banished for over a century by the hearing establishment concerned with the deaf. The long and short of *my* part in this story is that recently studies began to emerge showing that American Sign Language shares the complexity of patterning characteristic of spoken languages and therefore warrants the same kind of scientific examination. This meant that I could begin to relax in my advocacy. Besides, I needed a change. My own change-of-life pointed the way. I had gone into early menopause at the age of forty-five because I was so overworked and tired. Why not make a documentary film about menopause? I have medical training, so I was fairly up-to-date on the physiological effects of menopause and female aging. It was the dominant medical attitudes that needed exposure, the attitudes that tell us we are "deficient" and "diseased"—much like the deaf—only *our* "disease" begins when we can no longer make babies. Friends have asked me, whom would I be addressing? Menopause is a well-kept secret, something you don't want to know about unless you're a woman who is past her prime . . . over the hill . . . has seen better days . . .

CU of YVONNE R.*'s face center-frame. Her voice is muted behind that of*

YVONNE W. *(v-o):* . . . let herself go.

YVONNE R. *(sync):* Twenty-two percent of the children in this country live in poverty. . . . *Twenty-two percent!* Thirty-four million people live in poverty, and they are almost *all* women and children and black. Right? Fifteen million old women live on an amount of $5,000 a year or less—fifteen million old women in the richest country in the world! . . . So! what are we going to do, folks?

She is silent and looks at the camera.

YVONNE W. *(v-o):* Why do young women respond with such reluctance and dread? What do they fear?

Ten seconds pass.

Daytime. YVONNE WASHINGTON*'s apartment.* JENNY, *a white woman in her late fifties, is about to be interviewed by* YVONNE W. *(off-screen).*

JENNY *(v-o):* Where do you want me? Over here?

YVONNE W. *(v-o):* This is my workroom. Here, let me move this out of your way.

There is a blur of movement as YVONNE W. *in extreme CU crosses frame.* JENNY *sits down so that her face is in CU. The following dialogue is punctuated by three alternating images and two interwoven voices of* JENNY, *played by both Alice Spivak (*JENNY *#1 and #2) and Minnette Lehmann (*JENNY *#3).* JENNY *#1 has been shot in 16 mm;* JENNIES *#2 and #3 are transferred Video-8.* JENNY *#1 wears white pants and a gray cotton jacket over a black top.* JENNIES *#2 and #3 wear black leather jackets and bright red lipstick. If not otherwise noted, Alice Spivak's* JENNY *#1 is the speaker.*

JENNY: The problem with Caldicott is that she paralyzes us with horror rather than inspiring us to protest . . . (JENNY #2:) All that apocalypse and doom . . . *(She looks around.)* So Yvonne, what am I here for?

YVONNE W. *(v-o):* I thought I told you. I'm making a documentary about menopause.

JENNY: Menopause! Not *that* again. I thought you were going to interview me about my brilliant career *(laughs).*

Medical footage.

DOCTOR *(in garden):* Is her creative life over simply because she's reached the age of forty-five, or fifty, or fifty-five?

MCU, JENNY *in* YVONNE W.*'s apartment.*

YVONNE W. *(v-o):* Whaddya mean "Not that again?" Who's talking about it? Don't you know that menopause takes the prize for being the thing that the least number of people say they want to know anything about?

JENNY #2 *(speaking with* JENNY #3*'s voice):* Oh, it just seems like everytime

CU JENNY #3.

JENNY #3 *(sync):* I turn around I see an article on it somewhere.

YVONNE W. *(v-o):* Mostly in medical journals. In the mass media you don't hear about it that much. How about you? Did you have an easy time?

MCU JENNY #1.

JENNY: Not really. What kind of film are you making? If it's informational, I've done tons of research on the subject. *My* story's not that interesting. What you should do is start with what the word means. It's derived from the Greek and means "cessation of the month." And then you should go into the distortions that the doctors and shrinks have foisted on us. Like the psychoanalyst Helene Deutsch, (YVONNE R.'s *voice:)* that traitor to her sex, (JENNY:) who described menopause as "women's partial death: or the gynecologists who call it "a living decay" . . .

She continues to talk MOS.

DOCTOR *(v-o):* My present thinking is that the menopausal syndrome is a deficiency state analogous to hypothyroidism, in the sense that it can be treated, and treated effectively.

JENNY *(v-o):* . . . and then turned out to be in the pay of a couple of drug companies.

MS, JENNY #3, *who watches as* YVONNE W. *(off-screen) paces back and forth.*

JENNY *(v-o):* Let's face it, Yvonne, we live in a sexist culture that considers women old at an earlier age than men . . .

JENNY #3 *(with* JENNY #1's *voice):* Why are you so restless?

YVONNE W. *(v-o):* I hear you. And all of that will be in there. But what about you, Jenny? Did you have hot flashes?

MS, JENNY #1.

JENNY: Oh god did I have hot flashes!

YVONNE W.: For how long?

JENNY: Oh, it's been endless. And it's still going on. But we really do live in a culture that is terrified of aging. There's this poem by Eve Merriam:

During the following recitation, camera dollies to extreme left to reveal YVONNE W.*'s back as she stands leaning against the wall of books.*

Last night I dreamed of an old lover
I had not seen him in 40 years.
When I awoke
I saw him on the street
his hair was white,
his back stooped.
How could I say hello?
He would have puzzled all day
about who the young girl was
who smiled at him.
So I let him go on his way.

YVONNE W. *(moving out of frame to right):* That's nice. But Jenny, would you please tell me

YVONNE W. *sits down, back to camera, on a red Chesterfield couch in the foreground.* JENNY *is seated opposite her in the background.*

(sync): how long your hot flashes went on. Was it months, years, how long?

JENNY: *Five* years. It's been at least five years of that ridiculous sweating. I'm famous for suddenly throwing off half my clothes. But, Yvonne, really now, why talk about it? We'll just be reducing women to their biological processes all over again. Anatomy is destiny. When you're young they whistle at you, when you're middle-aged they treat you like a bunch of symptoms, and when you're old they ignore you.

YVONNE W. *(v-o):* They do, huh?

JENNY: Yeh. And besides . . . *(She continues to speak MOS)*

WOMAN'S VOICE *(from medical film):* I don't mind being middle-aged at all. I really don't.   .

JENNY *(sync):* But don't let me give you a hard time . . . Ask me as many silly questions as you want *(laughs)*. We go back a long way, Yvonne . . . and I probably owe you one, right?

YVONNE W.: Jenny, if you think you owe me something, that's fine with me. Frankly, you must know something I don't, or you have an unnecessarily guilty conscience. I have fond memories of dancing with you years ago and maybe we'll get into that later. But for now let's try and keep our personal history out of this, OK? First of all,

She gets up from couch and leaves frame-left. JENNY*'s gaze follows her movement.*

(v-o): when you talk about biology and "them," you're confusing biology with patriarchy. Just because some men invoke *our* biology for their own advantage doesn't mean *we* have to go along with them.

CU, JENNY #3.

JENNY #3: Keeping one's dignity as you enter menopause is like fighting city hall.

MCU, JENNY #2.

JENNY #2: Aren't you interested in my reminiscences about being a luscious young starry-eyed dancer in New York?

MCU, JENNY #1.

JENNY #1: I'm not trying to be funny. Aging has been such an emotional subject for me. No one ever told me how many hours of the day I'd spend mourning for . . . what? Myself? I don't know what . . . some part of me . . .

Interview with HELENE MOGLEN.

HELENE: That awareness of one's body, the sense of all kinds of things connected with one's girlhood and young womanhood. I think at that time it was very concerning for me. It's been quite astonishing to me since, though, how after my menopause was over how liberated I felt, and liberated I feel.

YVONNE R. *(v-o):* Liberated.

HELENE: I feel off the hook in all kinds of very surprising ways.

YVONNE R. *(v-o):* Such as?

HELENE: All of a sudden I feel like one of those wise women one read about in college in anthropology. I feel as though I've come into a special place, very free from needing to please other people in all kinds of ways.

MCU JENNY #2.

JENNY #2 *(yelling):* Why do you want to interview me? What about *black* women? Do you have any black women lined up? White women have been interviewing one another for years.

JENNY #1 *reaches for a low stool and places it beside her chair just in time to receive a tray (in CU) with coffee urn and cups brought in by* YVONNE W.*, whose response increases in volume as she draws closer to* JENNY.

YVONNE W. *(v-o):* Let me worry about that. Just because I'm African American doesn't mean I can't deal with anything but so-called "black" problems. Thanks . . . *(CU:* YVONNE*'s hands pouring coffee.)* Tell you what:

CU of YVONNE W. *holding a cup and saucer. Her face is on left edge of frame. Behind her, prominently centered, is a fancy CD player.*

YVONNE W. *(sync):* Let's do a trade-off. OK? If you tell me about your menopausal symptoms and your life as an aging

Very brief intertitle on word processor screen:

WHITE

woman, I'll listen to you talk about the period in your life when they whistled at you.

MCU, JENNY #2.

JENNY #2: Well! . . . Yeh, come to think of it. . . . Y'know, there's this incident—I know you'll be interested in—when I first came to New York and that I've never discussed with anybody. (JENNY #1:) In fact . . .

As she continues to talk, her voice fades out. She tears off her jacket, digs a fan out of her pocket, and briskly fans herself. Camera zooms in to CU, which goes out-of-focus and dissolves to

Daytime. A New York street lined with tenements. JENNY, *shot from behind, played by Alice Spivak and dressed the same as in the interview— white pants and black V-necked tee shirt—strides across the street past* CARLOS, *a tan Puerto Rican around thirty, and* STEW, *his African American friend, both of whom are seated on* CARLOS's *front stoop. A man walking in the opposite direction turns and whistles at* JENNY.

YVONNE W. *(v-o):* Hey! What's going on?

MCU of CARLOS *and* STEW.

CARLOS: There she goes, the new *blanquita.* I think she's a dancer or something.

STEW: She thinks her shit don't stink.

They both laugh and do a "low five." JENNY *enters her building, which is next door to* CARLOS's.

Hallway of JENNY's *building.* BRENDA, *a white woman around thirty, with short hair and dressed in men's pants and shirt, pokes her head out of the doorway of her apartment as* JENNY *walks by.*

Lotte Lenya's voice, singing "Mack the Knife" from The Threepenny

Opera, *floats from the interior of* BRENDA*'s apartment.*

BRENDA: Hey, ducks.

JENNY *(slowly turning):* You talking to me?

BRENDA: Yeh. Hi. You must be the kid who took over Jack Walton's apartment.

JENNY: Yes, I'm right over you.

BRENDA: Great. I'm . . .

Silence. They continue to talk MOS.

YVONNE W. *(v-o):* So what's her name?

JENNY *(v-o):* I can't remember.

YVONNE W. *(v-o):* Really! Why not?

JENNY *(v-o):* I don't know. I seem to have blotted it out somehow.

YVONNE W. *(v-o):* But we've got to call her something.

JENNY *(v-o):* OK, let's call her . . .

Jump-cut to a second take.

BRENDA: Great. I'm Brenda.

JENNY: I'm Jenny.

BRENDA: You want to stop by for a drink later?

Again the sound drops out though they continue to speak.

BRENDA *takes a few steps toward* JENNY, *who steps away. This is repeated, through the use of different takes, four times during the following v-o.*

YVONNE W.: What year did you say this was?

JENNY: '61, '62, somewhere around there.

YVONNE W.: But something's wrong here. It's *your* flashback . . .

JENNY: *Hot* flashback.

YVONNE W.: Whatever, and you look exactly the way you look now in 1989. You're even wearing the same clothes.

JENNY: So what? I can't be bothered trying to look the way I did then. And besides, I don't remember. Are you going to hold up this show for some expensive illusionism? Let's get on with it.

YVONNE W.: No one's going to believe this.

BRENDA *has by now entered her apartment and closed the door.* JENNY *walks down the hall away from the camera.*

BRENDA *'s livingroom later that same day.* JENNY *sits down in MCU on a black couch against overstuffed, tapestry-covered cushions. As the scene progresses other furniture can be seen: a wooden Eames chair, a black canvas-covered butterfly chair, a kidney-shaped coffee table on top of which are a* Life Magazine *and large turquoise bowl, a somewhat massive buffet/cabinet against a wall papered with a black-and-white photomural of bookshelves and books that covers most of the wall. Over the couch are three photos: a large print of the famous Andre Kertesz photo of a woman in black halter dress lying with limbs akimbo on a couch, and two small framed photos of Djuna Barnes and Virginia Woolf. During her opening lines* BRENDA *nervously changes chairs, finally settling in the wooden Eames opposite the couch.*

"Pirate Jenny," sung in German by Lotte Lenya, is heard in the background during most of the scene.

BRENDA: Have you met any of your neighbors yet? Lila is the great old dyke down the hall. She's a retired scenic designer who lives alone with her Yorkshire terrier. When I asked her, "Who's the sexy kid in the white ducks?" she told me you had moved into Jack's apartment.

Yeh, Jack and George split up, so Jack decided to move out to Hollywood to paint portraits of the stars . . .

JENNY: Yeh, he left this mural on the w . . .

BRENDA: They had a lot of nice things. Did they leave anything else?

JENNY: A 1910 toaster and a couple of lamps.

BRENDA: George will probably be coming around, just to get some salt rubbed in his wounds. I moved here two years ago to be near work. I'm a lab technician at Bellevue. The first decent job I've had. I'm only just beginning to get on my feet. I had huge debts. I don't have the apartment quite where I want it yet, but it's coming along. Do you like Lotte Lenya? What do you want to drink?

She jumps up and moves toward the buffet.

JENNY *(v-o):* Yes . . . uh . . .

CU tracking along top of buffet, revealing stack of records and miniature furniture, ending in BRENDA *'s hands putting ice and pouring vodka into glasses.*

I asked her about the Saturday night commotions that tore through the airshaft from the next building every weekend. In fact, the whole block sometimes had a carnivalesque air which I tried not to notice.

MS, JENNY *on couch.*

JENNY *(sync, sipping her drink):* Y'know, I don't own a pair of white ducks. Those were frontier pants.

"Deserie," a hit song from the late '50s, sung by The Charts, begins, and continues through the following two shots.

Daytime, WS of exterior of JENNY *'s and* CARLOS *'s buildings, followed by left-to-right tracking past exteriors of a tenement block. People saunter past and lounge on front stoops.*

"Deserie" ends.

Nighttime tracking—in opposite direction—of building facades. The street is now deserted.

A melange of sounds can be heard: sirens, laughter, screams, voices speaking a mixture of Spanish and English. When we are halfway down the block, "Deserie" fades up, continues until:

Four Hispanic male adolescents come into view, sitting on steps and mournfully monotoning:

> I'm satisfied.
> You're satisfied
> We're satisfied
> They're satisfied
> She's satisfied . . .

As camera zooms slowly toward them

their singing fades out and "Deserie" fades up. "Deserie" continues at lower volume as the following shot begins.

Night. Bedroom of JENNY's *apartment.* JENNY, *dressed in pale pink nightgown and blue-and-white striped bathrobe, is sitting up on a mattress that is on the floor. She is reading "The White Negro" and eating an apple. On the floor beside the bed are an alarm clock, lamp, phone, and small framed photo of Martha Graham performing in "Letter to the World."*

DIGNA's *voice, yelling in a mixture of Spanish and English from a neighboring apartment, begins to intrude on her consciousness.*

DIGNA *(v-o):* Help! Police! You mother fucker. Carlos! Don't touch me, man. Don't touch me . . .

DIGNA's *voice fades down.*

JENNY *returns to her reading.*

DIGNA's *voice becomes more strident.*

DIGNA *(v-o):* Police! Please help me. Help! He's killing me! . . .

JENNY *puts down her book and dials phone.*

JENNY: Brenda? Sorry to wake you. It's Jenny.

BRENDA *(v-o):* I'm awake. It's Carlos and Digna brawling again.

JENNY: Should we call the police?

BRENDA: Yeh, I guess it *is* more horrendous than usual.

Sounds of sirens, slamming cardoors, muffled voices.

BRENDA *(v-o):* There's the cops. Jesus, what a circus.

CU of JENNY *looking through Venetian blinds. Voices speaking in Spanish can be heard.*

DIGNA *(v-o):* He tried to kill me, that *cula Dios mio,* where are you taking me? Help, save me, *ayudame!*

DIGNA *in Bellevue. A Puerto Rican woman in her late twenties, she is wearing a blue-and-white seersucker hospital robe. She sits in front of a peeling, yellowed wall and addresses the camera in Spanish, which is translated in English subtitles.*

DIGNA: Victorian doctors used to say, "Religion and moral principles alone give strength to the female mind. When these are weakened or removed by disease, the subterranean fires become active, and the crater gives forth smoke and flame." *(She laughs)* Today religion and moral principles have been replaced by thorazine for the control of the female mind, especially the Latina female mind. Tell me, why are Puerto Rican women in this country more vulnerable to mental illness than the general population? Why do we not flourish here? Psychiatrists have different names for our condition. Most of you would be labeled manic-depressive. Me they call schizophrenic. The head honcho here asked me to name the presidents of the U.S., beginning with the current one and working backwards. Of course, he refused to speak Spanish. So I named a few presidents: Kennedy, Eisenhower, Truman, Roosevelt. Then I got stuck. And guess what. *He* finished the job. He went all the way back to Lincoln. He was very proud of himself. Imagine! A history lesson from the head shrink of Bellevue Hospital.

Daytime. CARLOS *and* STEW *seated on steps as before.* STEW *'s body is bisected by the right edge of frame.* CARLOS *addresses the camera mainly in English. When he speaks in Spanish, English subtitles appear.*

CARLOS: I was born in Fajardo, Puerto Rico, *un cariduro.*

STEW *(leaning into center):* Yeh, a hick.

CARLOS *(in Spanish):* None of us chooses the situation we are born into, not the time, the place, or the color we come in. *(in English):* I happen to be what my countrymen call *trigueño,* meaning that I was born with the same permanent tan the beautiful people spend millions to maintain. You know, racially speaking, being a Puerto Rican in New York City is totally different from the way we look at ourselves in Puerto Rico. Here we're caught between white and black. Here your skin color determines who you are. Not only are there no gradations, but if you look white but have a black Mama, you're still considered black. In Puerto Rico you'd be white. Here skin color precedes other kinds of identification. In Puerto Rico there are a lot more classifications than white or black skin. Besides color, there's class, facial features, and texture of hair. There are the *blancos,* for instance. My two brothers, my sister, and my mother are all *blancos.* Then there are the *indios,* or the Indians; the *morenos,* who are dark skinned with a variety of features, both Negroid and Caucasian; *negros,* who are like U.S. blacks. And there's the term *trigueño.* In Puerto Rico a black can become a *trigueño* by achieving economic status or becoming a friend. And he hasn't physically changed and isn't seeking escape from identification as a *negro. Hola!* Brenda, *qué tal?*

CARLOS *gets up and leaves frame. Cut to* BRENDA *'s back as she strides toward* JENNY *'s building.* CARLOS *darts in front of her, blocking her way.*

CARLOS: Do you know the cops took Digna away last night?

BRENDA: So that's what happened. Where is she now?

CARLOS: They took her to Bellevue.

BRENDA: Why her? It sounded like you were killing her.

CARLOS: Oh no, no. I didn't touch her. She was real drunk and jealous. We had a fight and she went *loca*. You work at Bellevue, don't you? Maybe you can get her out.

BRENDA: She's probably in the psychiatric ward. I don't know anyone there. I work in the laboratory. I don't think I can help you, but I'll think about it.

She goes into her building. CARLOS *shakes his head in a bemused way. Cut to MS of* STEW *still seated next door.* CARLOS *enters frame and sits down. He again addresses the camera. His Spanish is rendered in English subtitles.*

CARLOS *(in Spanish):* Like an angel of love, yes? She is my freedom and my bondage. Forbidden to me. Also her building—forbidden to me. Right next door, but I can't live there. It might as well be Sutton Place . . . *(in English):* The intermingled white, black, and tan world of Puerto Rico is foreign to people in the U.S. Puerto Rico is inhabited by people of many colors, and these colors are not associated with different ranks. My friend Stew was always riding me:

STEW: "You fuckin' yeller-faced bastard! Yuh goddamned Negro with a white man's itch! Y'all think that bein' Porto Rican lets you off the hook? Tha's the trouble. Too damn many you black Porto Ricans got yer eyes closed. Too many goddamned Negroes all over this god-damned world feels like you does. Jus' 'cause you kin rattle off some different kinda language don' change your skin one bit. Whatta y'all think? That the only niggers in the world are in this fucked-up country? They is all over this whole damn world. Man, if they's any black people up on the moon talkin' that moon talk, they is still Negroes. Git it? Negroes!"

Intertitle on word processor screen.

Piri Thomas, 1967

YVONNE WASHINGTON's *apartment as before.* JENNY *is still in the* "*hot seat.*"

YVONNE W. *(v-o):* What are you doing now, Jenny?

JENNY: "What am I doing now?" What're *you* doing now? Why are you interrupting my flashback? *You* know what I do. I drift.

YVONNE W.: Well, I mean, how do you support yourself?

CU: JENNY #2 *heaves a deep sigh.*

JENNY #1: I live on the remains of my parents' failed farming venture in the '30s. They sold off everything but a tiny wedge of land that—lucky for me—turned into a corner of a major intersection in southern California. So now it's leased to a Burger King. And me, a vegetarian . . . Y'know, it's funny. I had everything. Affordable housing; recognition in my profession; more than adequate income; the most unpressured teaching job you could imagine. I was so much better off on the whole than most of my artist friends. And I gave it all up. Or almost all of it. It was as though I wanted to do more than just retire; I wanted to throw it all away.

YVONNE W.: Everything but the Burger King. You say you drift . . . what do you mean? You're obviously not a bag lady.

JENNY: Well, in a manner of speaking I *am* a bag lady.

MS of desk with word processor. On the wall hang two large framed photos, each one a portrait of a young black girl. During the following monologue the camera scans the space around and under the desk. A cat licks itself. A suitcase, then a trash bag with blanket sticking out, can be seen under the table. When JENNY *herself finally comes into view again, her speech is way out of sync.*

(v-o): About a year ago I gave up the idea of a permanent address and decided to live a little dangerously. You have to sniff the wind more carefully, know when you've used up your welcome, especially when you're staying with family members. Not everybody is intrigued with my silences and obscure pieces of information. Do *you* want to know

that in the lifespan of the average white American there are twenty-three different sexual partners?

YVONNE W.: No kidding!

JENNY *(on camera, but out-of-sync):* Yeh. How many have you had? I've had thirty-two. Ha! I've had more colds than that. And who wants to know that Natalie Herzen spent the greater part of the year of revolution 1848 in a dangerous paroxysm of erotic excitement? *(sync):* And *this* ought to interest you: After menopause women don't have REM sleep anymore. What d'you think of that?

YVONNE W.: REM. You mean "rapid eye movement"?

Black-and-white footage of JENNY *"fleeing" as she looks behind her with a terrified expression on her face. Camera tracks from left to right, following her movement. In back of her is* BRENDA's *living room.* JENNY *and* YVONNE W. *are now both speaking in v-o.*

JENNY: Yeh, what happens in the first couple of hours after going to bed when you dream and have the most restful and deepest sleep. We don't get that kind of repose anymore. And we no longer dream. No wonder we're all so cranky.

YVONNE W.: I don't believe it.

JENNY: What?

YVONNE W.: That older people don't dream. *I* still dream.

Black-and-white footage. Two young black men are perusing the front page of the New York Times *"Help Wanted" section, which is pinned to the wall. As the camera tilts down and dollies back, we see first a sign:*

LOST:
MEMORY
MUSCLE
FRIENDS
HUSBANDS

LOVERS
DREAMING

then two young black women in bed. They are sleeping, entwined in each other's arms.

Why, just last night I had the weirdest dream.

JENNY: I've always known you're an exceptional woman. I'll bet men dream till the day they die. *I* sure as hell don't. And while I'm on the subject of loss, I could talk about lots more of that, like memory . . . but where were we?

The woman on the left suddenly sits up, a startled look on her face.

Reverse angle, her point of view reveals JENNY, *standing as though on the foot of the bed, returning the younger woman's gaze.*

YVONNE W.: Menopause.

Another reverse to the younger woman, still looking intently up at JENNY.

menopause.

JENNY: Ah yes: A week after Brenda had spoken to Carlos on the street . . .

DIGNA *as before, in Bellevue, in front of the peeling wall. She addresses the camera in English.*

DIGNA: Yeh. Why me and not Carlos? Why me beat up and why me in here? Victorian doctors used to make fine distinctions of complexion, spinal curve, and personality between those women who were merely assaulted and those who were actually murdered. Just like they distinguished between criminals and normal people. Would you ever dream that criminals and prostitutes have darker hair than you? How about my eyebrows? Does the way I tweeze my eyebrows make men unable to resist hitting me? And are my rages at Carlos more irrational than his violence toward me? I was no more out of control that night than he was. I just *acted* like a crazy woman. *(She pauses.)* "Peter Piker picked a pep of pickled peckers, how many pecks . . ." *(She breaks up, laughing.)* The latest development in proving women are biologically more prone to nuttiness than men is this test: They have you say this tongue-twister when you have your period and also when you don't have your period:

"Peter Pecker picked a pack of pickled . . ." Ha, ha, ha . . . I'm not menstruating and I still can't do it!

Nighttime. JENNY*'s bedroom. She is sleeping. A woman's screams propel her upright. She freezes. In the following sequence, all of the shots of* JENNY*'s bedroom are in color while those of* BRENDA*'s bedroom are in black and white.*

Nighttime. BRENDA*'s bedroom.* BRENDA *rolls over, turns on her bedside lamp and recoils in horror as she sees* CARLOS *standing stark naked beside the bed.*

BRENDA: *Jesus K. Christ!* What are *you* doing here?!

MS, CARLOS. *He moves toward her.*

(v-o): Oh no,

BRENDA *scrambles to the foot of the bed and throws him a bathrobe that is lying there.*

(sync): no you don't. Back off. Hold it right there. Here, put this on.

Reverse angle: CARLOS *receiving the tossed bathrobe.*

CARLOS: You're so beautiful.

MS, BRENDA *with* CARLOS*'s shoulder in the foreground.*

BRENDA: Oh sure. And you're so naked. Who the fuck asked you, anyway?!

She continues speaking MOS. Screams are heard, obviously not emanating from the on-screen BRENDA. *They continue into the next shot.*

JENNY*'s bedroom. CU of her bare feet pacing back and forth beside her bed. Camera follows her as she sits on bed and dials phone.*

BRENDA*'s bedroom. MCU of* BRENDA *as before.*

BRENDA: Oh sure. And you're so naked. Who the fuck asked you anyway?!

She goes to closet and takes a robe off of hook, glaring at CARLOS *as she puts it on. We see his back and also his reflection in a full-length mirror.*

Look, I'm going to make some coffee and we're going to talk this thing through. Just who do you think you are? You've got absolutely no right barging in here like this.

JENNY *(v-o):* Operator, could you get the police?

JENNY*'s bedroom. MCU of* JENNY *on the phone.*

(sync): My neighbor's in trouble. I think someone's broken in downstairs . . .

Energetic violins from the educational film lead into:

A succession of five white middle-aged male doctors from the medical film, all of whom address the camera. Each is identified by name in a subtitle. The first shot begins with a CU of an Impressionist-like painting of a field of flowers. Camera zooms back to reveal DOCTOR *in his white coat behind a desk.*

CHARLES F. FLOWERS, JR.: It's not an easy matter to treat the menopausal patient, because she's undergoing certain physical changes.

Same DOCTOR, *different scene.*

Women who are in their middle years and are premenopausal or menopausal have certain problems.

CHARLES W. LLOYD: And in the woman in the climacteric the relationship between endocrine changes and emotional stress is often quite obvious.

JUDD MARMOR: The way she faces up to these problems has an important bearing on what her menopause will be like.

ROBERT N. RUTHERFORD: The man's understanding and sympathy are particularly crucial at this time in a woman's life.

MS, interview with MINNETTE LEHMANN, *a white woman in her late fifties. She is seated at her kitchen table.*

MINNETTE: There's an assumption, there's a real assumption that what you're going to get is real.

YVONNE R. *(v-o):* What I get on here may not be the real, but your experience will be real.

MINNETTE: That's true.

YVONNE R. *(v-o):* Yeh, there is something real I'm after. For instance, how old are you?

MINNETTE: Oh, that's terribly real . . . Oh . . . forty-nine.

YVONNE R. *(v-o):* Alright . . . uh, you're lying!

MINNETTE *(laughing):* Well that's possible, isn't it?

YVONNE R. *(v-o):* OK, this is not going to be a real interview.

MINNETTE: But I'm menopaused, I am definitely menopaused. Not even menopausal. I'm menopaused.

YVONNE W.*'s apartment. CU of* JENNY, *who is smoking a cigarette.*

JENNY: The hot flashes began in my early fifties. They were really bad. Every ten minutes I would be drenched in sweat and then I'd be horribly cold. It was worse at night.

YVONNE W. *(v-o):* Did you try Vitamin E?

JENNY *(v-o):* Aah, Vitamin E didn't help a bit. I went to the doctor and he wanted to do a hysterectomy. He said he would take out everything but my playground.

YVONNE W.: Playground! What a hip gynecologist!

JENNY: Oh sure. *I* was horrified. Anyway, it was an offer I could and did refuse.

Intertitles on word processor:

> No one knows exactly what causes hot flashes. One reason is that scientists have been unable to detect hot flashes in animals. No middle-aged monkey is revealing her secrets.

> The intervals lengthen on my menstrual calendar: "28 days, 27 days, 30 days" is now giving way to "54, 76, 92, . . ." The dependability of seasons is replaced by . . .

Footage from medical film: A middle-aged WOMAN *in sheath dress and beehive hairdo sits at desk in an office. She speaks—MOS—to the camera.*

JENNY *(v-o):* About a year later my periods stopped. The hot flashes continued, but now I had pains in my vagina and pulling sensations there. The doctor said I had atrophic vaginitis and wanted to prescribe estrogen replacement therapy. I didn't like his attitude. He was barely civil,

WOMAN *in office gets up and moves to the left. Camera tracks with her as she goes to a coffee machine and pours a cup of coffee, all the while addressing the camera MOS. The following intertitle is superimposed over her image during this maneuver:*

> The most remarkable thing was the silence that emanated from friends and family regarding the details of my single middle age. When I was younger, my sex life had been the object of all kinds of questioning, from prurient curiosity to solicitous concern. Now that I did not appear to be looking for a man, the state of my desires seemed of no interest to anyone.

Intertitle fades out. WOMAN *continues addressing the camera MOS.*

JENNY *(v-o):* . . . very offhanded and unsympathetic. I went to another doctor,

Dissolve to DOCTOR *in garden.*

DR. JUDD MARMOR *(sync):* Under these emotional stresses she is likely to show emotional changes.

JENNY *(v-o):* who got annoyed at my questions.

MARMOR *(sync):* She tends to withdraw from her husband . . .

JENNY *(v-o):* By that time I was taking a very small dose of estrogen . . .

MARMOR *(sync):* . . . irritability . . .

JENNY *(v-o):* . . . and synthetic progesterone.

MARMOR *(sync):* . . . fretfulness . . .

JENNY *(v-o):* But the pains continued.

MARMOR *(out-of-sync):* . . . crying spells . . .

JENNY *(v-o):* I couldn't have sex . . .

MARMOR *(out-of-sync):* . . . insomnia . . .

JENNY *(v-o):* . . . and I was conscious of that area all the time.

Interview with MINNETTE *in her kitchen.*

MARMOR *(v-o):* . . . and so forth.

MINNETTE: . . . and it would be anger, or I'd have to say, "Now you're getting just a little excited, more than usual. What is this?" And it was physiologic.

YVONNE R. *(v-o):* That's probably what's happening to me. I was always kind of irritable. Now I'm even more irritable.

MINNETTE: I've always been irritable too. I'm now much less irritable.

YVONNE R.: Now that you're out of it.

MINNETTE: I mean, but less irritable than ever. And that is a delight. Not that I can't *get* irritable, but I was on edge a lot.

Interview with JENNY *in* YVONNE W.*'s apartment. She is seen over* YVONNE W.*'s shoulder in the foreground.*

JENNY: I'm off hormones now. I got scared off because they couldn't tell me about the future. One doctor told me, "You're too emotional. If you weren't so emotional, you'd be better off."

MCU. Interview with CATHERINE ENGLISH ROBINSON *in her living room. She is an African American in her late fifties.*

CATHERINE: Male gynecologists don't give you too much information. They would refer you to a book, but they're not able to sit and talk to you. And you have a lot of questions. You don't know what to expect; you hear a lot of stories. So you want someone to kind of talk to you, tell you what to look forward to and what is a symptom of menopause and what is not. And I guess maybe they can't give you the information because they don't know. They know medical theory. But none of them have been through it or have it to look forward to. So I feel there's a gap there.

MCU, interview with JENNY *in* YVONNE W.*'s apartment.*
Her voice is slowed down and deep.

JENNY: Yvonne, do you realize what you've unleashed? I hate going on about my goddamned body

Jump cut to panning movement from her body to the word processor on the table beside her chair. The titles on the screen scroll simultaneously with JENNY*'s v-o.*

like this. The good feminist in me wags a finger at my belly-aching. "Jenny, all you're doing is confirming what men already think, that our bodies are, by definition, defective and need fixing."

Intertitles on word processor:

> All of a sudden she didn't know how to dress. The body had filled out in this funny way. Her weight was the same but her shape had changed. Exercise didn't make the same dents anymore. And when she wore lipstick she looked like a transvestite. Then the veins and the swollen ankles . . . and the breast biopsies. And she couldn't even *stand* in anything but flat heels anymore, let alone walk. Raging hormones? What about those raging floods when your periods are phasing out? You bloody up everything.

JENNY *(in normal v-o):* So the medics try to "fix" us with hysterectomies and hormone replacement therapy so we'll stay feminine forever.

Hallway of JENNY*'s building.* JENNY *comes down stairs at far end and* *walks toward camera and* BRENDA*'s door. She is wearing her bathrobe.*

A woman's screams are heard.

Intertitles on word processor:

> By age 50, 31% of U.S. women will have had a hysterectomy.
>
> Hysterectomy is the most frequently performed operation in the U.S., double the rate of frequency in the U.K.
>
> Hysterectomies are performed most frequently in the southeast U.S. and least often in the northeast, and garner $800 million a year in gynecological fees.
>
> There is a popular saying among gynecologists that there is no ovary so healthy that it is not better removed, and no testes so diseased that they should not be left intact.

Screams are heard while the last intertitle is still up.

Hallway as before, JENNY *again walks down stairs and this time reaches* BRENDA*'s door, where she pauses, then retreats and pauses at another door halfway down the hall.*

JENNY *(v-o):* Has anyone ever suggested putting men on lifelong doses of testosterone in order to make them stay "masculine"? Why is the aging process perceived as so much more threatening to *women's* sexuality than to men's,

MCU of JENNY *inclining her ear to door.*

MAN'S VOICE: What we don't know won't hurt us.

Footage from medical film. A man enters DR. RUTHERFORD'*s office, shakes hands with him across desk. Both sit down.*

JENNY *(v-o):* . . . when in actuality it's the men who have more difficulties in bed later in life.

RUTHERFORD *(v-o):* We find out that his wife's emotional problems may be related to this particularly trying period.

MS of DR. RUTHERFORD *over shoulder of* HUSBAND. *He speaks MOS.*

JENNY *(v-o):* Yet they retain for themselves the myth and masquerade of virile masculinity long after women are seen as having shut down.

CU of HUSBAND.

Energetic orchestral strings accompany the following v-o.

DR. MARMOR *(v-o):* The glow from estrogen may no longer be apparent. Moreover, her libido

MCU MINNETTE LEHMANN *in her kitchen as before. She speaks MOS.*

may begin to decline at this time.

MINNETTE *(sync):* Once sexuality isn't physical, it doesn't mean it isn't. It's weird, I know, but I like to be in a room full of testosterone, no doubt about it.

YVONNE R. *(v-o):* You know, women produce testosterone.

MINNETTE: I know, the whole crowd does. And I like that. I can feel it. And I can feel when I'm in situations that are libidinousless, or without sexuality, and they're just as repressive as they ever were.

Intertitles on word processor:

> What happens to the libido? Her beloved GYN answered some questions: "Yes, testosterone, the male sex hor-

mone, is produced by women, and—yes—testosterone production increases somewhat after menopause. However, since the libido is in the head as much as in the hormones, the exact role testosterone plays in female sexuality is unclear."

. . . But, if not testosterone, something besides her head was making her think about sex all the time.

YVONNE W.'s *apartment. MCU of* JENNY.

JENNY: Y'know, I hate to admit it, but I just can't get used to our screwed-up

Found color footage from a 1950s Hollywood movie: a group of adolescents is partying. A girl in very tight pants and top is "boogying" by herself.

morality that denies middle-aged women the right to be beautiful, loving, and idealized by men.

YVONNE W. *(v-o):* Idealized! You mean, like young women? That's what got us into this mess in the first place!

Hallway outside of BRENDA'*s apartment.* JENNY *stands outside of* BRENDA'*s door as the screaming continues.*

BRENDA *(v-o):* Help! Police! He-e-lp!

Nighttime. Very wide black-and-white overhead shot of BRENDA'*s living-room, now revealed as a set in a very large space. Crew members stand around, while production assistants work in the hall area.* BRENDA *leans against the wall next to the buffet.* STEW *is seated on sofa next to* WHITE MAN X, *who speaks what* STEW, *"the ventriloquist," mouths. In the course of the speech, the camera cranes in to CU of* STEW. *The two men gradually switch roles, so that by the end, it is* STEW *who is speaking, and* X *is silent. (For the remainder of the film, all of the scenes in* BRENDA'*s apartment are in black and white.)*

WHITE MAN X: Yes, I became a rapist. To refine my technique and modus operandi, I started out by practicing on black girls in the ghetto—in the black ghetto where dark and vicious deeds appear not as aberrations or deviations from the norm—and when I considered myself smooth enough I crossed the tracks and sought out white prey.

X AND STEW: Rape was an insurrectionary act. It delighted me that I was defying and trampling upon the white man's law, upon his system of values.

STEW: and that I was defiling his women, and this point, I believe, was the most satisfying to me because I was very resentful over the historical fact of how the white man has used the black woman. I felt I was getting revenge. And I wanted to send waves of consternation *(CU of* STEW*)* through the whole white race. After I returned to prison I took a long look at myself and, for the first time in my life admitted . . .

His words fade down behind those of YVONNE W.

YVONNE W. *(v-o):* Jenny, why are you telling me all this? I don't need to hear how Eldridge Cleaver raped to save the black race! He made a much bigger contribution than inflaming white paranoia.

MS of BRENDA *leaning against the wall, her arms folded across her chest.*

BRENDA: The problem with men is their dignity is located in their balls.

MCU of CARLOS *seated on the couch.*

CARLOS: *guffaws.*

MS of BRENDA. *She moves toward the camera, turns away, then turns back, passing through "noirish" shadows along the way.*

BRENDA: You think I'm dying for it, don't you? Next you'll be telling me I want to be raped. But you don't know a damn thing about me. Can you even conceive that I might have *liked* you if . . .

CU of BRENDA*'s back as she sits down in the foreground in the Eames chair. It faces the couch on which* CARLOS *is seated in MCU. He stares intently at her, not speaking, as camera zooms slowly in to extreme CU of his face during the following v-o.*

CARLOS *(v-o):* She has an avid curiosity about my sexual endowments. She enjoys imagining the fucking that goes on among blacks and Latinos on this block. She thinks we are "looser" and less inhibited because we come from the steaming tropics. What's weird is *she's* the one who kept her shades up and walked around with no clothes on.

CARLOS *(sync):* When you look at me you see a dark continent, something unknown, exciting, frightening, exotic, different.

MS of BRENDA *rocking back and forth in a child's rocking chair.*

BRENDA: Hey, I'm supposed to be the dark continent. Freud called women a dark continent. And when you look at me the word lesbian might never have been invented. Now you listen, you doctor

Series of right-to-left swish-pans that ends in MCU of WHITE MAN X *seated on the couch.*

BRENDA *(v-o):* lawyer Indian chief, you engineer ayatollah shudder in the loins, you landlord Lenny Bruce chairman of the board, you . . .

Her voice fades down.

YVONNE W. *(v-o):* So who is this dude? This is all very confusing.

JENNY *(v-o):* I'm just trying to point out that rapists come in all colors.

YVONNE W. *(v-o): Thank* you, ma'am. *Thank* you!

BRENDA*'s voice fades up.*

BRENDA *(v-o):* . . . you engineer ayatollah shudder in the loins, you landlord Lenny Bruce chairman of the board, you party chairman, chief justice, raving queen, you gang of chancellors.

CU of BRENDA *in the rocking chair, rocking furiously.*

(sync): you head of sanitation.

Reverse-angle two-shot of BRENDA *and* WHITE MAN X. *He is seated on the right, holding a miniature coffee cup and saucer. At the beginning of the scene she pours coffee from an urn. A large projection of an aerial view of mid-Manhattan fills half the background. In the dimly lit recesses beyond the set, people move about performing tasks of some kind.*

BRENDA: As man conquers the world so too he conquers the female. You're no different from Genghis Khan, one of the first guys to make a direct connection between manhood, achievement, conquest, and rape.

Extreme CU of BRENDA *in profile.*

BRENDA: Man equals human, hero, the active principle of culture, the establisher of distinction, the social being, the mythical subject.

Extreme CU of X *in profile.*

BRENDA *(v-o):* Woman equals immutable matter, procreative earth, landscape, monster, Sphinx, Medusa, Sleeping Beauty, inert obstacle to his transformative striving.

Brief, sequential shots of FAITH, SHIRLEY, JENNY, VIVIAN BON- NANO *(a Hispanic woman in her mid-forties),* CLAUDIA, *another woman from the medical film,* AUDREY GOODFRIEND *(a white woman in her late sixties), and* GLORIA SPARROW *(a white woman in her mid- fifties). All of the women speak MOS.*

BRENDA *(v-o):* As women we are trained to be rape victims. At an early age we hear the whispers: *girls get raped.* Not boys. Every three min- utes a woman is beaten. Every five minutes a woman is raped. Every ten minutes a little girl is molested. Half of all rape victims are total strangers to their attackers.

MS, GLORIA SPARROW *sitting in a backyard.*

Another 30 percent are slightly acquainted. The statistics are silent on rape by husbands.

WOMAN'S VOICE: I can't believe that, Gloria!

GLORIA *(sync):* Why? What do you mean?

WOMAN'S VOICE: You were your father's darling!

Intertitle on word processor, simultaneous with its utterance in v-o by BRENDA:

> One out of every four
> women in the U.S. is
> introduced to sex
> through rape.

BRENDA *(v-o):* Most rapists don't have as political a motive for their acts as you have. Most rapists are of the same race as their victims.

Intertitle:

> 95% of rapes are
> black-on-black or
> white-on-white.

MCU, overhead. STEW *and* BRENDA *lie on the floor with their heads toward the camera.* BRENDA *rests on one elbow.*

BRENDA: Do you think it matters to the victim what the motive is? Sadism or politics? And anyway, I don't think you're as special as you make out. Your politics smacks of sadism like all the rest.

Screams are heard.

Color. Corridor as before. A man and woman in bathrobes now stand with JENNY *outside of* BRENDA's *door.*

Black-and-white MCU of CARLOS *seated on couch in* BRENDA's *living-room.*

CARLOS: The black man among his own in the twentieth century does not know at what moment his inferiority comes into being through the other. In talking about this problem with black friends, together we protested, we asserted the equality of all men in the world. And then the occasion arose when I had to look into the white man's eyes. An unfamiliar weight burdened me.

Daytime panorama. (This and the following shots in the park are in color.) On the far side of a pond a WHITE MAN IN BERMUDA SHORTS *stands watching his three dogs cavort at the water's edge.*

CARLOS *(v-o):* The real world challenged my claims. In the white world the man of color encounters difficulties in the development of his bodily schema. Consciousness of the body is solely a negating activity. It is a third-person consciousness. . . .

MLS, CARLOS *sitting and smoking on a park bench. A* WHITE MAN IN A SUIT *and carrying a briefcase walks by.* CARLOS *continues to speak in v-o.*

provided for me by the other, the white man, who had woven me out of a thousand details, anecdotes, stories.

LS, edge of pond. A PREGNANT WHITE WOMAN *in a white summer dress is throwing breadcrumbs to off-screen ducks while a* FIVE-YEAR-OLD GIRL *beside her blows bubbles with a bottle and wire loop. The* BUSINESSMAN *from the previous shot walks down the path behind them and out of the frame.* CARLOS*'s v-o continues. At the beginning of the shot the* WOMAN *points to something off-screen.*

"Look, a Negro!" It was an external stimulus that flicked over me as I passed by. I made a tight smile.

Cut to ANOTHER WHITE MAN, *walking his dog down a path. Camera follows them as they pass the* MOTHER *and* CHILD *by the lake, stays on* MOTHER *and* CHILD *as* MAN *and dog leave the frame.*

"Look, a Negro!" It was true. It amused me. "Look, a Negro!" The circle was drawing a bit tighter. I made no secret of my amusement

. . .

CU of CHILD *blowing bubbles.*

"Mama, see the Negro. I'm frightened."

MLS, CARLOS *on bench.*

CARLOS *(sync):* Frightened! Frightened! Now they were beginning to be afraid of me. I made up my mind to laugh myself to tears, but laughter had become impossible. I could no longer laugh, because I already knew that there were legends, stories, history.

Black-and-white CU of CARLOS *on* BRENDA*'s sofa. Camera zooms in to CU during following v-o.*

CARLOS *(v-o):* I moved toward the other . . . and the evanescent other, hostile but not opaque, transparent, not there, disappeared.

Black (no) image.

Nausea . . .

CARLOS *on park bench as before.*

(sync): I was responsible at the same time for my body, for my race, for my ancestors. I subjected myself to an objective examination, I discovered my blackness, my ethnic characteristics, and I was battered down by tom-toms,

A 1940s cartoon of Florida alligator menacing a black infant.

(v-o): slave-ships, cannibalism, intellectual deficiency, fetishism, racial defects, and above all else, above all: "Sho' good eatin'." On that day,

MCU, CARLOS *on park bench, smoking.*

(v-o): completely dislocated, unable to be abroad with the other, the white man, who unmercifully imprisoned me, I took myself far off from my own presence, far indeed, and made myself an object. But I did not want this revision, this . . . this thematization. All I wanted

was to be a man among other men. I wanted to come lithe and young into a world that was ours and to help to build it together.

Intertitle on word processor (simultaneous with its uttered v-o):

I wanted to come
lithe and young into a
world that was ours
and to help to build it
together.
Frantz Fanon, 1940

Daytime, street, CU of DIGNA. *She is wearing a summer dress and addresses the camera in English. The neighborhood ambience is extremely noisy.*

DIGNA: Many people back home tell you how wonderful life is here. There's television and the movies; they give another impression. Anyway, I never been glamorous or anything like that, and when Carlos proposed, I couldn't believe it. I saw a chance to get away, to see what was going on in other places, to live in New York, another kind of life. At home it was always so easy; with the sound of the first rooster crowing, I would open my eyes and start the day. I see the morning mist settling like puffs of smoke over the range of mountains that surrounds the entire countryside. Sharp mountainous peaks covered with many shades of green foliage that change constantly from light to dark, intense or soft tones, depending on the time of day and the direction of the rays of the brilliant tropical sun.

As camera begins to zoom back, we see that she is leaning against a blue 1960s convertible.

I take the path following the road that leads to my village. I inhale the sweet and spicy fragrance of the flower gardens that sprinkle the countryside. The country folk in every mountain village on the island of Puerto Rico pride themselves on their flower gardens.

A new voice is heard: It is DIGNA*'s off-screen voice, which slowly begins to override her on-screen voice. The street sounds—children's voices, traffic,* *horns—that had previously all but drowned her out, slowly recede, replaced by the "idyllic" quiet of her new voice.*

Oh, Papi's flower garden! There were bright yellows, scarlet and crimson hues, brilliant blues, wild purples; every color imaginable flourished on the plants and shrubbery that blossomed in my father's flower garden. I feel the soft, cool, gentle morning breeze as I stand by the road and dig my bare feet into the dark moist earth.

Intertitle on word processor:

Nicholasa Mohr, 1988

MS, black and white. BRENDA *on her couch. She is silent for about ten seconds.*

BRENDA: *Damn!* Why'd you have to say I'm beautiful? I don't need that kind of stuff from the likes of you.

The face of YVONNE RAINER *enters the frame, in CU, her mouth smeared with lipstick as at beginning of film. She addresses the camera and then leaves frame.*

YVONNE R.: She is the kind of woman who was never desired by men.

STEW: Hasn't anyone ever told you that before?

BRENDA: No *man* has told me that.

Reverse angle, MCU of STEW *in wing chair. Behind him is the studio space cluttered with lights and equipment.*

STEW: They should have.

BRENDA *(v-o):* It just doesn't matter to me what men think of my looks.

STEW: Then why'd you bring it up?

MS, BRENDA.

BRENDA: *Women* find me beautiful. That's what matters to me. But why am I even talking to you about this? *(She leans forward and speaks in an intense whisper.)* Your desire has always been the death of us.

STEW *(v-o):* Eldridge Cleaver said:

Reverse angle, MCU STEW.

(sync): "If a lesbian is anything she is a frigid woman, a frozen cunt, with a warp and a crack in the sky-high wall of her ice. She is allured and tortured by the secret intuitive knowledge that the walking phallus, symbol of the Supermasculine Menial, can blaze through the wall of her ice, plumb her psychic depths, melt the iceberg in her brain, detonate the bomb of her orgasm, and bring her sweet release. (In case you're wondering, that phallus is me.)"

MS, BRENDA, *laughing hysterically.*

Reverse, STEW, *also laughing.*

BRENDA *(v-o):* You're putting me on.

STEW: Maybe, maybe not.

YVONNE W. *(v-o):* Jenny, you're not going to let him get away with that, are you?

MCU of BRENDA.

BRENDA: Venus, ever since they knocked
        your block off
        your face is so vacant
        waiting to be moved in on
        by men's imaginations.
        How could anybody love you?
        having the ugliest mug in the world,

Corridor as before (color). JENNY *stands with outstretched arms as though holding up the walls of the narrow passage. There are now five (white) people in bathrobes behind her.*

the one that's missing.

Almost immediately camera tracks left-to-right into apartment (image changes from color to black and white), rhyming its movement with CAR-LOS*'s as—left-to-right—he backs* BRENDA *"up against the wall," pushing her swiftly and somewhat roughly across the thirty-foot width of the space. This happens repeatedly, sometimes in MCU, sometimes in CU, alternating slow motion and normal speed.*

BRENDA *(v-o):* Is it time to invoke the mothers who held us—or refused to hold us? Or is it time to name the common enemy? Our blackness, femaleness, shit, and blood dictate the moves of white men.

(sync): By the age of four the white man knows what the score is.

(v-o): By then the universe is radically split along lines of goodness and badness. In both, what is good is pure, clean and white and what is bad is

(sync): impure, dirty, smelly, and black.

(v-o): What is good in the world comes from the mind and what is bad comes from the body. In the culture of the West, the necessity for the white male infant to repudiate both his magical preoccupation with shit and his fantasized oneness with the mother create

(sync): the dual aversion to blacks and women.

(v-o): In contrast with the light color of the body of the Caucasian, the dark color of feces reinforces the connotation of blackness with badness. And since this dark brown color is derived from blood pigments, since in fact blood is the only internal bodily substance which is dark,

(sync): you the black, and I, the female,

(v-o): share the stigma imbedded in ideas of shit and blood, with their

MS, JENNY *in* YVONNE W.*'s apartment.*

JENNY (*speaking with* BRENDA*'s voice*): association of blackness, evil, danger,

CARLOS *slams* BRENDA *against the wall in slow-motion with a resounding crash. Her lip movements mime the final words.*

(v-o): and worthlessness.

MS, JENNY *in* YVONNE W.*'s apartment.*

YVONNE W. *(v-o):* What an obnoxious idea!

JENNY: What's obnoxious?

YVONNE W. *enters the frame and sits down on couch in the foreground, her back to the camera.*

YVONNE W. *(sync):* How shit gets connected with blackness-as-badness. What happens between black people and *their* shit?

JENNY: But she's clearly talking about the racist conditioning of *white* people in the *West.*

YVONNE W.: I didn't hear anything about *people* in there. It was white *men* she was dishing the shit to. And even so, your shit theory doesn't tell us when and how this particular alienation took hold.

She lies down, disappearing into the couch, only her Converse-clad feet visible frame-right. Immediately the camera begins to track left, arcing around the end of the couch to bring YVONNE W.*'s head into view toward the end of the following monologue.*

Did you know that racism didn't exist before Columbus stumbled upon North America? Before Europeans began to think about expanding their empire they didn't have notions of racial—or genetic—superiority. Religious superiority, maybe, like what propelled the Crusades, but not genetic. They had fantasies of wealthy black kingdoms somewhere in the East Indies, and, in their minds, these kingdoms were culturally superior to their own. It wasn't until they needed cheap labor to extract wealth from their colonies that they had to justify economic exploitation in terms of racial superiority. Before the era of European empire there was always a fluid assimilation between conqueror and conquered. Alexander the Great and Genghis Khan may have been sexists, but they weren't racists. It's capitalism, pure and simple, that's given us racism. So much for shit.

She pauses, then suddenly sits up, framed in CU.

But what's *your* investment in this psychoanalytic stuff? I won't go so far as to say it's total rubbish, but I do think it occupies much too big a place in your story.

MCU, JENNY.

JENNY: I guess I'm attracted to it because it's so elemental. Alimentary. *(laughs)* It holds out the promise of an ultimate explanation for racism, its earliest formation in the human psyche. I dunno, it gives me a much greater feeling of power and understanding than your historical, economic explanations.

Camera tilts down and tracks toward couch, revealing along the way an inert form lying on the floor under crumpled newspapers, finally settling in MCU on YVONNE W. *by the time she's saying "You've put the egg . . ."*

YVONNE W. *(v-o):* But the psyche itself is the product of external forces, like history and economics. Economics is the greatest single factor that *produces* the psyche, like homelessness pushes people over the edge into madness. Economic relations *reproduce* the family interactions that in turn incubate the psyche. *(sync):* You've put the egg before the chicken. And another thing: You've let Brenda off the hook.

JENNY: What d'you mean?

YVONNE W.: You've let her make this dubious alliance with Carlos against white men through the common stigma of their dark bodily secretions, and she does this without once implicating *herself* in the racist system. White women always manage to use their own victim status as a way of pleading innocent to the charge of racism, but *she's* enjoying life in that exclusive white building right along with you.

So please, get your ass back in that apartment. You have more work to do!

MCU, JENNY.

JENNY: No-o-o! I can't. I just can't. I'll only fall deeper into the soup.

YVONNE W *(v-o):* Hey, that's a new note: self-pity.

JENNY: Don't expect me to get it right. Just telling you this story in its barest form took all of my gumption. I'm scared of you now in ways I never was before.

MCU YVONNE W.

YVONNE W.: I don't expect you to "get it right." I guess I'd just like you to put yourself in my shoes so I don't have to explain everything. *I'd* like to forget about racism just as much as you. The difference is, you can . . . and I can't.

Series of intertitles on word processor screen begins:

WHO SPEAKS?
QUOTIDIAN
FRAGMENTS:
RACE

Music begins: Amelia's aria, Scene 1, Act 1, from Verdi's Simon Boccanegra. *It is a very scratchy recording.*

I

During my 1940s childhood my mother hired a series of black cleaning women who came once a week to clean the house. Mary Ellen would carefully cut the crusts from the sandwiches that my mother prepared for her lunch and leave them on the plate. Mama, who never allowed us to leave food on our plates, thought Mary Ellen was "putting on airs." Submerged in feelings of social inferiority, my mother knew the state of things all too well. If her own position of white, lower-middle-class housewife was implacably fixed, what right had the black cleaning-woman to mime the upper crust?

2

One day during my first year in high school I was taking the bus home from school. A black woman who had sat down beside me watched as I leafed through the pages of a *National Geographic*. As I paused at a color photograph of an African man dressed in traditional warrior garb, the woman remarked, "What a handsome man." Her simple utterance was a revelation to me. This was my first encounter with self-hood from a black perspective, with a black person's sense of being-in-the-world. Here was no strange, alien creature. Here was a handsome man.

3

In my early 30's I was in an intensive care unit after passing the critical stage of a serious illness. Theresa, the Puerto Rican day nurse, was trying to haul me out of bed and into a chair for the first time. I was so weak my legs wouldn't support me. As she struggled, I felt an inexplicable contempt for her. Some days later, after I had been transferred to a ward, my neighbor in the adjacent bed spoke admiringly of Theresa. When she had been in intensive care, Theresa had cared for her "like an angel."

4

Roy Wilkins said somewhere that the most he could ever hope to be was a permanent recovering sexist. Is "permanent recovering racists" the most *we* can ever be?

5

A woman who is just entering menopause meets a man at a conference at the University of El Paso. They hit it off. Later, after hearing his lascivious remarks about a much younger woman, she is shocked at having misinterpreted what she had thought was mutual sexual attraction. Toward evening, from the hilltop heights of the university, a Mexican-American student points out to her the sprawling shanties of Juarez across the Rio Grande. In the gathering dusk she realizes she is on two different sides of two frontiers: Economically, she is on the advantaged side overlooking a third-world country. And sexually, having passed the frontier of attractiveness to men, she is now on the *other* side of privilege.

Night. ROBERT*'s bedroom (color).* ROBERT *sits on the edge of the bed, his bare back to the camera. He is wearing only his pants and, as the scene begins, we hear the thud of his shoes hitting the floor.*

YVONNE W. *(v-o):* Who the hell is that?

Camera keeps him in frame as he bends over JENNY*, who is under the covers. They embrace passionately.*

JENNY *(v-o):* That's me, silly. Don't you recognize me?

YVONNE W.: Oh for Chrissake, not you—*him!*

JENNY: Oh! That's Robert, the assistant D.A. who handled the case.

YVONNE W.: What case?

JENNY: Brenda pressed charges against Carlos for attempted rape.

Hallway outside BRENDA'*s apartment.* JENNY *pounds on* BRENDA'*s door.*

JENNY *(in her best basso profundo):* OK. Open up in there. This is the cops!

The door opens and JENNY *pulls a terrified* BRENDA *out of the apartment.*

Daytime. ROBERT'*s office (color).* ROBERT *and* BRENDA *sit on either side of his well-appointed desk. He is in his early thirties, tall and imposing though not conventionally handsome, impeccably suited, very self-assured. At the beginning of the scene he lights a cigarette with an elegant lighter. He is very much in command, but not overtly patronizing.* BRENDA *too is self-possessed, not at all nervous, even when describing her frightening experience. In the establishing shot of the scene the camera dollies from wide to MCU of* ROBERT.

ROBERT *(after a long, leisurely exhalation):* And then what happened?

MS of BRENDA *over* ROBERT'*s right shoulder. As she speaks, camera dollies right-to-left behind him, ending with* BRENDA *seen over his left shoulder. An American flag can be glimpsed in the background.*

BRENDA: Something woke me up. I didn't know what, I was half asleep and reached over and turned on the light. And there you were, standing beside the bed, bare-assed naked. I started to scream. Maybe I yelled "Get out of here." I'm not sure. And you said—and I'm not sure of the sequence—"You're very beautiful. I want to talk to you. Don't be afraid." It all went very fast. I kept yelling. My bed is wedged in a corner of the room, so I couldn't get out. You were blocking my way. Then you hit me very hard on my left breast. It must have been then that Jenny rang the bell. You immediately ran into the kitchen and must have crawled back across the airshaft into your apartment. All I could think of was getting out of there.

The phone rings.

MCU ROBERT. *He sits dumbfounded, staring at her for a few moments before answering the phone.*

ROBERT: Excuse me. Yes? . . . Yes . . . Great. That's all we need to know. Let's throw the book at him. He'll never do his filthy act in this town again. *(He hangs up.)* Now, you've said that you had spoken to him previously in the street. How many days or weeks before the assault had this taken place?

MCU of BRENDA *over* ROBERT'*s left shoulder. Camera begins to track clockwise in a half circle, panning, in the process, from* BRENDA *to members of the crew, who sit immobile in the shadows off-set, finally settling on* ROBERT. *He is listening intently, his cigarette burning down to a butt.*

BRENDA: Wearing my voluminous flannel nightgown, I knelt before the small wood-burning stove, trying to see why the fire was so fragile. I felt huge and awkward in that position, aware of my rump and falling breasts, but the cold night air demanded that the fire be encouraged to burn at a brisker pace. My younger lover, small and tight in her body, sat on the couch watching me. I did not like what I thought she saw. I did not like the bigness of my ass, the weight of my body on my knees, and then just as I worked very hard to accept my lack of appeal, she said in a low firm voice, "You look very fuckable that way."

I froze, caught in that moment of self-hatred by the clarity of her desire. I stopped all movement, awed once again by the possibilities of life. I knew she was walking toward me. I felt her stand behind me, felt her hands shape my nightgown to my curves. I heard her breath come quicker, and still I did not move. She grew impatient and reached under the gown, piling up its lengths on her arm like a fisherman pulling in his nets, and then against all my fear, she entered me. The fire blazed up, and so did my hope as I finally left the burden behind me and rode her hand with all the grace love had ever given me.

ROBERT *is transfixed, showing no reaction until his cigarette burns his fingers, at which point he hastily stubs it out in the ashtray.*

Intertitle on word processor:

Joan Nestle, 1987

CU of ROBERT'*s hand stubbing out cigarette.*

JENNY *(v-o):* He called me in as a witness for the prosecution. The defense attorney was a real schmuck.

Courtroom (color). JENNY *is on the witness stand, being cross-examined by the defense. The mise-en-scène is indicated only by an encircling spotlight on* JENNY *and the direction of her gaze as she addresses the* DEFENSE AT-TORNEY *(downward, frame left) and the* JUDGE *(upward, frame right). On the wall behind her is a large photo of W.C. Fields before a judge.*

DEFENSE *(v-o):* Miss Doe, do you live in an apartment?

JENNY *(sync):* Yes, I do.

DEFENSE: What floor is your apartment on, Miss Doe?

JENNY: The second floor.

DEFENSE: Do your windows face the street, Miss Doe?

JENNY: Yes.

DEFENSE: Can people on the street see you when you are at your windows, Miss Doe?

JENNY: I suppose so.

DEFENSE: Yes or no, Miss Doe.

JENNY: Yes, I suppose so.

DEFENSE: Miss Doe, did you at any time prior to the incident you have described ever have occasion to appear at your windows?

JENNY: What do you mean?

DEFENSE: I mean just what I said, Miss Doe.

JENNY: Well, what does that have to do with anything?

JUDGE: Please answer the question.

JENNY: Sometimes I look out of my windows and sometimes I wash my windows.

DEFENSE: And what did you wear when you washed your windows, Miss Doe?

JENNY: For heaven's sake, what difference does it make?

JUDGE: The witness will kindly answer the questions as asked, without commentary.

JENNY: I wore clothes.

DEFENSE: What I am asking, Miss Doe, is, were you ever in a state of incomplete attire when you washed your windows? In other words, were you indecently dressed?

JENNY: No, I was not indecently dressed.

DEFENSE: What were you wearing, Miss Doe?

JENNY: I was wearing . . .

YVONNE W.'s *apartment. MCU,* JENNY. *She is seated in the "interviewee's chair," wearing a shocking-pink, off-the-shoulder, see-through dress. The lighting is hot and garish.*

JENNY *(v-o):* a dress!

(sync): There's this Lenny Bruce schtick: After his performance at a club in a small midwestern city, a middle-aged couple invited him to have a drink with them at their table. As Bruce put it, "The woman was wearing one of them see-through dresses, only ya don't wanna."

ROBERT*'s bedroom as before.* ROBERT *and* JENNY *are fucking, "spoon-fashion," on their sides. At the beginning of the shot* ROBERT *is having an orgasm. It is hard to tell what* JENNY *is experiencing.*

JENNY *(v-o):* So what do I do now that men have stopped looking at me? I'm like a fish thrown back into the sea, still longing to be hooked. Women like me never get used to it. It's hard to admit that I still want them to look. Don't think I'm proud of having been a woman that men look at. It's a chronic disease that you never get over.

ROBERT *rolls over on his back. Clutching the blanket around herself,* JENNY *sits up and addresses the camera. The effect is slightly ludicrous, but also touching.*

JENNY *(sync):* My biggest shock in reaching middle age was the realization that men's desire for me was the linchpin of my identity.

Interview with JENNY *as before. She is dressed as at the beginning of the film.*

JENNY: Suddenly the things you used to do and didn't even know you were doing don't seem to work anymore. Is my smile so different now? Maybe my smile has been dampened by my sweaty palms. Did you ever shake someone's hand when you were in the middle of a hot flash?

YVONNE W. *(v-o):* Are you going to finish the story?

JENNY: Which story—the race story or the change-of-life story? And now we have yet another possibility: the class story. Yvonne, don't tell me you're getting fed up with menopause already?

YVONNE W.: No, of course not. But now that you've got me

Clip from the climax of Tiger Shark *(Howard Hawks, 1932), printed backwards: the thirty seconds or so in which Edward G. Robinson has fallen into the water and is rescued from a shark's attack.*

hooked, I'd like to know how your flashback turned out.

JENNY *(v-o):* Well, there's not much more to tell. I was so pissed at the defense attorney that I perjured myself and said I saw Carlos in Brenda's apartment. The truth was that I couldn't possibly have seen him from the hallway, and we didn't go back into the apartment until the police showed up a few minutes later, so by that time, if he had been in there, he would've had plenty of time to escape. Carlos was sentenced to three or four months in jail and disappeared from the neighborhood. The assistant D.A. asked me out on a date, and we embarked on a six-month love affair. It was great while it lasted. The upper middle class was a total turn-on for me. I wouldn't have admitted it then, but . . .

Daytime. WS, DIGNA, *now dressed as Carmen Miranda, in a red, white, and black tiered, ruffled dress and a turban full of fruit, still leans against the blue convertible.* JENNY *and* ROBERT *enter frame-left.* JENNY *is wearing her "interview clothes."* ROBERT *wears a navy blazer, white shirt, and paisley silk ascot. He opens the car door for* JENNY, *then goes around to the driver's side and gets in. In this and the following scenes, they are totally oblivious to* DIGNA's *presence.* DIGNA *continues to address the camera, in English.*

DIGNA: She never saw Carlos again and she never saw me at all. Not like her mother, who was an intuitive expert on class, Jenny took her own social status for granted. Which meant pretty much ignoring it. Social distinctions were invisible to her, as I was invisible to her. Jenny was such a dummy when it came to class, a *tabula rasa,* unable to recognize, much less examine, her own blind spots.

ROBERT *starts the car.* DIGNA *hoists herself into the back seat and continues to speak as the car pulls out of the frame.*

Like the limits of social mobility. Her father was a house painter and she didn't go to college.

MCU of JENNY *and* ROBERT *in the front seat of the convertible. They are having a gay old time as she stuffs blueberries into his mouth as he drives and he tries to bite her fingers. Their hilarity is all MOS.* DIGNA *addresses the camera over their shoulders from the back seat.*

DIGNA: But why should I concern myself with *her*? Ordinarily I'm not an envious person, but here is this big fine car right in front of my house. What was I to think? Should I want to take her place in the rich man's car? Jenny thought she was free and unencumbered by such things. She wouldn't have admitted to being impressed by Robert's Harvard education, elegant manners, and professional status. How could she predict that not recognizing her own social disadvantage would be her undoing? Jenny was no Emma Bovary. Oh yes, so much fun, all this *(she gestures).* There is more that distinguishes the upper from the lower classes than bread crusts left on a plate. The number of heart attacks, for instance: *(pointing to* ROBERT*).* He is much less likely to die from a heart attack after making love than Carlos. A coca-colonial diet doesn't lead to long life expectancy . . .

ROBERT *and* JENNY *break up in (sync) laughter.*

Reverse angle. The camera is now located behind the car. We can see that the car is being towed by a truck, in the back of which sit the DIRECTOR, ASSISTANT DIRECTOR, SOUND RECORDIST, SCRIPT SUPERVISOR, *and* ASSISTANT CAMERAMAN. DIGNA *twists around in the back seat and again addresses the camera.*

DIGNA: . . . This country has the highest infant mortality rate in the industrialized world. Some people's stories have premature endings. Jenny's tale is no exception. Her disappearance from Robert's story will happen almost as quickly as Carlos's exit from hers. You'll see: Robert will get tired of her drunken displays of affection at social gatherings, and six months from now he'll dump her. But don't worry. I won't allow myself to be disappeared from Jenny's life like Carlos and Brenda. I'm going to hang around.

Music begins: Chet Baker singing "My Funny Valentine."

Succession of shots. ROBERT *and* JENNY *in a restaurant;* J *modeling a ball gown in front of* R *and then running to sit on his lap.* R *and* J *dancing,* R *and* J *in bed.* DIGNA —*in her summer dress*—"*hangs around*" *in every shot, watching.*

JENNY *(v-o):* To Robert I must have represented some kind of kooky Bohemian plaything. He was still sowing his wild oats and fancying himself an occasional *artiste*. He had an easel set up in his duplex with a permanently unfinished oil painting on it.

Chet Baker's voice surges up: "*You are my favorite work of art,*" *then subsides to background.*

We did things I've never done before or since. He took me to a charity ball at the Waldorf Astoria in his mother's mink stole after picking out a ball gown for me. Such *haute bourgeoisie* shenanigans made me ignore things that have since come back to haunt me.

DIGNA *is now sitting with her legs propped on* ROBERT'*s bed, smoking and looking off-screen (toward the head of the bed) in a contemplative mood. Camera pans along bed and comes to rest on* JENNY *and* ROBERT, *who is nuzzling her neck affectionately.*

YVONNE W. *(v-o):* "Oat bourgeoisie"? Is there something called "Wild Oat bourgeoisie"?

JENNY *(v-o) (laughing):* No, no, no. "h-a-u-t-e," *high* bourgeoisie. You know what I mean.

Daytime. JENNY *and* ROBERT *walk down a street in the Village toward the camera.* DIGNA *accompanies them.* ROBERT'*s gaze follows a young woman who has crossed their path.*

ROBERT: You know something?

CU of ROBERT.

You can always tell how a woman feels about herself just by looking at her legs.

Camera pans in CU to JENNY *and* DIGNA. JENNY *looks blankly at the camera;* DIGNA *looks from the off-screen woman to* JENNY'*s face.*

LENNY BRUCE'S VOICE: Really weird . . .

Interior of a nightclub. CU of ROBERT'*s hands playing with keys on a red-and-white checked tablecloth.*

> . . . OK, "an accident victim who lost a foot in an accident, who made sexual advances to a nurse while in an ambulance taking him to the hospital."

His voice fades to background.

Camera zooms out to reveal JENNY *and* ROBERT *laughing while watching the off-screen* LENNY BRUCE. DIGNA *is sitting at their table, dressed as in preceding scene. It is dark and smoky.* DIGNA *addresses the camera, in English.*

DIGNA: Jenny shut up like a clam.

BRUCE'S VOICE: There's a big difference between men and ladies.

His voice fades to background.

DIGNA: Isn't it amazing? All the ways in which we agree to inferior status in our daily lives. She made no objection, *not even to herself.* She didn't even ask herself the question: Must a woman's feelings about her *self* depend on a man's assessment of her *body?* The doors of her thought-storage tanks clanged shut. In total abjection, she handed over the keys.

LENNY BRUCE'S VOICE: Guys can detach and ladies can't.

MS, clip of LENNY BRUCE *performing.*

BRUCE *(sync):* A lady can't go through a plate glass window and go to bed with you ten seconds later. When they don't feel good they don't feel good. But *guys* can have head-on collisions with Greyhound buses, disaster areas, fifty people lying dead on the highway. On the way to the hospital in the ambulance the guy makes a play for the nurse.

MS, ROBERT, JENNY, DIGNA *as before.* R *and* J *explode in laughter, along with general audience laughter.* DIGNA *looks "meaningfully" at the camera.*

BRUCE *(v-o):* She goes, "How could you do a thing like that?" "I got hot." "You got hot!" How could he get hot, his foot was cut off? "I got horny, I dunno."

BRUCE *performing, as before.*

(sync): You don't understand where they're going. The appellate court's going to look at this: "Can you make any sense of this?" "Shit, no." And there's a difference, you know, between

He turns to the wall and pantomimes drawing on a black board.

a big piece of art with a little shit in the middle, a big piece of art, a little shit in the middle, a big piece of art. Then a big piece of shit with a little art in the middle . . .

His voice fades to background.

JENNY *(v-o):* Robert's office would subsequently mount a legal vendetta against Bruce after we broke up. I could hardly believe it when I read about it in the *New York Post.* They became Lenny Bruce's East Coast scourge.

YVONNE W. *(v-o):* What did you talk about when you were together?

JENNY *(v-o):* Art, movies, the usual New York cultural things. The *New York Times* art reviews of John Canaday. I took him to far-out music and dance events. All I remember of our conversations are some remarks about blacks and lesbians.

YVONNE W. *(v-o):* What kinds of remarks?

YVONNE W. *'s apartment, MCU* JENNY *in the "hot seat."*

JENNY *(sync):* Remember that '50s sociologist . . . what's 'is name? . . .

YVONNE W. *(v-o):* Reisman?

JENNY: No . . . Shockley! William Shockley.

YVONNE W.: Oh no, not that nutty physicist!

JENNY: Yeh, his theories about race and congenitally inferior intelligence were going around. I remember Robert arguing that Negroes *are* different; they have longer arms than whites.

They both laugh.

JENNY: Another time he said he had figured out that Brenda was a lesbian because she didn't lower her eyes when she uttered the word "breast."

CU of her face. She demonstrates lowering her eyes as she says:

"He hit me across the breast." A straight woman would have been more modest.

YVONNE W. *(v-o):* How could you put up with him? Didn't you protest?

JENNY: Oh god, let's get back to menopause, shall we? I've told this whole story hoping to find an answer to that very question. Who was that woman who put up with such vicious twaddle? If I argued, I didn't argue very hard. Being loved by him was more important than anything else. I was ready to sell my soul for a mess of pottage . . . a mass of penis. Yvonne, really, this is too painful. Why don't *you* try it? Y'know, I think it's about time we changed places. You've been behind that camera too long, gloating at my discomfort.

YVONNE W.: I haven't been gloating.

JENNY: You've been lurking. I'm tired of being your whipping boy. C'mon, get your ass out from behind that camera. It's your turn to be in the hot seat.

Camera zooms out as she gets up and leaves frame. We see only the empty chair and bookshelves as sounds of a tussle are heard, along with giggles, squeals, and shrieks from both of them.

YVONNE W.: No! No! No! No!

CU and MCU, hand-held camera. They fight it out over and around the leather couch. It is a kind of good-natured charade, not too serious, but very physical. During the tussle a few words can be heard.

YVONNE W.: What do you want from me? Absolution?!

JENNY: Who has the Macintosh and the CD . . . VCR . . . CAPITAL!

YVONNE W.: CAPITAL?! And who has the Burger King?!

CU of CATHERINE ROBINSON, *a middle-aged African American woman.*

CATHERINE: Well, we're traveling, which is something that we both like to do. What gives me pleasure? Going out to eat and not having to cook. Truthfully and selfishly, my youngest son has just finished his first year in college, so he was away all winter, and I just enjoy having the house to my husband and I after cooking for a big family. To shop for two, to cook for two, to have to wash dishes for two: *That's* an enjoyment for me. I'm enjoying—you know—this period of just he and I. You know, you love your children, you enjoy them, but then, now the rest of this life is for *me.*

MCU of YVONNE W. *sitting in the chair vacated by* JENNY.

YVONNE W.: Jenny, there's one thing I'm curious about. Did you ever make it with Brenda?

JENNY *(v-o):* Hell no, I was terrified of women.

Numerous shots of the "wrap party." All of the actors and crew, and some of the interviewees are present in shifting combinations and groupings.

Undifferentiated cacophony of voices is heard, which lasts throughout the credit sequence that follows.

Credits rise from bottom of frame.

Jenny	Alice Spivak
Yvonne Washington	Novella Nelson
Brenda	Blaire Baron
Carlos	Rico Elias
Digna	Gabriella Farrar
Stew	Tyrone Wilson
Robert	Dan Berkey
Signer	Claudia Gregory
"Helen Caldicott"	Yvonne Rainer
White Man	
in Brenda's apartment	Mark Niebuhr
Jenny's double	Minnette Lehmann

Interviewees
(in order of appearance)
Faith Ringgold
Shirley Triest
Helene Moglen
Minnette Lehmann
Catherine English Robinson
Evelyn Cunningham
Gloria Sparrow
Audrey Goodfriend
Vivian Bonnano

Doctors
(in order of appearance)
Judd Marmor
Charles W. Lloyd
Charles F. Flowers, Jr.
Robert N. Rutherford
Judith Weisz

Two-shot from medical film: DR. LLOYD *and a woman who is identified in a subtitle as* DR. JUDITH WEISZ. *They are seated at a conference table.*

LLOYD: Judith, it looks as though we're making a lot of progress. It looks as though the rights of women to be first-class citizens are coming along pretty fast. What's this going to mean to us?

CU of DR. WEISZ.

WEISZ: There is a danger that while abandoning the old stereotype, we replace it with a new one. That is, the woman who may be perhaps married, without children, not married who devoted a great deal of her energies to developing a career and fulfilling herself outside her home, who comes to you at menopause and then, the stereotype would be trying to attribute her problems to, say, her regrets about not fulfilling her basic biological role,

MS, interview with EVELYN CUNNINGHAM, *a seventy-year-old African American woman, in her apartment.*

whatever that may be.

EVELYN: Children? No, never had children. Never particularly wanted children, I'm very happy to report. I say that because for many years, you know, one could not say "I don't want children." That was a no-no. I feel so good now to freely say I never wanted children. I never wanted the responsibility.

YVONNE R. *(v-o):* Yeh, when you're young it's embarrassing to say that. You have to be careful who you say it to.

EVELYN: Are you telling me?! You get in deep trouble. "What kind of woman is she?" You know, oh, wow, it's really awful. It was years before I could say that. But no children.

MCU GLORIA SPARROW, *a white woman in her late fifties, seated at a dining table.*

YVONNE R. *(v-o):* How has your anarchist background informed your feminism?

GLORIA: I can remember that my mother's hero was Emma Goldman. And I can remember that my father's comrades laughed at her, laughed about Emma Goldman and made fun of her in exactly the same way that I remember, decades later when I was here at Cal. in the anthropology department in U.C., all these male anthropologists laughed at Margaret Mead.

MCU of AUDREY GOODFRIEND, *a white woman around seventy years of age, sitting in a wildly overgrown yard.*

YVONNE R.: But your own relation to change . . . Did they think that it would happen in their lifetime?

AUDREY: I don't think they really did. I think that people who remain anarchists generally can't expect change in their lifetime. And I think that one of the reasons that some of the more libertarian aspects of the SDS and those times went down so rapidly is because people had to see change right away, and if you didn't see change right away, you might as well look out for yourself. The notion that anarchism is a philosophy and it's a way of life and a way of interpreting what happens around you stays with you forever whether you're actively involved in something or not. I'm certainly not very actively involved . . .

YVONNE R.: But it has sustained you.

AUDREY: It has sustained me.

Another sequence of credits crawls upward, this time in silence.

Director, Writer, Editor	Yvonne Rainer
Director of Photography	Mark Daniels
Assistant Director	Christine Le Goff
Production Manager	Kathryn Colbert
Art Directors	Anne Stuhler
	Michael Selditch
Sound Recordist	Antonio Arroyo
Second Assistant Director	Robin Guarino
People in dream	Sybil Simone
	Wanda Phipps
	Rick Perry
	Maurice Stewart

People in hallway	Shirley Soffer
	Christopher Hoover
	Leann Brown
	Kevin Duffy
	David Schulman
Boys on stoop	Wilson Leon Gamboa
	Dino Guglietta
	J. Jeffrey Ortiz
	George Vallejo
Whistling man	Daniel Lopez
Woman and Child in park	Katy Martin
	Sally Jo Brand
Man with briefcase	Michael Selditch
Man with dog	Stanley Crawford
Young Woman on street	Jennifer Rohn
Defense Attorney's voice	William Raymond
Judge's voice	Michael Taylor
Production Coordinator	Carol Noblitt
Design Coordinator	Nancy Swartz
Casting Consultants	Natalie Hart
	Daniel Swee
First Assistant Camera	Tony Hardmon
Key Grip	Luis R. Perez
Gaffer	Tom McGrath
Script Supervisor	Michael Taylor
Second Grip	Frank Dellario
Videography	Ellen Spiro
	Yvonne Rainer
	John Canalli

Second Assistant Camera	Adrian Misol
Extra Electrics	Luke Eder
	Ethan Mass
	Rex D. West
	Peter Walts
	Liz Friers
Sound Boom	Julie Wild
Props	Cynthia Smith
Location Manager	David Welch
Costume Designer	Alexandra Welker
Hair/Makeup	Patricia Schenker Regan
Assistant to the Art Directors	Simon Leung
Assistant Makeup/Costumes	Eve-Laure Moros
Photo Mural/Production Stills	Vivian Selbo
Photos on Yvonne Washington's wall	Carrie Mae Weems
American Sign Language Consultant	Pearl Johnson
Sound Editor	Lisa Prah
Editing Assistance	Susan Conley
	Roddy Bogawa
Video Editing/ Additional Sound Recording	Mary Patierno
Carpentry	John Figley
	John F. Jones
	Joel N. Nicholas
Translation	Pedro Cosme-Prado

MCU FAITH RINGGOLD.

FAITH: So I think, somehow or another, that women as they get older have to not take on the look, the manifestations, whatever it is . . . don't take that role on. I just don't know all the ways to do it, because the whole idea of thinking about it is new to me. But you don't have to do certain things just because you're older. Do what you want to do. Dress any way you want to dress, go anywhere you want to go . . .

Another sequence of "wrap party" shots, lasting about two minutes, followed by

Intertitle on Macintosh screen:

UTOPIA
The more impossible
it seems, the more
necessary it becomes.

More shots of wrap party.

MS, VIVAN BONNANO *in* YVONNE W.*'s apartment. She is a Cuban woman in her late forties.*

VIVIAN: And now I think I can deal with it a bit better. It's a very un-comfortable thing, it's not at all pleasant. It's embarrassing. You sud-denly break out in a horrible sweat and you wake up in the middle of the night and your sheets are soaked. It's not nice, but I hope it will be over soon. It's much better, I think, than when my mother went through it. She was convinced that she was going to go mad. That's what happens when you have the change, you go crazy. So my mother was convinced that she was going to go crazy. But now, talk-ing to friends and seeing that they're going through the same thing that I'm going through, it's a lot easier to take. And I imagine soon they'll have TV commercials about menopause. They have them about everything else. So, it's fine. I can deal with it a bit better, but I don't like it.

MS, YVONNE WASHINGTON *herself is now in front of the camera, in the "hot seat."*

YVONNE W.: I try to monitor when my hot flashes occur. I'm watch-ing a video cassette of *Sweet Sweetback's Baadasss Song.* "Why does an embodiment of black protest have to be a stud?" flashes through my mind, and along comes a hot flash. I'm on the subway thinking about a friend. "Forget that family crap," I think. *Flash* . . . Ready to leave, I put on my coat in an overheated room. Instantly I am so hot, I must tear it off. . . . Reading about the Supreme Court's latest set-back to civil rights. One of the Justices is quoted as saying: "The fact that low-paying, unskilled jobs are overwhelmingly held by blacks is no proof of racism. *Flash.* . . . Thinking about what I could have said, should have said. *Flash.* . . .

The body manifests itself in new ways. In the Montreal airport en route to New York, I approach U.S. immigration. Suddenly I am burning. Sure that my sweat shows, I remember what the agents look for: signs of nervousness, sweating. My heart skips a beat. The agent asks for more than usual. I must recite my date of birth as she checks it against my driver's license. I falter, almost reverse the 24 and 34. She hands me back the license, and says, "Have a good trip."

Remaining credits rise.
Party voices can be heard in background.

Production Assistants: Marion Appel, Rachel Barrett, Hilary Brougher, Lenora Champagne, Susan Conley, Theo Dorian, Rob Fritz, Christopher Hoover, Takahiro Kataishi, Rachel Krantz, Craig Marsden, Martha Nalband, Lisa Pino, Catherine Saalfied, Rebecca Schreiber, Linda Yee

Opticals: Cynosure, B. B. Optics; Negative Cutting: One White Glove/Tim Brennan; Lab: Du Art; Sound Mix: Sound One/ Reilly Steele; Camera: Film Friends; Grip and Electric Equipment: Electric Feat; Dollies: Blake Production Systems; Caterer: Upstairs/ Downstairs

Quotations and Literary Sources: Lefty Barretto, Susan Brownmiller, Lenny Bruce, Dr. Helen Caldicott, Eldridge Cleaver, Oliver C. Cox, Frantz Fanon, Piri Thomas, Judy Grahn, Heresies Collective #6, Calvin C. Hernton, Joel Kovel, Harlan Lane, Teresa de Lauretis, Nicholasa Mohr, Joan Nestle, Clara E. Rodriguez, Ntozake Shange, Elaine Showalter

Film Clip from "Lenny Bruce" Courtesy of John Magnuson Associates, San Francisco

"My Funny Valentine" (Lorenz Hart/Richard Rodgers) Courtesy of Warner/Chappell Music, Inc.

"Seeraeuberjenny" Used by permission of Stefan Brecht and European American Music Corp., Agent for the Kurt Weill Foundation for Music, Inc.

"Deserie" (Leslie Cooper/Clarence Johnson) Courtesy of Longitude Music Co.

Chocolate Box Label Courtesy of Janette Faulkner's Collection "Ethnic Notions"

Special Thanks to: The Kitchen, Lauren Amazeen, John Figley, The Lesbian Herstory Archives, New York City Mayor's Office of Film, Theatre and Broadcasting

Additional Thanks: Joanne Akalaitis, Maurice Berger, Donna Binder, Vivian Brown, Maureen Burnley, Rudeen Dash, Lilly Diaz, June Ekman, Lynn Elton, Martin Elton, Claire Glover, Tami Gold, Thyrza Goodeve, David Kaufman, Alexander Kluge, Kate Lambert, Beni Matias, Nancy Meehan, Leland Moss, Sheila McLaughlin, Nelli Perez and the Center for Puerto Rican Studies, Mark Rappaport, B. Ruby Rich, Faith Ringgold, Lapacazo Sandoval, Judy Simmons, Dr. Nelly Szlachter, Polly Thistlethwaite, Eva Weiss

Special gratitude to the following for their support and criticism: Joan Braderman, Trisha Brown, Martha Gever, Ernest Larsen, Sherry Millner, Belle Rainer, Ivan Rainer, Bérénice Reynaud, Martha Rosler, Michele Wallace, Carrie Mae Weems

This film has been made possible by funding and awards from: New York State Council on the Arts, National Endowment for the Arts, Rockefeller Foundation, John Simon Guggenheim Foundation, New York Foundation for the Arts, American Film Institute, Brandeis University

In Memoriam: Ronald Bladen, Lyn Blumenthal, Claudia Gregory, Michael Grieg, Leland Moss, "Louie"

MURDER and murder

This script from the film (16 mm, color, 113 minutes, released in 1996) was previously published in *Performing Arts Journal* 55, 19, no. 1 (January 1997).

Here is a list of some of the abbreviations used in the film script:

CU—close-up

ELS—extreme long shot

MCU—medium close-up

MOS—without sound

MS—medium shot

MW—medium wide

POV—point of view

sync—the visual image is synchronized with the soundtrack

v-o—voice over

Daytime. Early fall. Very wide shot, an almost deserted beach. The theme music from Jaws *begins. Steadycam begins to move at a rapid pace toward two tiny figures who, as we get closer, are revealed as two white women playing with a frisbee. They are the ghosts who haunt the film.*

JENNY, *the older of the two (in her early sixties), is wearing a brown 1915 bathing costume. Although her legs, which are clad in brown stockings, are grossly swollen, she moves with agility.* YOUNG MILDRED *is around eighteen and wears sunglasses, a straw hat, and an unbuttoned man's shirt over a turquoise, gingham, two-piece outfit consisting of pedal-pushers and midriff-baring sleeveless blouse.*

MS, low-angle. JENNY *and* YOUNG MILDRED *look off-screen into the distance. Music fades down as they speak.*

JENNY: Uh-oh, here they come.

YOUNG MILDRED: Hey Jenny, let's give them a run for their money. Let's get into the act.

Reverse angle. JENNY *and* YOUNG MILDRED *run away from camera toward steadycam crew that is moving toward them.*

MCU of JENNY. *There follows a kind of cat-and-mouse game as* JENNY *and* YOUNG MILDRED *try to get themselves "framed" and the cameraperson tries to avoid them.*

JENNY *(to camera):* My name is Jenny Schwartz. I was born in 1896. In 1915 I live on Hinsdale Street in East New York with my parents. If you're looking for my daughter Doris, she's over there. *(pointing)*

Camera pans in the direction in which JENNY *points.* YOUNG MILDRED *plants herself in front of camera.*

YOUNG MILDRED *(to camera):* My name is Mildred Davenport. I was born in Scarsdale, New York, in 1942. I just graduated from high school.... *(offscreen)* Jenny Schwartz is dead.

Camera evades YOUNG MILDRED *and moves toward two middle-aged white women sitting on the sand.* DORIS, *in her early sixties, is speaking to*

ALICE, *who appears to be in her mid-forties.*

JENNY *(offscreen):* Mildred, I'm as real as you are.

YOUNG MILDRED *(offscreen):* OK, so you're a ghost. But *I'm* alive, be-cause I'm going to be fifty when I get together with Doris.

JENNY *(offscreen):* And I'm going to be seventy-eight when I die. So what? *(now shouting to camera crew)* Don't believe anything Doris says about me.

YOUNG MILDRED *(offscreen):* Why should she talk about you? You're long gone. It's me she's obsessed with.

JENNY *(offscreen):* But I'm her mother!

Dissolve to MW of DORIS *and* ALICE.

DORIS: Maybe I was delusional. It was one A.M., a warm night. I stopped at a shop to buy fish and chips and ate it as I strolled the mile from the theater to my hotel. I was all alone and felt relaxed in a way I hadn't felt for months, even years, like my body belonged to me, and I belonged on that street. I had no doubt about my right to be on that street all by myself savoring my fish and chips late at night. It was a kind of bliss.

ALICE: Doris, you've changed the subject.

DORIS: Oh yeh, you want to know what it's like with Mildred.

CU ALICE *and* DORIS.

ALICE: I don't mean to pry, but yeh.

DORIS *(thinks for a bit):* You know, Alice, never in my wildest dreams, my most far-out fantasies, did I ever come close to imagining that I would one day be able to say—with the utmost conviction—I *love* eating pussy.

Cut to wide shot of the ocean. A frisbee sails across the frame followed by
JENNY, *running after it.*

JENNY: As long as she's happy.

Music—Herbert Clark's "From the Mighty Pacific"—*begins. Title—a
film by Yvonne Rainer—followed by Joanna Merlin, Kathleen Chalfant,
Catherine Kellner, Isa Thomas, MURDER and murder and other opening credits, each supered over a separate shot depicting* DORIS *and (adult)*
MILDRED *smiling or scowling in various vacation settings. The last shot
doesn't quite mesh with the others:* MILDRED *and* DORIS *in profile on either side of a kitchen table craning toward each other in confrontation like
a couple of gargoyles.*

Night. DORIS's *two-room "cold-water" apartment. CU of inside of bathtub.* DORIS *is cleaning the tub. She is humming "Sentimental Journey."
She covers the bathtub with its lid, then goes into the hallway connecting
the two rooms. She stands in front of a mirror and examines herself as she
tries on a tailored jacket. She then goes into the tiny bedroom/study, which
is only large enough for a loft bed, desk, chair, and clothes pole under the
loft-bed. The room is stuffed to the ceiling with memorabilia, photos, boxes,
papers, books. A conspicuous item of furniture is an old beat-up wooden
office chair whose ripped leather back is patched with silver gaffer tape.*
DORIS *examines some photos on the desk, practices some poses, notices the
presence of the camera, and then, seating herself on a stool, addresses the
camera.*

DORIS: I'm not going to apologize for the mess. I was sixty-three last
week. Yeh, I know what you're thinking, but you'll just have to take
my word for it. I always thought reaching sixty would be a watershed
of some kind. Little did I know. I mean here I am, a grandmother. I
have a seven-year-old granddaughter and a wonderful daughter who
hates my guts. She's still living with her husband, so I don't have to
have too much responsibility for their child. I can't quite believe that
at my age I'm barely earning a living as a part-time art school teacher.
And they don't pay health insurance. I don't even have a credit card.
And now to top it off I'm with a woman. Can you beat that? I fall in
love with a woman after being alone for fifteen years and liking it.
Am I asking for trouble or what? I've sometimes thought that what I
need is an adoring young wife to clean up my messes. Or at least I

should have had a muse for some of those years. All the *male* artists of my generation had muses. So did I ask to fall in love with a waspy, high-minded, stubborn, well-off professional dyke who's more than ten years younger than me, more successful, and already is offering to pay some of my bills? Do I need this at my age? . . . Maybe I do.

Daytime. Manhattan Street. ALICE *is talking into a pay phone. A man stands in the foreground, waiting for the phone.*

ALICE: Y'know, Claire, I think Doris loves being a lesbian even more than being with Mildred. . . . OK, bye.

ALICE *hangs up and leaves. Phone rings.* JEFFREY, *a thirty-five-year-old black gay man who had been waiting, picks up the receiver.*

JEFFREY: Hi, this is Jeffrey . . . Huh? . . . I think it's great, but some people are going to be weird about it. Do you know what she said to me? "Now Doris can be the oppressed person she's always wanted to be." . . . OK, bye.

JEFFREY *hangs up. Phone rings. A* WOMAN *next in line takes her turn.*

WOMAN: I think she just got tired of feeling oppressed as a woman. At least feeling oppressed as a lesbian will be new and different.

WOMAN *hands receiver to next in line and leaves.*

WOMAN #2: Gossip, gossip, gossip. What's Mildred going to feel about all this?

WOMAN #2 *exits frame.*

Title:

FALLING IN LOVE AGAIN

Interior, MILDRED'*s loft. Night. CU of* MILDRED, *a woman in her mid-fifties. Her facial expression is ambiguous. Her head is resting on the arm of a couch. She wears an unbuttoned white shirt. A hand enters the frame and camera follows its caressing passage over* MILDRED'*s face, then her exposed left breast and belly revealed by unzipped pants. Just as camera—and hand—reaches her pubic hair,*

Cut to MS reverse of DORIS's *face and clothed torso, seated on the edge of the couch, her gaze focused intently down toward* MILDRED's *head just visible from behind and resting on the same arm of the couch. There is some half visible movement of* DORIS's *arm. In the background on a TV monitor is a scene from the beginning of Kubrick's* The Shining *(Jack Nicholson and family in the car heading for the hotel: "Dad, I'm hungry." "Ya shoulda eaten yer breakfast.")*

DORIS: When you get dressed up in a butch way I'm utterly thrilled. I think, "My lover is an unabashed dyke."

CU of MILDRED *as before.*

MILDRED: You have to be an unabashed dyke to be thrilled by one.

MILDRED *turns to the camera and speaks in a languid fashion.*

MILDRED: I knew this wasn't going to be easy. But I also knew it was what I wanted. We'd find a way. After seven years with Clara and eight years of loneliness and flirtation, I figured I could handle anything. This is serious business. She doesn't fool around. I'm going to have to play my cards right; I don't want to screw up. . . . Court jesters were always male. Even as fools they were accorded dignity. But when a woman plays the fool she's made to feel like an idiot. There's no dignity in the role for us. . . . Don't ask me any more questions. I don't feel like being interrogated. . . . You'll find out about me soon enough. . . . Just remember that when Doris claims to know what I'm thinking, she's probably wrong.

Title:

PMS: PRE-murder SIGNS

Night. Interior of DORIS's *"cold-water" apartment.* YOUNG MILDRED *is taking a bath in the kitchen tub.* JENNY *perches on the edge of the tub. She wears the same 1915 bathing outfit throughout the film.*

YOUNG MILDRED: Why will I have to get married? If I'm going to end up a lesbian, why do I have to go through all this stuff with a man?

JENNY: Patience, Young Mildred. It won't last long. What else can you do? You're still in 1960. How many lesbians do you know? No woman is coming out of the woodwork to sweep you off your feet. Besides, your husband's going to be a nice guy!

YOUNG MILDRED: The person I really want to marry is his mother. He had a great mother.

Sound of key turning in lock. JENNY *hastily pulls tub cover over* YOUNG MILDRED. *Jump-cut to* JENNY *sitting down on edge of tub and* YVONNE *flipping the tails of her tuxedo jacket as she sits next to her. She addresses the camera.*

YVONNE: I'm the director, Yvonne Rainer. What's Stanley Kubrick been doing lately? He lives in England, eats well. Lives well. Maybe has an English wife. You have to have a wife to live in England. To live well, anyway. As a North American.

Sound of key turning in lock. MILDRED *and* DORIS *enter.*

Even when YVONNE, JENNY, *or* YOUNG MILDRED *are in the same frame with them,* MILDRED *and* DORIS *never acknowledge their presences.* DORIS *crosses frame and goes to bedroom.* MILDRED *puts bag of groceries on tub, forcing* JENNY *to move to other side of* YVONNE.

DORIS*'s study. CU of her hands putting mail on the dilapidated chair. Tilt up to MS of* DORIS.

DORIS: Did you lock the door?

MW of kitchen as before with all three "ghosts" on the tub, now including YOUNG MILDRED *wrapped in a towel and drying her hair.*

MILDRED: Of course I locked the door. What do you take me for, an idiot? I know the ropes around here. Did I lock the door!

MILDRED *tosses a half-eaten sandwich she has found on the tub into a garbage can.*

DORIS*'s study. MS of* DORIS *sitting in her chair, sorting mail.*

DORIS *(v-o):* Caught her at it again.

Kitchen. MS of YVONNE *sitting on the end of the tub.* JENNY *and* YOUNG MILDRED *are in profile behind her.* YVONNE *addresses camera.*

YVONNE: Holier-than-she, Doris doesn't respond, but tucks her companion's outburst away for future reference or ammunition. Like the elephant, she will remember. Mildred feels vindicated.

Series of shots: MCU's of MILDRED *and* DORIS, *their speech sometimes on screen, sometimes off, as they prepare for bed, brush teeth, make tea, put on pajamas, etc.*

DORIS *(off-screen):* We're very different people.

MILDRED, *in the hallway, removes a pink padded hanger from her bag and hangs up her jacket.*

MILDRED: Yes, you're more judgmental than I am.

DORIS *(filling kettle at sink):* And you're more secretive.

MILDRED *(in bedroom, removes blouse):* You're inflexible.

DORIS *(brushing teeth at kitchen sink):* What!? Look who's talking. . . .

MILDRED *(puts on pajama top):* You never want to come to my house.

DORIS *(toothbrush in mouth):* That's not true. It can't be true.

MILDRED *(hangs up blouse):* And when you're there you always want to leave.

DORIS *(walks down hall with teacup):* That's not true either.

Bedroom, top of loftbed. MILDRED *climbs up ladder and crawls into bed. She is carrying the* New York Times Sunday Magazine *open to the crossword puzzle.*

MILDRED: You don't have to be defensive. It may not be true, but that's the way I feel. Why can't you accept my feelings? And another thing: You never let me make love to you.

Bedroom. MS of DORIS *in bed beside* MILDRED, *who is doing the crossword puzzle.*

DORIS *(blows her nose):* Bullshit. You make love to me plenty. But why don't you ever say my name when you make love to me? I love the sound of your voice.

MILDRED *(in a whiny, sarcastic voice): A* my name is Anna. I come from Alabama. I live on Altona Street, and I eat apples. *B* my name is Betty. I come from Bakersfield. I live on Bickford Street, and I eat bananas. *C* my name is Cindy . . .

Ironic saxophone riff segues into beginning of next shot. Day. Busy New York City street with corresponding sound. MW of MILDRED *and* DORIS *standing at two adjacent public phones.* YVONNE *leans against one of the phone cubicles and addresses the camera.*

YVONNE: After days of acrimonious and analytic phone calls, a theory of communication emerges:

MILDRED: You're always leaving.

YVONNE: should have been expressed ten months earlier as

MILDRED: I feel bad when you leave so abruptly. Could you prolong or give advance warning of your goodbye?

YVONNE: And

DORIS: You never say my name

YVONNE: should have been expressed as

DORIS: It would make me feel good if you would address me by name more frequently.

Medium two-shot of MILDRED *and* DORIS. *They are silent for about ten seconds.*

MILDRED: I don't know.

DORIS: What don't you know?

MILDRED: I just don't know.

MS of YVONNE, *still leaning against phone booth. She addresses the camera.*

YVONNE: Stanley Kubrick's wife knows her place and how to function in it. She can see the misery coming on a mile away and avert it. Stanley never even has to think about it.

Archival footage; POV from a seat on a Roller Coaster around 1920. JENNY *and* YOUNG MILDRED *are in the foreground with their backs to the camera flailing and shrieking as though they are on the ride.*

Daytime. Exterior of a small rustic summer cabin. JENNY *and* YOUNG MILDRED *are prostrate on the floor of the porch, leaning against the front door and gasping for breath.*

YOUNG MILDRED: I can't believe you did that kind of thing back then.

JENNY: Steeplechase Park is our favorite, although you do meet some pretty low elements there. But when I go with three or four girlfriends, we always have fun. We tumble around in the Barrel of Love, then do the Dew Drop and the Razzle Dazzle. Good Heavens, where have those names come from? You'd never know I died from Alzheimer's.

YOUNG MILDRED: Were you working?

JENNY: Of course I'm working. I've been a pieceworker in a corset factory for the last two years. I work nine hours a day and make six dollars a week. I turn four dollars over to my mother and keep two dollars for myself. And out of that I pay union dues and membership in the Women's Self-Education Society. . . . When I had Doris that all came to an end.

Sound of car motor.

JENNY *and* YOUNG MILDRED *look in the direction of sound.* DORIS *and* MILDRED *drive up in a car.* DORIS *gets out, opens trunk, removes a canvas bag and throws it on the ground. She stands gazing toward the cabin with a grumpy expression.* MILDRED *goes to* DORIS *and tries to embrace her.*

DORIS: I've got to get out of here. I'm going for a walk.

DORIS *breaks free and rushes down the drive.* MILDRED *looks after her, shrugs. Camera pans to follow her as she goes toward the cabin.* JENNY *and* YOUNG MILDRED *are standing on the porch gazing in the direction of* DORIS'*s exit.*

YVONNE *(v-o):* Their first travel venture. The trip was horrendous. The one gyrates and rebounds out of obsessive concern for her companion's happiness. The other feels smothered, always ready to flee, suffocated by ordinary demonstrations of affection that come, in the course of a day in the tiny cabin, about every half hour, or hour, or two hours.

Same day. A dirt road, flanked by trees, stretches away from the camera. DORIS *is rapidly retreating into the distance.* JENNY *and* YOUNG MILDRED *follow her at a slower pace. Camera dollies behind them.*

JENNY: The shorter work day brought me my first idea of there being such a thing as pleasure. It was quite wonderful to get home before it was pitch dark at night and a real joy to ride on the cars and look out the windows and see all the bustling people in the street. When I was a pieceworker I would fool around, tell jokes, talk with the girls. And I would sing.

JENNY *begins singing "Fatal Wedding." ("While the wedding bells were ringing . . .") First shot of archival footage of a 1930 garment factory with hundreds of women workers at sewing machines. Succeeding shots show CU's of single women at work.* JENNY's *singing fades out during the following v-o.*

JENNY *(v-o):* Three o'clock, a-quarter-after, half-past! The terrific tension had all but reached the breaking point. Then there rose a trembling, palpitating sigh that seemed to come from a hundred throats, and blended in a universal expression of relief. In my clear, high treble, I began the everlasting "Fatal Wedding." That piece of false sentiment had now a new significance. It became a song of deliverance, and as the workers swelled the chorus one by one, it meant that the end of the day's toil was in sight.

JENNY's *singing fades up during the end of the above series. Dirt road as before.*

MCU of JENNY *and* YOUNG MILDRED, *who joins in the last refrain ("Just another fatal wedding, just another broken heart").*

WS. YOUNG MILDRED *and* JENNY *move toward camera down the road as it emerges from the woods.*

YOUNG MILDRED: Were you ever attracted to a woman?

JENNY: Oh, I dunno. I love my girlfriends. I guess I just never thought much about it.

YOUNG MILDRED: What about Doris? Did you ever think that she might be a lesbian?

JENNY: Good Heavens no. I expected her to find a husband, just like I did, and not fool around much beforehand.

Landscape. Same day. YOUNG MILDRED *and* JENNY *walk into the foreground with their backs to the camera. Before them a vast golden meadow reaches toward a lake ringed by trees. In the far distance the tiny figure of* DORIS *stands with her back to the camera, looking at the lake. The scene suggests a Casper David Friedrich painting. There is a suitcase at* DORIS's *feet, which she eventually opens. She removes a number of boxes of different shapes and sizes.*

CU of DORIS's *hands trying to fit the brown paper-wrapped boxes back into the suitcase, without success. She stands. Camera tilts up to reveal* JENNY, YOUNG MILDRED, *and a* MAN *in a rowboat way out on the lake. The* MAN *is rowing.*

JENNY *(v-o):* Several of my girlfriends belonged to the Bachelor Girl's Social Club, which organized dances and excursions for working girls. Once a big group took a ferry to Coney Island. This was in the days before the subway went out there. It was supposed to be a day trip, but a man

WS of lake. The rowboat glides into frame, left-to-right, then out. A young MAN *in collarless shirt and straw hat rows.* JENNY *and* YOUNG MILDRED *are seated in the stern.*

JENNY *(v-o):* I met on the ferry persuaded me to stay behind when everyone left. We went out on the lake in a rowboat and

CU of oar moving in and out of water. The sun is setting behind the trees.

JENNY *(v-o):* He told me that women with thick ankles are very sensuous. That night we went to sleep in separate tents. I became so aroused I went into his tent

MW of JENNY *and* YOUNG MILDRED *seated in boat from over-the-shoulder of* ROWING MAN. *The boat is stationary.*

JENNY: and we had a sexual relation. I always blamed the chaperone for allowing me to stay behind.

YOUNG MILDRED: Wait a minute. If you went to Coney Island how come you ended up on a lake? And were your legs always so swollen?

JENNY: Getting pregnant with Doris did in my legs. They called it milk leg then. You don't see it anymore. The quacks have made *some* progress.

Archival footage of roller coaster POV, accompanied by ecstatic shrieks.

Title:

PUBLIC ADDRESS

Night. A corner of MILDRED'*s half-renovated (or half-"deconstructed") loft. Her desk-top is very neat, in contrast to the cavernous space behind her, and in contrast to the congestion of* DORIS'*s apartment. Boxes and building materials are in evidence in the background.* MILDRED *is seated in a director's chair behind the desk. She finds some music on the radio that she likes and tries to make herself comfortable, then fetches a bed pillow from a pile of objects behind the desk and arranges it to support her back. It slips out the back of the chair, taking the canvas flap with it, which then results in the arms of the chair crashing down to the sides. After reassembling the chair, she finally settles down to work at her Powerbook.* DORIS *enters from the deep space behind* MILDRED. *She is all high energy and enthusiasm. They kiss perfunctorily.*

DORIS: Vancouver was fabulous. Bookstores, water, mountains, lovely people. And you know what? *Lesbians are everywhere!*

DORIS *exits frame right.*

MILDRED: And homeless people. *(loud)* Maybe you've just begun to notice . . . How'd your act go over?

DORIS *(off-screen):* Oh you know, the usual mix. But I came up with a new shtick. You wanna see?

MILDRED: Sure.

MILDRED *removes her glasses and closes her lap-top. Fanfare of music.*

Cut to WS of proscenium stage. DORIS *is standing in the center of it, wearing a leather mini-skirt, heavy boots, torn fishnet stockings, smeared lipstick, and a bustier with huge gold coils over her breasts.* DORIS *presents a "performance" that consists of a series of stylized poses and the following monologue (from Kathy Bates/Annie Wilkes in* Misery).

DORIS: When I was growing up in Bakersfield my favorite thing in the whole world was to go to the movies on Saturday afternoons for the

. . . the cliffhangers. My favorite was *Rocketman.* And once it was a no-brakes chapter, and the bad guys stuck him in a car on a mountain road and knocked 'im out and welded the door shut and tore out the brakes and started him to his death and he woke up and tried to steer and tried to get out but the car went off a cliff before he could escape. And it crashed and burned and I was so upset and excited and the next week you better believe I was first in line and they always start with the end of the last week. And there was Rocketman trying to get out and here comes the cliff and just before the car went off the cliff he jumped free. And all the kids *cheered.* But *I* didn't cheer. I stood right up and started shouting. "*This* isn't what happened last *week.* Have you all got amnesia? They just cheated us. This isn't fair. He didn't get out of the cockadoody car!"

WS of MILDRED *at her desk.* YOUNG MILDRED *perches cross-legged on a corner of the desk, while* JENNY *sits on a stool to her right. The two ghosts applaud, while* MILDRED *does not.* DORIS *enters.*

DORIS: So whaddya think?

CU of MILDRED *looking perplexed.*

MILDRED: Um . . . let's see. A recuperation of history; a cry of outrage at the deceit of illusion. It's hard to say . . . OK, you know what I think? I think it's about confrontation, pure and simple.

MW, reverse angle. DORIS *is standing at the desk.*

DORIS *(defensively):* Recup . . . confrontation? What d'ya mean? Well, maybe, but there are plenty of reasons . . . oh, let's drop it.

She exits frame left. Camera dollies left as JENNY *moves into* DORIS*'s position.* YOUNG MILDRED *remains on the desk.*

JENNY *(to* YOUNG MILDRED*):* Y'know, she did these strange performances in the backyard when she was ten years old, and I never took them seriously.

DORIS *(off-screen):* What did *you* do while I was away?

MILDRED: I wrote.

DORIS *(off-screen):* Read me something.

MILDRED: Oh, you don't want to hear.

YOUNG MILDRED *sniggers impishly.*

Reverse LS of DORIS *as she re-enters wearing sweatpants, shirt, and no make-up. She sits in* MILDRED*'s now-vacated chair. Boxes are stacked in the background.*

DORIS: I do; I do.

WS of MILDRED *on the stage.*

MILDRED *(reading):* "And already the hallmarks of the famous Flanner style were present: the ironic flourishes, the polysyllabic wit, the taste for glittering, catachrestic, sometimes macabre description. Attracted by anything theatrical, outré, or baroque, Flanner perfected a prose to match—full of spectacular figures, mordant turns of phrase, adamantine alliteration, and a sinuous, burnished beauty."

WS shot of DORIS *in* MILDRED*'s chair flanked by* JENNY *and* YOUNG MILDRED *in their own director's chairs.*

DORIS: Wow.

MS of DORIS *and* MILDRED *on stage.* MILDRED *gets up from her chair.*

MILDRED: Mmm . . . earrings.

DORIS: Whaddya mean "earrings"! I've been wearing earrings since long before I ever met you. I just wear them more infrequently now.

MILDRED: Oh. Then it means something when you *don't* wear them.

MS of JENNY *and* YOUNG MILDRED *watching the new "performance." They exchange puzzled looks.*

MS of DORIS *and* MILDRED *onstage as before.*

DORIS: Why can't you say you missed me?

MILDRED: Who says I can't?

DORIS: Well, you haven't.

MILDRED: You didn't ask. And even if you do now I won't.

DORIS: Why not?

MILDRED *doesn't reply. Her face gets moodier and moodier until she looks about to cry.*

DORIS: I said, why not?

MILDRED *glares away from her, silently shaking her head.*

Reverse MS of YOUNG MILDRED *and* JENNY, *watching.*

YOUNG MILDRED *(incredulously):* She's still acting just like me!

JENNY: Whady you expect?!

LS of DORIS *now alone on the stage.* MILDRED's *desk is in the foreground. She and the ghosts are gone.*

DORIS *(shouting):* Now come on, Mildred, don't give me the silent treatment. Say something. What'd I do now? What's wrong? I can't stand it when you don't talk.

DORIS *abruptly leaves the stage, clumping down the steps toward* MILDRED's *desk.*

YVONNE *(v-o):* As my mother was descending into Alzheimer's

MS of TV monitor on MILDRED's *desk.* YVONNE *appears on monitor.*

YVONNE: —they called it brain deterioration then—I brought her to see a performance of mine. During the solo I named all the proper nouns in my early life. I can still recite the litany of grade school teachers: Anderson, Dettner, Barrett, Myers, Pepina, King, Mac-Carthy, Kermoian. My mother said "That's ancient history." Sometimes my life feels like one ancient history piled on another. It's enough to curdle the blood. I never used to be ruled by fear, caution, amnesia, and its bedfellow—obsession with the past. Maybe I'm being too hard on myself. Let's just say they're ruling me today. . . . Today I wouldn't be caught dead hitchhiking like Madonna, nude on that highway with purse and plastic heels and scarred abdomen and aching hip joints and single breast.

MS of DORIS *with the remote, changing the channel.*

Closer shot of the monitor.

YVONNE: I'd like to address the woman who said, in my presence, probably quite unaware of my changed—maybe I should say "evolved," *(thinking to herself)* yes, evolved sexual preference, or should I say evolved sexual "orientation," or leave out "evolved" . . . anyway this woman was talking about her grown children, and she said, "I'm just happy they didn't turn out to be junkies or gay." . . . YOU KNOW WHO YOU ARE!

MS of white middle-aged WOMAN *at pay phone (on the monitor).*

WOMAN: I'm just happy they didn't turn out to be gay or have breast cancer.

MS of white middle-aged MAN *at pay phone (also on the monitor).*

MAN: I'm so glad they didn't turn out to be HIV-positive or black.

MCU of YVONNE *on monitor.*

YVONNE: Anything is possible in the homophobic racist unconscious of heterosexual white parenthood.

OFF-SCREEN MALE VOICE: Ms. Rainer, really. That's over the top.

YVONNE: And those smug biological parents are the worst!

MS of DORIS *looking at the TV incredulously.*

DORIS: Is that PBS?!

Title:

GAINING

Morning. MILDRED's *bedroom. In the background can be seen a portable clothes rack and a large partition consisting of paint-spattered plastic sheeting.* MILDRED *and* DORIS *are lying under a floral-print sheet at opposite ends of a bed, heads propped on pillows.* DORIS's *feet rest on* MILDRED's *breasts. Her toes play with her lover's nipples. The camera dollies and pans back and forth between them.*

DORIS: Well, *your* credentials as a bonafide lesbian have never been in question.

MILDRED: No, that's not true. My old girl friend always said I wasn't the real thing because I'd had sex with men. Not only that but I had been married.

DORIS: You mean she never fucked a man, even once? That's pretty extreme, isn't it?

MILDRED: I'd say it's fairly common.

DORIS: Oh Christ, they'll never let *me* into the club, after my lifetime of copulation. And here I'd thought all I had to do was give up wearing two identical earrings.

MILDRED: What club? There is no club. Let's face it, you're a lesbian, like it or not.

DORIS: How do you know?

MILDRED *(laughing):* I don't sleep with straight women.

DORIS: I was straight when you first got involved with me.

MILDRED: No you weren't. A straight woman wouldn't have behaved the way you did.

DORIS: You mean, at the Clit Club? How did I behave? Tell me again, my love. Tell me about the rabbits and the chickens.

MILDRED *(laughing):* The way you came on to me. Only a lesbian would have behaved like that.

DORIS: OK, I'm a lesbian. I'll take your word for it . . . for now.

Title:

LOSING

Street in front of MILDRED's *loft building. Day.* MILDRED *and* DORIS *are returning home from somewhere. They walk toward the camera.* DORIS *is walking a bicycle.*

DORIS: My mother had this wonderful old dog named Emma . . . Emma . . . G . . . begins with a G.

MILDRED: Goldman . . . A dog? I thought Jenny was allergic.

DORIS: Emma Goldman. And she had this great trick. She had these two . . . two . . . she would fetch a blue or red . . . *(gesticulates wildly)*

MILDRED: What?

DORIS: She would fetch . . . you throw it in the air . . . you know . . . Whadyacallit. *(gesticulates in exasperation)*

They have reached their building. MILDRED *unlocks the door and holds it open for* DORIS *and her bicycle.*

MILDRED: Frisbee!

DORIS: Yes! Frisbee! Sometimes I liked Emma Goldman more than my mother.

They enter the building and close the door. There follows a series of words that initially appear all together, but no sooner does the spectator begin to read than each word successively disappears at a slightly faster pace than is comfortable for a fairly nimble reader. The effect is that the reader feels "pursued." The only word to escape erasure is "metastasize," which remains when all the others have vanished. Dixieland-style music is heard throughout.

> frisbee, Raquel Welch, bandolier,
> Lady Chatterley's Lover, Joseph
> Losey, Lee Remick, accelerator,
> Swarthmore, To Live and Die in
> L.A., metastasize, brown study,
> Lazy Legs, sterilization, Jack
> Palance, sapphist, Yasir Arafat,
> rappel, ill-fated, wrong-headed,
> profiteer, reify, colloidal.

Title:

SINGING DIFFERENCE

Night. DORIS*'s kitchen. The first of many statistics crawls right-to-left across bottom of frame. Camera moves from MS of* YVONNE, *who is sitting on the bathtub, to* MILDRED *chopping potatoes at the table, finally settling on* DORIS, *who has crossed the kitchen to the stove. The full impact of the following information falls on her image.*

Crawling title: There are 1.8 million women in the U.S. who've been diagnosed with breast cancer. One million others have the disease and do not yet know it.

MS of YVONNE *on the tub, surrounded by stacks of newspapers.*

YVONNE: Pat Robertson opposes equal rights amendments. He warns against "a socialist, anti-family political movement that encourages women to leave their husbands, kill their children, practice witchcraft, destroy capitalism and become lesbians."

View through the door of DORIS*'s apartment.* MILDRED *and* DORIS *are cooking at a three-burner counter-top gas stove.* MILDRED *is preparing* boeuf bourguignon *while* DORIS *cooks tofu, carrots, and kale.*

MILDRED: Doris, could I have some of your carrots?

DORIS: No, that's all I have to eat.

MILDRED: Oh, come on. *(looks in* DORIS's *pot)* What's that?!

DORIS: That's tofu; it's very good for you. Tell you what—why don't you try some of this. *(She puts some kale into* MILDRED's *pot.)*

MILDRED: Doris, stop it, just stop it. *(She pulls the kale out and drops it into* DORIS's *pot.)*

DORIS: Don't do that. It's full of butter.

MILDRED: Wash it off!

DORIS: Wash it off?! Oh yuck!

YVONNE *steps into the foreground and leans against the door frame, her arms crossed and palms flattened against her chest, thumbs visible, macho style.* MILDRED *and* DORIS *move back and forth between table and stove.*

YVONNE: At least Pat Robertson has mentioned us. When members of the House of Lords decided in 1921 not to amend the antihomosexual Criminal Law of 1885 to include acts of "gross indecency between women," it was not because they deemed the threat of lesbianism inconsequential—quite the contrary—but because they were afraid that by the very act of mentioning it, they might spread such unspeakable "filthiness" even further. Thus was the lesbian transformed into a legal phantom in the U.K.

YVONNE *walks through the kitchen as* MILDRED *and* DORIS *sit down at the table. The following repartée takes place in individual CU's.*

DORIS: We made it!

MILDRED: Look, I'm putting your kale right in the middle of my plate.

DORIS: For God's sake Mildred, give it a rest.

MILDRED: What do you mean, you're the one who's always talking about food.

DORIS: Me!

MILDRED *breaks into song, to the tune of "Let's Call the Whole Thing Off."*

MILDRED: You crave kale and I love potatoes
    You devour tempeh and I eat tomatoes
    Kale, potatoes
    Tempeh, tomatoes
    Let's call the whole thing off.
    You say couch and I say sofa
    You say sponge and I say loofa
    Couches, sofas
    Sponges, loofas
    Let's call the whole thing off.

DORIS *(loudly):* Jane Spratt could eat no fat, her wife could eat no lean.

MW of the two of them.

MILDRED AND DORIS: But between the two of them they licked the platter clean.

They subside and eat in silence. MCU of DORIS.

DORIS *(v-o):* Sometimes when I look at her I see some kind of laboratory animal, which is an awful irony: her father used to own a prescription drug company.

MCU of MILDRED.

MILDRED *(v-o):* I've got to finish grading those papers tonight. I'm going to leave right after dinner.

MCU of DORIS.

DORIS *(v-o):* Me and my extreme prioritizing of the body and physical health. Ex-dancer, ex-survivor of multiple medical crises, I monitor my body like a piece of fine machinery.

MCU of MILDRED *lighting up a cigarette.*

MILDRED *(v-o):* And if I can get up an hour earlier tomorrow I'll go to the library and take care of my footnotes.

MCU of DORIS.

DORIS *(v-o):* Not that I always take optimal care of it, but I watch over its every vagary, hiccup, shift, and sputter. It is, in many senses, my life's work. She, an achieved—and continually aspiring—intellectual, ignores her body, or tries to, of course unsuccessfully. The body of the mid-life female refuses to be ignored by the brain that inhabits it.

WS of MILDRED *and* DORIS.

MILDRED: I'll wash the dishes.

MILDRED *starts to clear the table.* DORIS *grabs* MILDRED'*s plate, which contains her uneaten kale.* MILDRED *leaves frame.* DORIS *remains seated, picking at remaining food. Title crawls across bottom of frame.*

Crawling title: One out of four women who are diagnosed with breast cancer die within the first five years. Forty percent will be dead within ten years.

Daytime. Wide shot of facade of Columbia University Library.

MILDRED *(v-o):* This was something that concerned Joan Rivière as early as 1929.

Daytime. Interior. MS of empty podium in front of blackboard upon which is printed:

JOAN RIVIÈRE: "Womanliness as a Masquerade" first published in The International Journal of Psychoanalysis, vol. 10 (1929)

MILDRED, *speaking continuously, steps into frame to stand behind podium. She wears the same clothing as in previous scene and reads from her notes.*

MILDRED: She wrote, and I quote: "She delighted in using her great practical—and masculine—ability to aid or assist weaker and more helpless women, and could maintain this attitude successfully so long as rivalry did not emerge too strongly. But this restitution could be made on one condition only; it must procure her a lavish return in the form of gratitude and 'recognition.' . . .

Cut to DORIS*'s kitchen as before. MW of* MILDRED *washing up; she starts to remove her apron.* DORIS *enters, putting on a sweater and holding a pair of scissors.*

DORIS: How does it look?

MILDRED: Pretty good for ten bucks.

DORIS: Could you cut off the tag?

DORIS *hands scissors to* MILDRED, *who starts to cut off the sales tag.*

DORIS: Cut it as close as you can . . . there's another one . . . oh and this dangling piece of yarn . . . careful, *careful,* not too close or it'll unravel.

MILDRED*'s face registers irritation.* DORIS *exits.* MILDRED *starts to put on her jacket.*

MILDRED: You owe me ten bucks.

Reverse angle. DORIS *comes into the kitchen from the hallway.*

DORIS: What!? Where are you going? I thought it was a gift!

MILDRED: I thought I wasn't supposed to give you any more gifts.

DORIS: But it was so cheap.

MILDRED *(embracing her):* I'm joking.

DORIS: You're so serious. How am I to know?

MILDRED: Well, you are a bitch, you know. You still haven't thanked me for the gloves.

DORIS *backs away from* MILDRED *and looks at her appraisingly.*

DORIS: You want more than gratitude.

They stand, glaring at each other.

MILDRED *(v-o):* "The recognition desired was supposed by her to be owing for her self-sacrifices; more unconsciously what she claimed was

Cut to MS of MILDRED *at podium as before.*

MILDRED *(sync):* recognition of her *supremacy* in *having* the penis to give back. If her supremacy were not acknowledged, the rivalry became at once acute; if gratitude and recognition were withheld, her sadism broke out in full force and she would be subject (in private) to paroxysms of oral-sadistic fury, exactly like a raging infant."

MCU of MILDRED.

MILDRED *(v-o):* Oh dear, which one of us is she talking about?

MS of YOUNG MILDRED *and* JENNY *whispering in the back of the classroom.*

YOUNG MILDRED: What are we doing here?

JENNY: The head is the first sense to go, I always said. You have to keep improving your mind. When I was your age I went to evening school and lectures. Once I heard Emma Goldman speak. And once I heard Galli-Curci sing.

YOUNG MILDRED *rolls her eyes. Music segues into the next scene.*

Title:

GENERATIONAL TWIST

Day. A Ladies' Room with three stalls, all of them occupied.

1ST WOMAN *(v-o):* What'd you do last night?

2ND WOMAN *(v-o):* I went bowling.

1ST WOMAN *(v-o):* How'd you do?

2ND WOMAN *(v-o):* I scored sixty-five. Not bad, considering I hadn't done it for awhile.

1ST WOMAN *(v-o):* Have you talked to Amelia lately?

Sound of flushing. DORIS *emerges from middle stall and washes her hands.*

2ND WOMAN *(v-o):* No, but I heard . . .

1ST WOMAN *(v-o):* Well, they were going to just do a biopsy and then all of a sudden everything had changed and they did a lumpectomy.

More flushing. DORIS *dries hands and leaves before the women can be seen. Music fades out. Interior of restaurant. Daytime. Medium two-shot of* DORIS*'s daughter* FLO *and son-in-law* JIM, *both in their mid-thirties, seated at a table in front of a window.* FLO *is wearing high CEO drag: beige tailored jacket, designer scarf, gold earrings, heavy make-up. Just outside the window two white middle-aged homeless women are sitting.*

JIM *(to* FLO*):* What do you call yourself? You call yourself a heterosexual, don't you?

FLO: I don't call myself anything. No one asks.

MCU of DORIS.

DORIS: You don't have to. Everyone knows. Where's the coffee?

MCU of FLO.

FLO: I guess the word is for women who've always been that way. You've always been with men. It doesn't apply to you.

JIM *(off-screen):* Listen to her. She can't even say the word!

FLO *(snapping at him):* I've said it once and that's enough!

WS of all three, including homeless women outside window.

DORIS: I thought you were being protective of me, saving me from the Christian Coalition or something worse.

M two-shot of FLO and JIM.

FLO: Protect you?

Waiter brings coffee. Cut to WS. Waiter tries unsuccessfully to shoo homeless women away from window. DORIS looks at them; FLO, oblivious, takes out a cigarette and indicates JIM should light it. The discussion resumes when the waiter has left.

JIM *(to FLO):* It does apply to her if other people call her that.

M two-shot of FLO and JIM.

FLO: Now look who can't say the word! *(she turns to DORIS)* How have other people responded?

DORIS *(off-screen):* Someone said, "It's better than being alone." And Jim, weren't you the one who told me that I was willing to settle for less?

JIM: Not me. I might have thought that, but I wouldn't have said it. *(looks from one to the other)* OK, Doris. What are we talking here? Homophobia? Is that what you're trying to pin on us?

MCU of DORIS.

DORIS: Maybe a wee bit. Have you told any of your friends?

MCU of JIM.

JIM: Well, no. I have to admit that I had an opportunity to bring it up the other day with my parents. They were talking about my sister Cathy. They're afraid she might be a lesbian. She's stopped shaving her legs and she's going to Hampshire College.

M two-shot of DORIS *and* FLO. *They laugh.*

JIM *(off-screen):* I just couldn't bring myself to mention your situation, though it would have been perfectly appropriate.

DORIS: Why couldn't you bring it up?

JIM: I was uncomfortable.

FLO: Why?

CU of JIM.

JIM *(bristling):* I don't have to know why I was uncomfortable. I just was.

M two-shot of FLO *and* DORIS.

DORIS: Sounds to me like you're both a little uncomfortable.

FLO: Maybe we are.

Title:

IDENTITY POLITICS

DORIS*'s study. Day. CU of bookshelf containing books about history of homosexuality, interviews with older lesbians, gay and lesbian films, etc.* ALICE*'s hand selects a book (* Inside Out. *She will read an excerpt from D.A. Miller's "Anal Rope").*

MS ALICE.

ALICE: Are you studying how to be a lesbian? *(reads)*
   ". . . straight men *need* gay men, whom they forcibly recruit (as

the object of their blows, or, in better circles, just their jokes) to enter into a polarization that exorcises the 'woman' in man through assigning it to a class of man who may be considered no 'man' at all. Only between the woman and the homosexual together may the normal male subject imagine himself covered front and back."

Hm. The straight man as a ham sandwich . . . So where does the lesbian fit into all this?

MILDRED's *classroom as before.* "MURDER and murder" *is printed on the blackboard.*

MILDRED: Why is it so difficult to see the lesbian, even when she is there quite plainly, in front of us? In part because she has been "ghosted"—or made to seem invisible—by culture itself. It would be putting it mildly to say that the lesbian represents a threat to patriarchal protocol. Western civilization has for centuries been haunted by a fear of "women without men"—of women indifferent or resistant to male desire. Precisely because she challenges the authority of men so thoroughly, the "Amazon" has always provoked anxiety and hatred.

Halfway through the above lecture marching band music can be heard in the background. It surges up as MILDRED *finishes and ends abruptly before* YOUNG MILDRED *speaks.*

Back of classroom. JENNY *is snoring into her folded arms.* YOUNG MILDRED *pokes her.*

YOUNG MILDRED: Jenny, wake up. How do you expect to improve your mind if you fall asleep?

JENNY *(groggily):* Ooh, I have to go now. My mother is calling me.

Carousel music fades up.

Coney Island. Day. MS of MILDRED *who continues her lecture on the carousel. She is astride a horse that moves up and down.*

MILDRED: The vagina requires penetration to induce sexual pleasure in that area. Lesbians use whatever is at hand, including fingers, dildos, cucumbers. The dildo suggests hegemony when it is used for humiliation and submission. Otherwise it is the instrument of the lover who provides pleasure.

Cut to the back of the classroom, where JENNY *and* YOUNG MILDRED *are now very attentive and erect, in fact, open-mouthed with amazement. There is no break in the soundtrack. Cut to* MILDRED *on the carousel.*

MILDRED: Much depends on *who* is using it and *how* it is used: for pleasure, humiliation, power, submission, or any combination of these. To generalize and collapse all of these into "emulating men" misses a great deal of nuance. But, I should add, even among lesbians some years ago the dildo was considered politically incorrect.

CU of carousel animals revolving past the camera. Carousel music surges up, segues into next shot.

LS of DORIS *and* ALICE *leaning against a railing on the boardwalk at Coney Island. The ocean is behind them.*

MS reverse of DORIS *and* ALICE. *They lean on the railing in front of them. The Coney Island Parachute Jump looms behind them.*

DORIS: There were more men out there making the advances than women. But women never quite disappeared from my fantasy life.

Flashback. The fitting room of a lingerie shop in Manhattan. A young saleswoman brings brassieres to DORIS *(age 63) who is trying one on in the dressingroom.*

DORIS *(v-o):* Around 1960 I was trying on brassieres in a little lingerie shop on 57th St. The saleswoman comes into the dressingroom to help me into a Hollywood Vassarette push-up number. She handles my breasts as she adjusts the fit. This scene appears in my masturbatory fantasies for the next ten years or so, then somehow disappears until I disinter it for Mildred thirty years after the fact. Frankly, I think most women, if left to their own devices, could go either way. . . . Weren't you ever in love with a woman?

ALICE *(v-o):* Sure. But whenever I fell in love with a woman I would run into the

DORIS's *study. MCU of* ALICE.

ALICE: arms of a man. . . . I've been in love with many women, but there was never anything . . . *genital* about it. Last night I went to a party with all these wonderful women. But it was a sexual excitement I felt, not . . . genital. But I'm still curious about what made you take the leap.

ALICE's *POV.* DORIS *walks toward camera from the kitchen and down the hall until her body blocks the lens.*

DORIS: Mildred and I had been theater buddies for a few years. One day she called me up and invited me to the Clit Club, said she was doing field work. I said I would think about it. I was scared. And then I read an essay by a student of mine; an essay about sexual identity which culminated in a peculiar daydream.

Music: Aretha Franklin, "Eight Days on the Road"

Title:

AS YOU DESIRE ME

DORIS *(v-o):* It was about her difficulty in finding appropriate erotic images for her masturbatory fantasies.

Night. Steamy, red-lit interior of the Clit Club. Hand-held camera pans from three women laughing and seated around a table studded with beer bottles to various women dancing in the packed club.

DORIS *(v-o):* She was so torn between women and men that instead of one fantasy, she would produce this weird amalgam of mix 'n match bodies, heads, and genitals. After reading that I thought, "Hey this isn't my story. I know what I want. I want Mildred." So I immediately called her up and we made a date. The first thing I noticed was that she was wearing the socks I had given her.

MCU, from bartender's POV, of two white women, one in her early forties, the other around thirty-five, as they sit down at the bar.

YOUNGER WOMAN: Let's go back to my place.

OLDER WOMAN: I don't feel ready.

YOUNGER WOMAN: You mean you want to stay here longer?

OLDER WOMAN: No, I mean I'm not quite up for it.

YOUNGER WOMAN: What will make you feel up for it?

OLDER WOMAN: Look, there's something you should know about me, about my body.

YOUNGER WOMAN: What's wrong with your body? You look fine to me.

Camera dollies past them along the bar and stops at two young African Americans.

WOMAN #3: Five years ago I got together with a forty-year-old who looked thirty and now that she's entered menopause she's become a forty-five-year-old who looks fifty.

WOMAN #4: And you still look twenty-five. But so what? Do you want her to stay young forever?

WOMAN #3: I want her to *look* young forever.

Camera moves to end of bar. Two white women in their early thirties are talking. They seem to be a bit drunk.

WOMAN #5: You'd think that dykes would be more savvy.

WOMAN #6: That's like wanting women to be better politicians than men. There are all kinds of dykes, honey.

WOMAN #5: I think woman *are* better politicians than men, in the best sense. But I just can't tolerate racism in a lesbian. I mean, at this point in history, at this point in history, it just pissed me off, her saying, "You don't stand a chance if you're white."

Music surges up: Etta James, "Don't Cry Baby."

CU of MILDRED *and* DORIS *swaying on the dance floor. Camera tilts up as they draw together. Ambient sound and music fade out as* MILDRED*'s v-o begins.*

MILDRED *(v-o):* On that first night we went to her house, but she was drunk to the point of not feeling well, so I went home around 3 A.M. I dreamt I crossed the Rubicon carrying a large suitcase. On the far shore I opened it and found there was room for several more objects. I picked up some stones and put them in. They fit perfectly.

DORIS *(v-o):* I dreamed I was a young man. I had been

Interior. Dusk. MW of a large open window which frames the facade of a building across the street. A barren but brightly lit loft interior can be seen through a window of the opposite building.

DORIS *(v-o):* working out in a gym and was now in the changing room. A handsome young man stood very close to me. We started a casual conversation.

MS of DORIS, *with the shadows of the window frame across her body, sliding down the wall to a sitting position and closing her eyes.*

DORIS *(v-o):* "Do you come here often?" I think I was the one who asked, even as each of us knew what was on the other's mind.

Dusk. WS, from street level, of facade of a building. A YOUNG ASIAN MAN *leans out of a second-story window and peers across the street.* DORIS, *dressed in a man's suit, joins him.*

DORIS *(v-o):* In unspoken consent we went to a room with a bed. We were now in Japan or a Japanese-like place.

LS of MILDRED*'s loft.* DORIS *and* YOUNG ASIAN MAN *walk toward* *the stage in the background. Camera tracks behind them. They mount the steps and, fully clothed, lie down on a mattress and embrace.*

DORIS *(v-o):* I heard Japanese being spoken in the distance. The door remained open. We talked while embracing on the bed. Someone outside the room closed the door. My partner suddenly became so impassioned that he came. We talked some more. His penis again grew hard in my hand. I asked him if he wouldn't mind fucking me. For some reason I specified "in the vagina." Suddenly confusion reigned. The order of things vanished.

ELS. DORIS *and* YOUNG ASIAN MAN *are in the background on the stage. A table laid out with checked table cloth is in the foreground.* MIL-DRED *and* JEFFREY *are seated at opposite sides of the table, eating.* YOUNG MILDRED *and* JENNY *are also seated at the table, playing cards. A clamour of voices is heard as ambient sound.*

DORIS *(v-o):* We were surrounded by chattering people. I was forced to admit that I had totally forgotten that I was a man and didn't have a vagina. How could I have forgotten such a thing? My companion became disgusted with me. I discovered he was German. He had had a heavy German accent all along but I was doing so much of the talking that I hadn't noticed. With all those chattering people around I had been mounting elaborate arguments for my pansexuality and the vagina I may or may not have had, or once had, or might have again. It was all a dodge to avoid

CU of hands playing cards.

DORIS *(v-o):* anal penetration. If I had a vagina he wouldn't have to go in "that other way." I think that's when he got disgusted with me.

JEFFREY *(off-screen):* I was closeted on both fronts

MS of JEFFREY *from over* MILDRED's *shoulder.*

JEFFREY: as far as my parents were concerned. So I had the onerous task of telling them that I was gay and HIV-positive all at once. I don't recommend that strategy for anyone.

Reverse MS of MILDRED *from over* JEFFREY*'s shoulder.*

MILDRED: She's told her daughter and son-in-law about the two of us, but I don't think she's told them about her breast cancer. God, she's barely discussed it with me. It drives me a little bananas. She'll bend my ear till the cows come home about food, bodies, AIDS, sex, money, aging, you name it, but when it comes to a disease that's threatening her life, she's all privacy and information, as though it's happening to someone else or she's reading the newspaper.

JEFFREY *(off-screen):* It's called denial.

MILDRED: I feel so excluded. She's acting like she may not even want me to go to the hospital with her. What am I? Her enemy?

MS of JEFFREY *and* YOUNG MILDRED *and* JENNY *leaning in so the three of them form a chorus.*

JEFFREY, YOUNG MILDRED, *and* JENNY *(in unison):* Of course not!

MCU of MILDRED.

MILDRED: Sometimes I want to throttle her.

MS of the threesome as before.

JEFFREY, YOUNG MILDRED *and* JENNY *(in unison):* Kick her when she's down!

MCU of JENNY.

JENNY: So, Young Mildred, how's it going to come out?

MCU of YOUNG MILDRED.

YOUNG MILDRED: I'm able to foresee just a few steps at a time. Doris is going to let me come to the hospital. She'll call my name when she's waking up from the mastectomy, and I'll bring her home three days later.

Reverse high-angle LS. The foursome at the table can be seen in the background, now watching the "performance." The YOUNG ASIAN MAN *gets up from the bed and removes "paraphernalia from his body."* DORIS *stands in foreground, looking up at camera.*

DORIS *(sync):* We were now alone on a rooftop. He had been lying on top of me, face to face. He got up, moved away. He then removed all this paraphernalia from his body: a tongue ring, belts and clothespins that had been attached to his skin. As I was waking up I was filled with remorse and guilt. What was I going to tell Mildred? Technically I hadn't had sex with him, but I had certainly wanted to. I decided that if she asked me, I would say no, I hadn't had sex with him.

Title:

CONJUGAL PLUNGE

Haircutting salon. Daytime. Very chic haircutter is cutting MILDRED*'s hair. She has an English accent.*

HAIRCUTTER: So how are you?

MILDRED: We've been looking for a place to live. Doris and I have decided to live together.

HAIRCUTTER: Oh, how wonderful. 'S funny, Doris told me you were looking, but she didn't say anything about it being for the two of you. What are you looking for, a two-bedroom?

MILDRED *(does a slight double-take):* Um . . . Things are so expensive out there we'll probably end up renovating my place.

HAIRCUTTER: At the moment, the fact that the entire complex network of advanced capitalist economy hinges on home-buying, and that the philosophy of home-ownership is intimately linked to the sanctity of the nuclear family, shows how completely the uterine norm of womanhood supports the phallic norm of capitalism.

Title:

THE CITY SPEAKS

Music over title and following sequence. There is no audible dialogue. MILDRED *and* DORIS *walk down the steps of a museum. The footage has been optically printed so they appear to move at twice normal speed. They pause as* MILDRED *anxiously searches for something in her bag. They argue as they descend the steps. CU of two pairs of hands gesticulating. Camera tilts up to reveal* MILDRED *trying to put a token into the slot of a tall revolving turnstile. It sticks. They argue. They ascend the subway stairs. Cut to* MILDRED *and* DORIS *at token vendor's booth, where* MILDRED *argues with the vendor and with* DORIS. *Subway platform, where* MILDRED *and* DORIS *wait for a train. A title crawls across the bottom of the frame:*

> The incidence of breast cancer among American women has
> been rising for the past thirty years. And those who should
> know, claim not to know why.

Interior of subway car seen through the open doors from the platform. MILDRED *and* DORIS *enter and sit down. Cut to a very young heterosexual couple sitting across from them. The girl is chewing gum and sits with both her legs across her companion's lap. Music ends before* DORIS *speaks.*

DORIS: What if we did that?

Unintelligible crackle of P.A. system. WS from platform through open door of subway car. Young couple, followed by MILDRED *and* DORIS, *leaves the train.*

Day. MILDRED *and* DORIS, *holding hands, walk past a gas station. A mini-van, leaving the station, lurches toward them aggressively rather than stopping short to let them pass.* DORIS *gives the young male driver the finger. He starts to get out of the car. They run.*

DRIVER: You're too goddamned happy!

Music (a languid section of Herbert Clark's "Sounds of the Hudson") begins. Day. MCU of a forty-year-old man weeping on a park bench. MILDRED *and* DORIS *observe him from nearby, then move off. During this shot a crawling title moves across bottom of frame:*

75% of breast cancers occur in women with no risk factors whatsoever.

MW. MILDRED *and* DORIS *sit down on a bench elsewhere in the park.*

WOMAN *(off-screen):* I didn't know gay people go through all that emotional stuff.

MILDRED *and* DORIS *exchange glances, get up, and leave frame. Cut to MW as they sit down on another bench.*

WOMAN #2 *(off-screen):* Lesbians can't get AIDS because their sexual activity is too infrequent and too boring.

Two middle-aged white men carrying briefcases—one in a tweed jacket with leather patches on the elbows, the other in a Burberry raincoat—pass by.

MAN: The lesbians are coming and they're going to be politically correct and make everyone miserable, and we're going to have to deal with every issue and won't get any work done.

Again MILDRED *and* DORIS *move. They pass two very old African-American women walking arm-in-arm in the opposite direction.*

WOMAN: I'll be damned if I let them treat me like an old tangerine skin cast out behind the ballroom.

Street corner. YVONNE, *in profile, wearing tuxedo, is standing, waiting for the light to change.* MILDRED *and* DORIS *walk into the frame between her and the camera.*

MILDRED: I remember the exact moments my mother taught me how to iron a shirt, write a check, darn a sock, parse a sentence.

MILDRED *and* DORIS *exit frame.* YVONNE *turns to camera.*

YVONNE: Statistics show that lesbians are chronic late returners of library books.

She exits frame.

Day. Bookstore. Camera tracks along a shelf of books in the Gay and Lesbian Studies Section. A hand removes a book. Pan to MS of FLO.

EMMA *(off-screen):* Mama, when are we going to get *my* book?

FLO: Just a few more minutes, Emma. We're looking for something for Granma's birthday and then we'll get something for you. *(to* JIM*)* I don't know whether to get her something on sexuality or breast cancer.

JIM: If I know Doris, she's taking care of her cancer research very well by herself.

FLO: Do you think she'll like this?

JIM *(reading book jacket):* "No Priest But Love: The Journals of Anne Lister 1824–1826." Sounds juicy. But what do I know?

FLO: She's gotten interested in lesbian history. Let's get it.

FLO *shoves the book into* JIM*'s hand, grabs the book that he has been reading, slams it onto a shelf and leads the way toward the front of the store, away from the camera.* JIM *follows her.*

JIM: Maybe now she won't come down on us for being homophobic.

They pass JENNY, *who has her eyes on* EMMA.

FLO: I think she's touchy because she's so new at it. She treats us like parents. Give her time. She'll calm down.

JIM *(turning):* OK, Emma,

Reverse MCU of JENNY *crouched, touching* EMMA*'s nose.* YOUNG MILDRED *stands behind them silently reading a book.*

JIM *(off-screen):* let's get you a book.

EMMA skips out, followed by JENNY.

YOUNG MILDRED *(reads aloud from* The Taming of Chance *by Ian Hacking):* Probability is *the* philosophical success story of the first half of the twentieth century. To speak of philosophical success will seem the exaggeration of a scholar. Turn then to the most worldly affairs. Probability and statistics crowd in upon us. The statistics of our pleasures and our vices are relentlessly tabulated. Sports, sex, drink, drugs, travel, sleep, friends—nothing escapes. There are more explicit statements of probabilities presented on American prime time television than explicit acts of violence (I'm counting the ads). Our public fears are endlessly debated in terms of probabilities: chances of meltdowns, cancers, muggings, earthquakes, nuclear winters, AIDS, global greenhouses, what next? There is nothing to fear (it may seem) but the probabilities themselves. This obsession with the chances of danger, and with treatments for changing the odds, descends directly from the forgotten annals of nineteenth-century information and control.

Title:

SHRINKAGE

*Night. The black-and-white footage in this sequence is from various '40s and '50s Hollywood movies (*Golden Boy, The Set-Up, Kiss of Death*). Wide shots of the boxing ring and crowd in a large arena. CU (color) of an old-fashioned steel microphone dropping into the frame. The* REFEREE, *an African-American woman about forty years of age enters in CU.*

REFEREE: This is it, ladies and gentlemen. Welcome to the main event, the title bout. In this corner we have Mildred Davenport, otherwise know as the Amazing Titania, 130 pounds and still growing.

WS of ring, showing MILDRED*'s corner and her* TRAINER, *a forty-five-year-old white man chomping a cigar.* MILDRED *prances and waves her arms with triumphant bravado. The* REFEREE *is dressed in high heels, skirt suit, and bow tie.*

Ringside. YOUNG MILDRED, JENNY, *and* YVONNE *sit next to each other on a scaffold.* YOUNG MILDRED *and* JENNY *are eating hotdogs and guzzling beer.* YVONNE *is wearing a flashy robe and bright red hand wrapping, as though she is the next contender. They all cheer.*

WS of ring as before. The REFEREE *continues her introduction.*

REFEREE: And in this corner we have Doris Schwartz, otherwise known as the Unphased Amazon, 135 pounds and stable.

DORIS *prances around, acknowledging roar of crowd. Cut to black-and-white footage of crowd. A man stands and wildly applauds. Crowd roars. WS of the ring as before. The* REFEREE *beckons to the fighters to come to the center of the ring.*

REFEREE: OK, ladies, I want a good clean fight, no rabbit punches, no punches below the belt, no clinches; and in case of a knock-down, go to a neutral corner. I want you to hug and have a good fight. OK, hug.

MILDRED *and* DORIS *punch right hands and go to their respective corners.*

The bell clangs. MCU, low angle shot from outside the ring of DORIS *seated in her corner and her* TRAINER, *a forty-year-old Asian woman dressed in floral print jacket and pearls.*

DORIS'S TRAINER: OK Doris, go out there and *don't fight*!!

DORIS *prances out into the ring. The crowd roars. CU of* MILDRED's *and* DORIS's *feet sashaying around the ring. The canvas is stenciled with breast cancer statistics.*

MCU of YVONNE *on the scaffold. She removes her left arm from the sleeve of the robe, revealing a mastectomy scar. During the following monologue we hear the sounds of pummeling taken from Hollywood fight sequences.*

YVONNE: Alright, I've been putting this off. I had been living an oblivious cat's life, only in my case I had five chances instead of nine. Five biopsies—I almost said lobotomies—five biopsies in eight years following up on that first diagnosis of lobular carcinoma *in situ.* Eight years ago they didn't call *in situ* carcinomas breast cancer. "A marker of higher risk," that first breast surgeon kept repeating, and I in turn repeated it like a mantra. "Not breast cancer, but a marker of higher risk." He wanted to take 'em both off. No breasts, no breast cancer.

I did my research, found a more conservative surgeon, and weighed the odds. Twenty to thirty per cent higher risk than the general population. At that time one woman out of every ten or eleven got breast cancer. Now it's one out of eight or nine. "You're more likely to die in a car accident," Dr. Love had said. Since I didn't own a car, I didn't know quite what to make of that.

Various shots of ring, spectators, and trainers, the two non-combatants moving warily around, jabbing, darting, shuffling, clinching. The REF-EREE *breaks up a clinch. The crowd cheers. The crowd boos.* RICHARD WIDMARK *screams from the stands.* DORIS*'s trainer pantomimes punches outside the ring. The bell clangs. Black-and-white shot of rich dowager looking shocked, followed by shot of very fat man munching popcorn.*

CU (color) of MILDRED *in corner with her* TRAINER. MILDRED *has a towel around her neck and looks exhausted.*

TRAINER: Just back off. Back off, stay down; stay on the defensive. Got it?

MILDRED: Gotcha.

TRAINER: It's nothing to worry about. You're doin' fine. Watch the jaw. Keep the chin up, watch the jaw, and stay down.

MILDRED: OK, down.

The bell clangs. MS of JENNY *and* YOUNG MILDRED *on scaffold. After* YVONNE*'s voice yells "ACTION!" they start screaming and gesticulating. MCU of* MILDRED *and* DORIS *jabbing and weaving, ending in another clinch.*

DORIS: You put too much soap in the wash. That's why your skin itches.

MILDRED: Don't you dare tell me how to do laundry. You're always throwing off the blankets and making me freeze.

DORIS: You wash the kitchen counter with that stuff and never rinse it off. You're trying to poison me.

Black-and-white footage of woman jumping up from her seat and scream-ing something.

CU of MILDRED *and* DORIS *in clinch as before.*

MILDRED: You're still putting the English muffins in the freezer.

DORIS: I have no rights here. You can throw me out anytime. I don't feel at home.

MILDRED: You don't support my work.

Black-and-white footage of two different groups of men jumping up from their seats and yelling.

CU of MILDRED *and* DORIS *in clinch as before.*

DORIS: You're not there when I need you.

MILDRED: You don't *tell* me when you need me.

DORIS: You expect too much of everybody.

MILDRED: You're always angry.

The phone rings. DORIS *goes to a corner (toward the camera) and answers it.* MILDRED *leans against the ropes in the background.*

DORIS: Hello. Yeh, that's me. Hi, how ya doin'? . . . No kidding. He sounds like the one for us. Thanks a lot. . . . Yeh, we'll be home tonight. Bye.

DORIS *hangs up. ML.* DORIS *turns and faces* MILDRED.

DORIS: Hey Mil, looks like we got a cat.

MCU of MILDRED.

MILDRED: It scares me how much I want you.

ML. DORIS *walks toward* MILDRED *(and camera).*

DORIS: Then we're a perfect match. There's nothing I desire more than to be wanted.

MCU of MILDRED.

MILDRED: You . . . you.

MCU of DORIS. MILDRED *walks into frame. They embrace.*

DORIS: How about dinner and a show?

The crowd roars. MCU of YVONNE *at ringside. Her teeth clench an enormous unlit cigar. In the course of her monologue she alternates holding up one of two 8×10 inch cards when she utters the word* murder. *"MURDER" is printed on one card and "*murder*" on the other.*

YVONNE: Women don't often *MURDER* each other. Why not? When it occurs or comes close to occurring we sit up and take notice, like that case of the mother of the high school cheerleader who allegedly plotted to have her daughter's rival's mother knocked off. There is *MURDER* and then there is *murder. MURDER* by homophobia; *murder* by social and legal abuse, repression, stigma. *MURDER* by DDT, PCBs, dioxin, by 177 organochlorines stored in our fat, breast milk, blood, semen and breath, by nuclear tests conducted in the 1950s. *MURDER* by electromagnetic fields. *MURDER* by breast cancer. And how must lesbians *murder* in order to survive? As children we fantasized *MURDERING* our sisters, our mothers, our newly born siblings. As adults we must learn to tolerate and work through the fantasized *murders* of our lovers. Thoughts can be *murderous,* but thoughts don't kill. The seeds of certain fruits are said to be toxic if eaten. When I was ten years old I saved up appleseeds with which to poison my older sister. I had heard it took a cup.

WS of MILDRED *and* DORIS *rolling around on the canvas, still wearing their gloves. The crowd cheers. The* REFEREE *begins the count. On "five" the "Ode to Joy" from the last movement of Beethoven's Ninth Symphony begins, segues into the following three shots: Day. WS of New York street and exterior of* MILDRED's *loft building. A moving van drives up, parks.*

*A man gets out and goes to back of van. MCU of back of van as man opens
sliding door to reveal* DORIS*'s battered chair. Another man appears to help
the first to remove it from interior of van and carry it to the front door of
building. Ringside. MS, camera tracks past* YVONNE, *then* JENNY,
finally settling on YOUNG MILDRED. JENNY *is ecstatic,* MILDRED *looks
despondent. Music fades down.*

JENNY: I never thought they'd get this far, did you?

YOUNG MILDRED *(to camera):* We're both afraid of things to come.
   Doris has fantasies of jumping ship. It hurts me to the quick. She
   tries to make us sound pretty dreary: Like, yes there is intellectual
   stimulation but she can get that elsewhere. And she gets so tired of
   my hair-splitting in discussions and what she calls my blanket show-
   stopper of "It's not that simple" which she accuses me of never bothering to explain. And, worst of all, she tells herself that when it
   comes to sex she can take it or leave it. And she gets sick to death of
   my don't's and my black looks, and irrationality and my feelings of
   being unloved. Someday she'll ask me why in her fantasy life she
   feels loved by me while in mine I feel unloved by her. I'll not have an
   answer. Another one of those impossible—leading, "not innocent"—
   questions. I know what she's getting at: Her father loved her and my
   father didn't love me. What presumption, I think. How condescend-
   ing, how patronizing, how complacent, how straight. How dare she?

JENNY *(embracing* YOUNG MILDRED*):* Mildred, my dear, don't worry.
   It's all going to work out.

WS of MILDRED *and* DORIS *lying on the canvas. The crowd roars. The*
REFEREE *continues the count: "Five, six, seven, eight, nine, ten." CU of
heads of* MILDRED *and* DORIS. *It now appears that they are making love.*
MILDRED *is behind* DORIS, *nuzzling and whispering into her ear.* DORIS
squeals.

MILDRED: Guess who I ran into yesterday?

DORIS *makes orgasmic sounds. She is in the middle of multiple orgasms.*

Cut to CU MILDRED *and* DORIS, *same framing but different lighting. As
the camera dollies back during the following dialogue we see that they are*

in their tee shirts and boxing shorts, sans gloves, and are lying on a dining room table. There is a life-size black-and-white photomural of kitchen cabinets and counter in the background.

MILDRED: Woody Allen. He was in the middle of a shoot right down the street.

DORIS *has another one.*

MILDRED: And then I brought the groceries home and put them away.

DORIS *has another one.*

MILDRED: Gee, it doesn't matter what I say to you, does it? *(sings)* Old MacDonald had a farm. . . .

DORIS *(in the middle of another one, laughs, then gasps out):* It's not the content, it's the voice. You know that.

YOUNG MILDRED *(v-o):* But then she comes home while I'm watching *Broadway Danny Rose* and it's the part where Woody Allen and Mia Farrow have been tied together prone on the table by the crazy Mafiosos and we laugh and hoot and look at each other with delight and I'm beside myself with love for her and climb all over her body.

Night. MILDRED's *and* DORIS's *loft.* DORIS *is at her computer.* YVONNE, *in tuxedo, is looking over her shoulder. Camera dollies around and tilts up to reveal a large blow-up of a 1916 photo of three women sitting on a beach. Instrumental version of "Fatal Wedding" fades in. Camera tilts down to CU of Powerbook screen upon which is printed:*

Far into her dotage, my mother—Jenny Schwartz—was looking at a photo of Marilyn Monroe. She said, "What beautiful breasts she has." When I described this to my then husband he remarked—in disbelief—"She sounds just like a man!"

New text on the Powerbook:

I've been having all these dreams in which I'm a man dressed in a tangerine suit. But I don't seem to have any success as a man. In one dream I even forget that I don't have a vagina. A real man wouldn't forget. I guess the Dan Quayle alter-ego I portray in my performances is a way of washing this masculine wash-out out of my hair.

Wide shot of YVONNE *seated on* DORIS's *desk, facing the camera. The whole left side of her tuxedo and shirt has been cut away so as to reveal her mastectomy scar. This will be her costume for the rest of the film. Behind her on the wall is fabric that is vertically striped in white, green, and orange, suggesting a carnival motif.*

YVONNE: So what caused this? Who's the enemy? My body? My behavior? All the peanuts I've eaten in my life? Not having enough fun? Having too much fun? Becoming a lesbian? Moving in with my lover? Do the women who live on Long Island, which has one of the highest rates of breast cancer in the country, cause their cancers, or is it the pesticide-poisoned water they drink? And what about the uranium miners in New Mexico and the people in Colorado whose town was built on uranium pilings? Did their cancers come from unresolved anger? Did the women who live downwind of the Hanford nuclear complex in Washington State exacerbate their cancers by eating too much peanut butter?

Camera tilts up to an opening in the wall that has been decorated to look like a Punch and Judy show. JENNY *and* YOUNG MILDRED *pop up in the Punch and Judy frame.*

YOUNG MILDRED: How is a tumor different from a lesbian?

JENNY: Ugh! I give up.

YOUNG MILDRED: One ages well and the other doesn't.

JENNY: What?!

YOUNG MILDRED: What did the lesbian say to her breast?

JENNY: I don't wanna know.

YOUNG MILDRED: That's it. That's what she said.

They pull out soft bladder-like clubs and beat each other over the head. A raspy burlesque show coda is heard, along with raucous cartoon-like sound effects. CU of computer screen.

In high school she was a jock, along with all these other girls. There was a lot of joking around in the locker room. Sex? No, a bit of fondling, sensuality, and jokes. And of all those women she was the only one who left that suburb and became a lesbian. All the rest married and had children. Back then it seemed, and still seems, so obvious to her that they were no different from her. Attracted to each other, enjoying each other's bodies, loving female physicality. Now maybe when they're older and divorced and their children are grown, some of them will become lesbians. But they sure didn't, they sure couldn't, when they were younger.

MS of YOUNG MILDRED *and* JENNY *peering through an open window, resting their arms on pillows.*

YOUNG MILDRED *(dreamily):* Just think of it: If in one year only one girl from every graduating class in every high school in the country becomes a lesbian, that means 33,000 lesbians! In a decade that would add up to 330,000. And in thirty years it would be a million!

JENNY: You really know yer numbas.

"September Song," sung by Lotte Lenya, begins. JENNY *and* YOUNG MILDRED *look into the distance.*

Another part of the loft. MCU of MILDRED *and* DORIS *dancing. In the far distance behind them we see the edge of a plastic partition, cables, lights.*

DORIS: Do you want to exchange versions of the last two days?

MILDRED: Maybe it's not such a good idea right now. We're both tired.

DORIS: You have such good sense.

They continue to dance.

DORIS: Why did it happen to me? Sometimes when I'm cooking I think of Sally. She was the one who told me about using wooden spoons in metal pots. She used to say, "Your pots will last longer." And sometimes when I enter a subway car I hear Roberta saying, "My mother taught me never to ride in the first or last car." She never was in a subway accident. And Sally's pots outlived her. Breast cancer got both of them.

Cut to another part of the loft. In the foreground, in front of a plastic partition, are piles of newspapers. Behind the partition shadowy figures hover. YVONNE *walks right-to-left behind the screen, emerges at the left side of screen. Camera pans right as she walks toward newspapers. Her monologue starts in voice-over as she starts to walk, then continues in sync following a jump-cut which finds her seated amidst the newspapers.*

YVONNE: Infiltrating tubulo-lobular carcinoma, well-differentiated, grade I, the tumor measures approximately 1.5 cm. It had not shown up on the mammogram. I repeat: It did not show up on the mammogram. It was revealed by a fifth biopsy. One day I didn't have cancer and the next day I did, and I didn't feel any different, in fact I felt in the pink. So what happened? It still hadn't penetrated that I had cancer. The breast surgeon didn't say, "You have cancer." After reporting the pathologist's diagnosis, she said, "I recommend a modified radical mastectomy." Period. It took a few days for me to be able to confront the reality. *(She pounds an adjacent pile of papers.)* I HAVE CANCER. It was obviously too late for recriminations. I had my left breast removed post-haste.

An off-screen commotion erupts: much banging of metal, crashing around, as if objects are falling from shelves. DORIS*'s voice mingles with coercive rejoinders from several other voices, male and female.* YVONNE *appears to be listening as camera tracks left. The shadowy figures continue to hover behind screen.*

DORIS *(off-screen):* Hey, what's going on, whaddya think you're doing? . . . No, it's not my turn. It was supposed to happen to *her,* not me. *She's* the one in the higher risk category. She's the one who smokes and drinks. I've been such a good girl; I eat my turnip greens and brown rice. . . . Get away from me, you creeps.

VARIOUS VOICES *(off-screen):* Come along, your time has come. . . Hold her down . . . This won't hurt. You'll be back on your feet in no time . . . Fighting will get you nowhere. It won't take long.

MCU of YVONNE *as before. She is holding a manuscript page. The following sequence jump-cuts between her reading from the page and addressing the camera.*

YVONNE: I'm a sucker for statistics. They make your head spin with the dizzying prospect that the body is a quantitative entity, and death can be determined with easy calculation.

In the United States breast cancer is the leading killer of women between the ages of thirty-five and forty-five. It is the leading cause of cancer death among American women ages twenty to fifty-four.

I find myself posing in ways that all my life I've seen men do. At first you feel a tremendous tautness across this area. . . .

That means 2.8 million women have breast cancer . . . and you have very limited mobility in your arm.

Of 182,000 women newly diagnosed with breast cancer in 1993, 46,000 will be dead in five years . . .

They give you exercises *(she demonstrates)* . . .

more than 75,000 will be dead in ten years . . .

and after a few months you regain almost full range of motion.

One out of nine women will develop breast cancer sometime in her life. That rate has more than doubled in the last thirty years.

That taut feeling, however, never quite disappears.

One out of three Americans will face some form of cancer. Of these, two out of three will die from the disease.

That taut feeling, . . .

The death rate . . .

however, never quite disappears . . .

from breast cancer has not been reduced in more than fifty years.
. . .

Yet there are some of us who escape . . . and some of us survive.

(She crosses her arms and takes the "macho" pose.)

Day. MILDRED *and* DORIS*'s loft. Camera pans from CU of Kleenex box and flowers sticking up from canvas bag to MCU of* DORIS. *Her right hand is feeling her left armpit. We hear approaching footsteps.* DORIS *abruptly starts sorting mail. The boxing ring is in the background.*

MILDRED *(v-o):* I thought you wanted to go to bed.

DORIS: I don't feel like it.

Camera pans to follow MILDRED *as she crosses behind* DORIS *and stands beside canvas bag.*

MILDRED: I don't like this. You're not letting me take care of you.

DORIS: What?! What do you want to do?

Camera tilts up to MCU of MILDRED.

MILDRED: Just let me take care of you. You know you aren't supposed
to carry anything with your left arm. When we left the hospital you
said you were tired and wanted to go to bed. And then you insist on
carrying this bag.

DORIS *(off-screen):* All I want to do is look at my mail. Look, if it had
hurt I wouldn't have picked anything up.

DORIS *pounds desk and stands up into the frame.*

DORIS: You are upsetting me!

They both leave the frame. It is empty for ten seconds. They return, make a bee-line for each other, embrace. DORIS *begins to sob uncontrollably.*

MILDRED: It's OK, love; it's OK.

DORIS: Oh God, I just felt your breast against my ribcage.

YVONNE's *voice begins reading cancer statistics. The image remains for ten or fifteen seconds.*

YVONNE *(v-o):* U.S. cancer death rates increased seven percent between 1975 and 1990. Breast cancer is the most commonly diagnosed cancer in American women today—more common than lung and colon cancer. Lung and breast cancer are now the leading killers of women. Thirty women die from breast cancer every hour. That's one every two minutes. By the year 2000 cancer will be the leading killer of everyone.

The v-o crossfades with sounds of rasping motor and male singing. Daytime. Exterior of a '50s station wagon. MS through the windshield of the driver, GEORGE, *a dissolute-looking white man in his early '30s. He is singing "Goin' to Chicago." A shimmering night impression can be seen through rear window. Before he finishes refrain, cut to side view of* GEORGE *and sixty-three-year-old* DORIS. *She wears a lavender angora sweater and is voraciously gobbling peanuts.*

GEORGE: "Goin' to Chicago; sorry but I can't take you. Goin' to Chicago; sorry but I can't take you, cuz there's nothin' in Chicago that a monkey woman can do."

DORIS: George, would you call me flat-chested?

GEORGE: No, I wouldn't call you flat-chested.

DORIS *stuffs tissues into her sweater.*

DORIS: How's that?

GEORGE: Wha'd ya do, put peanut shells in there? Doris, when we get to Albuquerque do you think you could call your mother and get her to wire some more dough? We're going to need it.

CU of DORIS.

DORIS: I'll do it if you stop calling me a monkey woman Jew.

YOUNG MILDRED *(v-o):* Doris and I are so different. Barely older than I am now, she'll run off with an alcoholic drifter. In some ways she's still the perennial bad girl;

Cut to an examination room of a gynecologist's office. Over DORIS *'s shoulder we see her hands holding an issue of the National Enquirer open to a blaring headline and picture:* Twenty-five-year-old Man Trapped in Toddler's Body. *A paper sheet is draped over* DORIS *'s lower body and her legs are bent.*

YOUNG MILDRED *(v-o):* but I'm not going to be a goodie two-shoes forever. I'll learn pretty quickly that *(now ironically)* marriage deprives one of worldliness and a coherent inner self.

A knock is heard. DORIS *'s off-screen voice says, "Come in." Nelly, her gynecologist, enters the room. She is a white woman in her early fifties, dressed in the usual white coat, unbuttoned to reveal a fashionable black dress. She stands at the narrow counter and writes in the folder she has brought with her.*

NELLY: Hell-lo, how are you today?

DORIS: I'm OK, considering. Nelly, before you see for yourself, I must tell you that I've had a mastectomy.

NELLY: Oh, so it finally caught up with you. Did Alisan do it?

DORIS: Yep.

NELLY: When did you have it and what did they find?

DORIS: In June. Infiltrating tubulo-lobular carcinoma, 1.5 cm, estrogen positive, all twenty-six lymph nodes negative.

(NELLY writes.)

DORIS: You're looking very elegant today.

NELLY: Oh, it's the lipstick.

DORIS: And the black dress and the necklace.

NELLY: No, it's the lipstick. I caught myself in the mirror and it's too much. I have to take it off. Have you seen an oncologist?

DORIS: Yes. He would have given me chemo if I had let him. I'm taking tamoxifen.

NELLY: Any side effects?

DORIS: A leaky twat.

NELLY: You should talk to him about that.

DORIS: He said to talk to you about it.

NELLY: OK, then I have to give you a D and C to look at the endometrium.

DORIS *groans.*

NELLY: But I'll tell you, if you're going to have breast cancer this is the best one to have. It's very slow-growing and very rare. So let's take a look in your vagina and see what's what. *(She inserts speculum.)* It looks very good in there. Much better.

DORIS: What about the atrophic vaginitis?

NELLY: It's all gone. That's the tamoxifen.

DORIS: We sound like a drug company commercial. So am I trading in my atrophic vaginitis for endometrial cancer and liver damage?

NELLY *(removes speculum):* No, no, no. But still we have to make sure. I want you to get a pelvic sonogram and then we'll see about the D and C.

DORIS: That's so painful. Will you put me out or give me a local?

NELLY: You, we must put out. I'll put you out with a baseball bat.

DORIS: I bet you will.

NELLY: So get your sonogram and then we'll talk. OK?

DORIS: Yeh. Bye, Nelly. Thanks.

NELLY *exits. WS of* DORIS *perched on the end of the table. The room is bare save for a standing scale in the background.*

YVONNE *(v-o):* Lesbians have a one-in-three risk of developing breast cancer. That's a two to three times higher risk of developing breast cancer than heterosexual women. Not giving birth increases a woman's risk by 80 percent. Lesbians with breast cancer have a mortality rate of 80 percent, compared to 25 percent for heterosexual women. Lesbians are also at a higher risk for cervical and ovarian cancer, because we're less likely to have children by the age of thirty.

Title:

RECONSTRUCTION

Early evening. A cocktail party in MILDRED *and* DORIS*'s house. MS.* MILDRED *holding two glasses of wine, sits down very close to* JEFFREY *on a sofa. A* MAN *is sitting on the back of the sofa between the two of them. His head is not visible. Behind them people mill in the crowded noisy room, and occasionally people pass between* MILDRED *and* JEFFREY *and camera.*

Fragments of a statistic can be seen stenciled on the wall behind them. The din gradually increases in volume so that by the end of the scene they have almost to shout to be heard.

MILDRED: You did say white, didn't you? I knew he was hostile, but to accuse me of *sexual harassment?* I *had* to give him a D. He did hardly any work and cut more than half the classes.

JEFFREY: It's preposterous. He can't possibly get away with it. You're out there, aren't you?

MILDRED: Of course. I've never made any secret of being a lesbian, and besides, it's been in my curricula for years. That's what's so perverse about the situation.

JEFFREY: He has to be some kind of nut.

MAN *sitting on back of sofa moves abruptly, bumping into* MILDRED. *CU of* MILDRED.

MILDRED: What a week. How was yours?

CU of JEFFREY.

JEFFREY: Not so good. I got my blood tests back. My T-cell count has gone down to 200.

MILDRED *(off-screen):* Oh, Jeffrey, I'm so sorry.

JEFFREY: This numbers game is weird. I feel fine.

MILDRED *(off-screen):* You look good. Are you still taking those drugs?

JEFFREY: No. They were fucking up my liver, so my doctor took me off of them. How is Doris doing? Is she back from her tour?

MS of MILDRED *and* JEFFREY.

MILDRED *(looking around):* She said she'd be here later . . . Doris is great. She's already working on a new performance. It's me who's doing all the wrong things. I keep irritating her by being so solicitous.

CU of JEFFREY.

JEFFREY: I wouldn't worry about that. She really needs you.

MW of a wall upon which someone is stenciling: In 1992 37-and-a-half million people in the U.S. had no health insurance. *Yvonne walks into the frame, turns around to face the camera and begins to speak as she cleans her glasses. Occasionally people walk by, not noticing.*

YVONNE: In the beginning you also get stabbing pains at the back of your armpit if you move in the wrong way. The surface of your skin remains numb for a long time. That's why you want to keep touching it, testing it, caressing it. It is your vulnerable place, your Achilles heel, the new love of your life, this absence, this flatness, this surgeon's gift. I could say I don't want my breast back. It's more complicated than that. It isn't that I don't miss it. It's just that I've gotten used to this asymmetry. I want it not to happen again. I want to live out my allotted time without disease.

CU of MILDRED *now standing beside a column.*

MILDRED: No, she'd never get breast reconstruction. She's too much of an exhibitionist to try to hide what's happened to her body. She wears her flat left chest like a medal. She doesn't even use a prosthesis most of the time.

MS of ALICE *and* JEFFREY.

ALICE: Audrey Lorde said that reconstruction and prostheses are merely another way of keeping women with breast cancer silent and separate from each other. What they don't tell women is that as you age one breast drops while the reconstructed one stays youthfully upright.

JEFFREY: Oh my god.

ALICE: "Oh my god" is right.

JEFFREY: Why can't women do whatever they're comfortable with?

CU of MILDRED.

MILDRED: I don't want to think about this anymore. My brother and sister died from cancer. Enough is enough.

YVONNE's *v-o begins intoning cancer death rates over the party ambience. As camera dollies backward away from* MILDRED, *party guests fill in the intervening space.*

YVONNE: In 1900 cancer accounted for only 4 percent of deaths in the U.S., but now accounts for 22–23 percent and is the second leading cause of death. One woman dies every twelve minutes from breast cancer. The percentage of women who survive five years beyond treatment after a mastectomy is 76.6 percent, up only 8 percent since 1970. Black women's five-year survival rate is 13 percent lower than that of white women. For women whose cancer has metastasized, the survival rate has held at 18 percent for the last fifty years.

Title:

OUT OF THE MOUTHS OF BABES

Evening. EMMA*'s bedroom.* DORIS *is reading the end of a story to her granddaughter. They are both leaning against the headboard of the bed.*

EMMA: Why is everyone getting poorer, Granma?

DORIS: Not everyone is getting poorer. Some people are getting richer.

EMMA: My friend Lincoln told me that everyone has gotten poorer. And Mama is always saying we're going to end up in the poorhouse.

DORIS: That's very funny, Emma. Florence talks like I used to talk. But look at me. Am I in the poorhouse?

EMMA: No, but Mama says she doesn't want to end up like you.

DORIS: I think she just doesn't want to get old. It's not so bad, getting old. You still have some good times even if things go wrong once in awhile.

DORIS *closes book, exits, returns and sits on edge of bed, facing* EMMA.

EMMA *(after a pause):* Did it hurt when they did your operation?

DORIS: A little, but they give you medicine that takes the pain away. You know, there used to be a tribe of women who took off one breast so they could hunt better with their bows and arrows. They were called Amazons.

EMMA *(thinks for a bit):* But how did their babies get enough to eat?

DORIS: Oh, they probably did OK on one breast. Maybe they just didn't grow up to be Amazons.

EMMA: They grew up to be kids.

DORIS: Right. They grew up to be kids.

Title:

GETTING AWAY WITH MURDER

Ironic musical riff on "Little Bo Peep" begins. WS, lobby of apartment building. MILDRED *and* DORIS *stand in front of an elevator. They are dressed for a masquerade party.* MILDRED *is wearing a rust-colored velvet Oscar Wilde get-up with ruffled shirt, top hat and cane.* DORIS *is dressed as Little Bo Peep, with cape, shepherd's crook, and snakeskin cowboy boots. Her head is encased in a Sylvester Stallone mask.*

Crawling title: Of the 140,000 toxic waste dumps in the U.S. over 60% are located in black or Hispanic neighborhoods.

Medium two-shot of MILDRED *and* DORIS. DORIS *is swaying while her muffled voice from inside the mask sings, "Little Bo Peep has lost her sheep."*

DORIS *(taking off her mask):* Ugh, I'm suffocating. Sometimes I feel like a toxic waste dump.

MILDRED: If you're going to take off the top of your dress, I'm leaving.

DORIS: I'll feel it out. I may not have the nerve.

MILDRED: This is supposed to be a pleasurable event. Why do you want to shock people?

DORIS: But I'm legal. It isn't as though I'd be exposing a sexual part of myself. And besides, if femininity is something we can put on and take off, like a prosthesis, a masquerade party is the perfect place to do it.

MILDRED: You're being perverse.

DORIS *(stubbornly):* No, I'm being real. My new chest is as much an artifice as this mask.

MILDRED: It's like wearing a sign. I mean that's the way people will look at you—it's like wearing a sign that says "My days are numbered."

Long pause. Cut to WS of lobby. Both women look troubled.

DORIS: Is that what you think?

MILDRED: On bad days I think that.

Screams are heard off-screen. JEFFREY *and* ALICE *rush in.* ALICE *wears a skeleton costume.* JEFFREY *wears a huge Afro wig and long lamé gown over D-cup breasts. There is much hilarity as they all exchange greetings. The elevator doors open to a fanfare of music and* YVONNE *emerges with a shopping cart full of merchandise. The foursome ignores her and piles in. Elevator doors close.* YVONNE *remains in front of elevator as she speaks. She now wears a large pink breast prosthesis over the otherwise bare left side of her chest.*

YVONNE: I never told you life was a party. I'm taking this drug called tamoxifen, brand name is Nolvadex. It's been around for almost ten years, but it's still experimental as far as I'm concerned because they don't know the long-term effects. It supposedly improves your five-year survival odds by 20 to 30 percent. Nolvadex is manufactured by a British company called Imperial Chemical Industries whose principal business is the production of synthetic chemicals. In fact they are the world's largest producer and user of chlorine, which is used to make paper, plastic, paint, and pesticides.

Series of jump-cuts as she takes various items out of the shopping cart and displays them for the camera: paper towels, Kleenex, notebooks, paint can, roach spray, plastic container. Raucous Dixieland-style music begins. Elevator doors open. COP/DOC #1 *in white coat, police hat, gun holster, with billy club and stethoscope—half cop and half doctor—forcibly ejects* YOUNG MILDRED *now wearing a diagonal ribbon labeled ESTROGEN over her blouse. They bump into* YVONNE *and overturn her cart with a great clatter and clanging of spilled objects. The ensuing melée is like a silent Keystone Cop movie, with many jump-cuts. The spatial framing remains constant, i.e. a wide shot of the lobby in front of the elevator doors.*

YVONNE *begins to clean up the mess of pestilent products.* COP/DOC #2 *hauls* JENNY, *wearing a ribbon labeled CHLORINE, out of the elevator. They jostle* YVONNE *as* YOUNG MILDRED *runs back into the frame, chased by* COP/DOC #1. *Both* COP/DOCS, *brandishing billy club and gun, pursue the elusive* YOUNG MILDRED *and* JENNY *around* YVONNE *and the shopping cart, which is again overturned. Finally the* COP/DOCS *manage to push* YOUNG MILDRED *and* JENNY *against the elevator doors. They gesticulate wildly, resisting blame for whatever charges are being pressed on them. The elevator doors open and* MILDRED, DORIS, JEF-FREY, *and* ALICE, *plus a half-dozen* WOMEN *wearing huge breast prostheses over wild costumes, burst out. There are a Brunhilde, a bearded bride, and various mismatched stereotypes. They all immediately attack the* COP/DOCS, *who are still chasing* YOUNG MILDRED *and* JENNY. *The whole mob surges back and forth.*

YVONNE *(v-o):* Residues of chlorine reside in the body tissues of people in all industrialized countries and have been found to disrupt the action of hormones in a woman's body. They enhance the activity of estrogen, and we know that high levels of estrogen are associated with higher incidences of cancer.

The masqueraders chase the COP/DOCS, *now with a great roar that replaces the music of the preceding footage.*

MS of JENNY *and* YOUNG MILDRED *clapping and laughing with glee.*

YVONNE *(v-o):* Every October for the past ten years Imperial Chemical Industries has paid for National Breast Cancer Awareness Month, also called "Beecam."

COP/DOC #2 *(who has been knocked down by some of the revelers):* BCAM's message is, "Early detection is your best protection."

YVONNE *(v-o):* Neat, wouldn't you say? First they give us breast cancer by polluting the environment;

COP/DOC #1 *is chased into the frame, trips and falls.*

COP/DOC #1: then we educate you to watch out for the early signs of cancer;

YVONNE *removes her prosthesis and stuffs it into his mouth. She and three others drag him off.*

JEFFREY *pulls* YVONNE *into the elevator just before the doors close.*

The two COP/DOCS *run from opposite sides, collide, try to get by each other. Women rush in, chase #2 off while others hold #1.*

YVONNE *(v-o):* and then they reap millions in profits from its treatment with the drug that they manufacture. Early detection is not only about saving lives.

COP/DOC #1: It means bigger profits.

A woman thrusts a pie into his face.

MS of elevator doors, which open to reveal YVONNE *bent over* JEFFREY *in a tango kiss.*

Title:

THE REST OF THIS LIFE

MILDRED *and* DORIS*'s kitchen. Night. MS.* DORIS*, at kitchen table, is laughing hysterically at* MILDRED*'s off-key attempt to sing-along to The Byrds' version of "Hey Mr. Tambourine Man." Camera pans to* MILDRED*, who is standing beside a stack of steel shelves housing CD player et al.*

She finishes singing and removes head phones. The ensuing six-and-a-half-minute scene consists of one shot, the camera tracking and panning to follow the characters' movements. The kitchen is bare. The glass-doored cabinets are empty; there are no pots hanging on the peg board above the stove, and plastic sheeting covers a piece of furniture—probably bookshelves. The gaffer's "tie-in" to the fuse box can be seen in a corner. The only visible kitchen paraphernalia is what is necessary for this meal.

DORIS *(off-screen):* What's to eat?

MILDRED: Chicken and chicken soup.

MILDRED *goes to refrigerator, removes a large bowl which she takes to the stove. She then ladles soup from a big pot into a smaller pot and starts slicing up chicken.*

MILDRED *(indicating the smaller pot):* Do you think you'll be wanting more than this?

DORIS *(goes toward stove to look):* Oh yeh.

MILDRED *ladles more soup and puts pieces of chicken into the smaller pot.* DORIS *sets the table with soup bowls, spoons, folded paper towels.*

MILDRED: Do you want more chicken in yours?

DORIS *(gets up to look in pot):* No.

DORIS *slices a piece of bread from a loaf she has brought to the table, eats it while reading a magazine. Camera pans to* MILDRED *leaning against the kitchen counter. Time passes as the small pot heats up. After awhile she ladles soup into a bowl, then takes the bowl to* DORIS *at the table.* DORIS *immediately begins to eat.* MILDRED *brings her bowl to the table, puts on her glasses, and opens a book.* DORIS *slumps over her bowl, gustily slurping.*

DORIS: Mm. I don't think it's as good as yesterday.

MILDRED: I haven't tasted it yet.

DORIS *finishes—*MILDRED *has hardly begun—and goes to the stove with her bowl. Camera stays on* MILDRED.

DORIS *(v-o):* Do you want some more chicken? I just want the other stuff.

MILDRED: OK.

DORIS *brings the small pot to the table, spoons out a few pieces of chicken into* MILDRED'*s bowl, leaves pot on the table, goes to the counter, gets her bowl and brings it back to the table. She ladles soup from pot into her bowl, then noisily slurps it up.*

DORIS: You know, this is the first meal we've had together in ages.

MILDRED: That's true, isn't it.

DORIS: Mmm, yes, it *is* as good as yesterday.

MILDRED: I think it's as good.

DORIS: I love the broth part.

DORIS *finishes off her soup, then picks up the pot and momentarily contemplates drinking out of it, thinks better of it, pours remainder of soup into her bowl, picks up bowl and drinks from it. They look at each other as the lights fade to black.*

End credits rise from bottom of frame. During the ensuing 3-minute crawl, DORIS *and* MILDRED *engage in v-o dialogue.*

DORIS: Today I read that one in five lesbians is likely to get breast cancer in her lifetime.

MILDRED: I thought it was one in three.

DORIS: Where'd you read that?

MILDRED: It might have been in that material I got from the Mautner Project in Washington, D.C., while you were in the hospital. I didn't want to show it to you. It's all speculation, you know. There's been so little research on lesbians and cancer.

DORIS: Are you saying lesbians are *not* more likely to get cancer?

MILDRED: No, I'm not saying that. Oh, these statistics make me tired. Lesbians, lesbians. Before you got involved with me you had a one in eight chance of getting cancer. The day after you seduced me did your chances jump to one in three?

DORIS: Hey, wait a minute.

MILDRED: Yes, I suppose some lesbians *are* at greater risk. For a lot of different reasons. Like, *some* lesbians don't go to doctors for things like birth control and Pap smears and mammograms. They can't get shared health insurance, for one thing.

DORIS: *And* they drink and smoke.

MILDRED: Yes, we do have more stress in our lives. And medical people are notorious for hostile or off-handed treatment of lesbians. So *some* lesbians stay away from doctors and get diagnosed at a more advanced stage of disease.

DORIS: So many ways to get messed up. Your numbers are even more terrifying than mine.

MILDRED: They're just numbers. Everyone has a different set of numbers. You can't live your life by numbers.

DORIS: But you can use the numbers as cautionary. Like, when did *you* last get a Pap smear and mammogram?

MILDRED: Oh, don't start on me now. I don't know, two or three years ago. Did you feed the cat?

DORIS: I fed him four times today! He's getting fat.

MILDRED: We're increasing his risk of feline kidney cancer. Goodnight, dear.

DORIS: Goodnight, Mildred.

A light switch is heard to click.

Cast in order of appearance

Jenny	Isa Thomas
Young Mildred	Catherine Kellner
Camera Crew	Sandy Hays
	Eileen Schreiber
	Betsy Nagler

Doris	Joanna Merlin
Alice	Alice Playten
Mildred	Kathleen Chalfant
Jeffrey	Kendal Thomas
Phone Woman #1	Elizabeth Cohen
Phone Woman #2	Linda Gui
Yvonne Rainer	Yvonne Rainer
Man in Boat	Jerry Fisher
Woman on T.V.	Rosalyn Deutsch
Man on T.V.	Robert Ubell
Ladies Room Voice #1	Lee Nagrin
Ladies Room Voice #2	Ernece Kelly
Flo	Jennie Moreau
Jim	Rod McLachlan
Homeless Women	Lee Nagrin
	Inez Bragagnolo
Waiter	Chris Field
Bra Saleswoman	Melina Jochum
Club Woman #1	Carolin K. Brown
Club Woman #2	Barbara Butcher
Club Woman #3	Jocelyn Taylor
Club Woman #4	Brigitte Barnett
Club Woman #5	Jones Miller
Club Woman #6	Sabrina Artel

Other Women at Club

Caroline N. Brown	Cathy Cook
Susana Cook	Linda Gui
Amy Harrison	Nanette Harty
Sharon Hayes	Priscilla Holbrook
Kimberly Horton	Suzan Hurwitz
Nora Jacobs	Ernece Kelly
Rosalynde LeBlanc	Shigem McPherson
Angie Oliver	Robin Warwick
Kate Wilson	Millie Wilson
	Kristine Wood

"Japanese Man"	Gordon Synn
Haircutter	Lorraine Massey

Subway Couple	Jhana Lowe
	Khan Lowe
Minivan Driver	Stephen Schmidt
Man Crying in Park	Dan Berkey
Men in Park	Bob Huff
	Dan Berkey
Women in Park	Yvonne Warden
	Ira Jeffreys
Offscreen Voice	Eileen Schreiber
Emma	Sasha Martin
Woman in Bookshop	Lorraine Martinez
Referee	Novella Nelson
Mildred's Trainer	John Hagan
Doris's Trainer	Patsy Ong
Moving Men	Craig Rosenzweig
	Chris Des Marais

Party Guests

Gregg Bordowitz	Carrie Cooperider
Chris Des Marais	Richard Elovich
Julie Finch	Su Friedrich
Thyrza Goodeve	Nancy Grossman
Linda Gui	Ernece Kelly
Mary Kelly	Elizabeth Kendall
Tiffany Monroe	Claire Pentecost
Kathryn Ramey	Jill Rubin
Catherine Saalfield	Diane Shapiro
	Julie Thaxter-Gourlay

George	Rainn Wilson
Nelly	Barbara Haas
Masquerade Revelers	Eunice Fein
	Ernece Kelly
	Jennifer Miller
	Lee Nagrin
	Katherine O'Sullivan
	Jennifer Romaine
	Bonnie Seiler
Cop/Doctor #1	Richard Elovich
Cop/Doctor #2	Bob Huff

Director	Yvonne Rainer
Casting	Heidi Griffiths
Director of Photography	Stephen Kazmierski
Production Designer	Stephen McCabe
Costume Designer	Linda Gui
Composer	Frank London
Line Producer	Stephen Schmidt
1st Assistant Director	Christine LeGoff
2nd Assistant Director	Melina Jochum
1st Assistant Camera	Mia Barker
2nd Assistant Camera	Eileen Schreiber
	Doray Donnet
Sound Recordist	David Powers
Art Director	Cathy Cook
Propmaster	Chris Des Marais
Script Supervisor	C. Leigh Purtill
Location Scout/Manager	Matthew Chilsen
Gaffer	Kristy Tully
Best Person	Deidre Lally
Key Grips	Kathryn Ramey
	Alice McDermitt
Best Grip	Karen Rodriguez
Swing	Simeon Moore
Production Manager	Jill Rubin
Office Coordinator	Julie Thaxter-Gourlay
Asst. Costume Designer	Diane Shapiro
Art Dept. P.A.'s	Carrie Cooperider
	Ashraf Meer
Boom Operators	Betsy Nagler
	Irin Strauss
	Jose Torres
	Lisa Van Houten
Steadycam Operator	Sandy Hays
Lead Man	Ken Bush
Make-up and Hair	Clare Bonser
Asst. Location Scout	Dake Gonzalez
Carpenters	Chris Des Marais
	Rob Knatlowitz
	Sally Sasso
Photo Mural	Vivian Selbo

Caterer	Susan Lawrence
Still Photographer	Esther Levine
Key Production Assistant	Craig Rosenzweig
Set Production Assistants	Sloan Eric Lee
	Camille J. Norment
	Simon Olson

Additional Production Assistants: Jenifer Berman, Annie Husson, Hellin Kay, Tiffany Monroe, Ivan Hurzeler, Scott Jordan, Marlon R. Lawe, Emily Schaeffer, Stephen Schaeffer

Editor	Yvonne Rainer
Sound Editor	Leo Trombetta
Assistant Editor	Robert Hall
Asst. Sound Editor	Julie Wang
Postprod. Supervisor	Christine LeGoff
Archival Research	Susan Hormuth
Script Consultant	Lynne Tillman
Music Consultant	Frank London
Legal Consultant	David Dretzin
End Credit Formatting	Jenifer Berman
Fiscal Sponsor	Women Make Movies
Boxing Coach	Angel Rivera
Prop Car	Leonard Shiller/
	Antique Autos
Ms. Chalfant's Haircut	Frederick Waggoner
Ms. Merlin's Haircut	Richard Stein

Locations: Den of Thieves, Liquor Store Bar, Devachan, Verso Books, Surf Avenue Carousel, Chelsea Parking

Roller Coaster Footage	Archive Films
Factory Footage	Library of Congress
Video Formatting	Christy MacKarell/
	Stable Films
Video Transfer	Du Art
	Colorlab-Baltimore
Opticals	B.B. Optics
Titles and Opticals	Cynosure
Negative Cutter	Tim Brennan

Laboratory	Du Art
Sound Mix	Sync Sound
Sound Mixer	Grant Maxwell
Music Recording	Tom Mitchell/K Studio
Drums	Newman Baker
Bass and Tuba	David Hofstra
Trombone	Jim Leff
Piano	Brian Mitchell
Cornet	Frank London
Additional Lyrics	John Greyson

Quote Sources: Judy Brady, Vivian Gornick, Stephen King, D. A. Miller, Joan Rivière, Terry Castle, Ian Hacking, Audrey Lorde, Kathy Peiss, Gayatri Spivak, Paula Treichler

Thanks: Jackie Allen, Donna Brogan, Lisa Cartwright, Elizabeth Cohen, Katherine Dieckmann, Veralynn Behenna, Jean Carlomusto, Ron Clark, Mark Daniels, Andrew Fierberg, Gleason's Gym, Lorie Hiris, Isaac Julien, Minnette Lehmann, Sheila McLaughlin, Maria Nardone, Open City Films/Joana Vicente/Jason Kliot, Robin Rausch, Katie Roumel, Alisa Solomon, Stephen Stanczyk, Dorothy Thigpen, Dan Walworth, Jill Godmilow, Amy Hobby, Terry Lawler, Tina London, Nabile Nahas, Mark Nash, Catherine Lord, Peggy Phelan, Dorothy Richardson, Share, Ellen Shapiro, Nathan Stockhamer, Christine Vachon, Lois Weaver

Special Thanks: Martha Gever and Jay Anania, Gregg Bordowitz, Su Friedrich, Barbara Kruger, Ernest Larsen, Sherry Millner, Belle Rainer, Robert Rauschenberg, Gay Block, E. B. Friedlander, Agnes Gund, Ellen Kuras, Lorraine Massey, Loretta Palma, Ivan Rainer, Michael Shamberg, Dr. Nelly Szlachter

From the Shores of the Mighty Pacific composed by Herbert L. Clarke, Gerard Schwarz, cornet, William Bolcom, piano, Nonesuch Records

Eight Days on the Road performed by Aretha Franklin, Jerry Ragovoy, music, Michael Gayle, lyrics, Warner/Chappel Music, Atlantic Records

Don't Cry, Baby performed by Etta James, music & lyrics by J. Johnson/S. Unger/S. Bernie, Warner/Chappel Music, MCA Records

September Song performed by Lotte Lenya, Kurt Weill, music, Maxwell Anderson, lyrics, Warner/Chappel Music & Hampshire House, Sony Music Licensing

Hey Mr. Tambourine Man music & lyrics by Bob Dylan, Special Rider Music

This film has been made possible in part by funding and awards from J.D. and C.T. MacArthur Foundation, Wexner Center for the Arts at Ohio State University, National Endowment for the Arts, New York State Council for the Arts, New York Foundation for the Arts, Astrea National Lesbian Action Foundation, Rockefeller Foundation, and The American Film Institute in association with The National Endowment for the Arts

In Memoriam
Shirley Triest
Nancy Graves

Filmography

1967   *Volleyball* (Foot Film) 16 mm, black and white, silent, 10 minutes

1968   *Hand Movie* 8 mm, black and white, silent, 5 minutes

        Rhode Island Red 16 mm, black and white, silent, 10 minutes

        Trio Film 16 mm, black and white, silent, 13 minutes

1969   *Line* 16 mm, black and white, silent, 10 minutes

1972   *Lives of Performers* 16 mm, black and white, 90 minutes

1974   *Film About a Woman Who . . .* 16 mm, color/black and white, 105 minutes

1976   *Kristina Talking Pictures* 16 mm, color/black and white, 90 minutes

1980   *Journeys from Berlin/1971* 16 mm, color, 125 minutes (won the Special Achievement Award from the Los Angeles Film Critics' Association)

1985   *The Man Who Envied Women* 16 mm, color, 125 minutes

1990   *Privilege* 16 mm, color, 103 minutes (won the Filmmakers' Trophy at the Sundance Film Festival, Park City, Utah, 1991, and the Geyer Werke Prize at the International Documentary Film Festival in Munich, 1991)

1996   *MURDER and murder* 16 mm, color, 113 minutes (won the "Teddy" Award at the Berlin Film Festival, 1997)

All of the above feature films are distributed by Zeitgeist Films, 247 Centre Street, New York, NY 10013; telephone: (212) 274-1989; fax: (212) 274-1644.

Selected Bibliography

Ahlgren, Calvin. "There's No Narrative to this Woman's Tale" (interview). *San Francisco Chronicle* (September 1985).

Albright, Ann Cooper. "Mining the Dancefield: Spectacle, Moving Subjects and Feminist Theory." *Contact Quarterly* 15, no. 2 (Spring/Summer 1990): 32–40.

Anbian, Robert. "Three Win Phelan Filmmaking Awards" (interview). *Release Print* 8, no. 9 (November 1990): 9

Anderson, Jack. "Yvonne Rainer: The Puritan as Hedonist." *Ballet Review* 2, no. 5 (1969): 31–37.

Arthur, Paul. "Desire for Allegory: The Whitney Biennials." *Motion Picture* 2, no. 1 (Fall 1987).

Banes, Sally. "The Aesthetics of Denial." In *Terpsichore in Sneakers: Post-Modern Dance.* Boston: Houghton Mifflin, 1980: 41–54.

————. "Lives of Performers: Annette Michelson Discusses Acting in *Journeys from Berlin*." *Millennium Film Journal,* nos. 7, 8, 9 (Fall 1980–Winter 1981): 69–84.

————. *Greenwich Village 1963.* Durham: Duke University Press, 1993.

Bassan, R. "Forme et ideologie chez Yvonne Rainer." *Revue du Cinéma*, no. 357 (January 1981): 129–30.

Bear, Liza, and Willoughby Sharp. "The Performer as a Persona: An Interview with Yvonne Rainer." *Avalanche*, no. 5 (Summer 1972): 46–59.

Berger, Maurice. "The Cave: On Yvonne Rainer's *Privilege*." *Artforum* 29, no. 3 (November 1990): 27–28. Reprinted in Maurice Berger, *How Art Becomes History.* New York: Harper Collins, 1992: 114–22.

————. "Minimal Politics: Performativity and Minimalism in Recent American Art" (catalogue essay for exhibition). *Issues in Cultural Theory*, no. 1, Baltimore: Fine Arts Gallery, University of Maryland,1997: 1–35.

Berman, Susan. "Yvonne Rainer." *Ms* (April 1975): 40–44.

Bernard, Jami. "Finding Humor Behind a Tumor" (review of *MURDER and murder*). *Daily News.* (June 20, 1997).

Blumenthal, Lyn. "On Art and Artists: Yvonne Rainer." *Profile* 4, no. 5 (1984).

Borden, Lizzie. "Trisha Brown and Yvonne Rainer." *Artforum* 4, no. 5 (1984).

————. "Yvonne Rainer: 'This is a story about a woman who . . . .' Theater for the New City." *Artforum* 11, no. 10 (June 1973): 80–81.

Briggs, Kate, and Fiona MacDonald. "Three Possible Endings: An Interview with Yvonne Rainer." *Photofile* (Australia), no. 30 (Winter 1990): 28–33.

Brinkmann, Noll. "Was is fiktionswürdig? Gedanken zum Klimakterium im Hollywoodfilm un zu Yvonne Rainers *Privilege*." *Frauen und Film*, nos. 50–51 (June 1991): 72–83.

Brooks, Linda. "*Paris is Burning, Privilege, Queen of Diamonds*: Sundance Film Festival, Park City, Utah" (review). *Art Papers* 15, no. 6 (November–December 1991): 114–15.

Brown, Georgia. "Flash Points" (review of *Privilege*). *Village Voice* (January 15, 1991).

Bruno, Giuliana. "La mela di Adamo." *Filmcritica,* 37, nos. 365–66 (June–July 1986): 361–62.

Buckley, T. "The Screen: *Journeys from Berlin/1971.*" *New York Times* (February 11, 1980): C16.

Camera Obscura Collective. "Yvonne Rainer: An Introduction." *Camera Obscura*, no. 1 (Fall 1976): 53–70.

————. "Appendix: Rainer's Descriptions of Her Films. " *Camera Obscura,* no. 1 (Fall 1976): 71–75.

————. "Yvonne Rainer: Interview." *Camera Obscura,* no. 1 (Fall 1976): 76–96.

Carroll, Noel. "Interview with A Woman Who . . ." *Millennium Film Journal* nos. 7, 8, 9 (Fall 1980–Winter 1981): 37–68.

———— "Film." In *The Postmodern Moment.* Edited by Stanley Trachtenberg. Westport, CT: Greenwood Press, 1986: 118–19.

Castle, Frederick, "Occurrences: To Go to Show Them." *Art News* 67, no. 4 (Summer 1968): 34–35.

Chin, Daryl. "Add Some More Cornstarch; or, The Plot Thickens: Yvonne Rainer's *Work 1961–73. Dance Scope* 9, no. 2 (Spring 1975): 50–64.

Christie, Ian. "Lives of Performers." *Monthly Film Bulletin* 44, no. 520 (May 1977): 101.

Coco, William, and A.J. Gunawardana. "Responses to India: An Interview with Yvonne Rainer." *The Drama Review* 15, T-50 (Spring 1971): 139–42.

Copeland, Roger. "Toward a Sexual Politics of Contemporary Dance." *Contact Quarterly* 7, nos. 3–4 (Spring–Summer 1982): 45–51.

———— and Marshall Cohen. *What is Dance?* Oxford: Oxford University Press, 1983.

Crow, Thomas. *The Rise of the Sixties.* New York: Harry Abrams, 1996.

Dargis, Manohla. "Talking Pictures" (review of *The Films of Yvonne Rainer*). *The Independent* (July 1990): 16–18.

Dawson, Jan. "A World Beyond Freud." *Sight and Sound* 49, no. 3 (Summer 1980): 196–97.

de Baecque, Antoine. "Yvonne Rainer: Le style, c'est l'emotion." *Cahiers du Cinema*, no. 369 (March 1985): 41–42.

de Lauretis, Teresa. *Alice Doesn't: Feminism, Semiotics, Cinema.* Bloomington: Indiana University Press, 1984.

———. "Strategies of Coherence: Narrative Cinema, Feminist Poetics, and Yvonne Rainer." In *Technologies of Gender: Essays on Theory, Film, and Fiction.* Bloomington: Indiana University Press, 1987: 107–26.

DeMichiel, Helen. "Rainer's Manhattan." *Afterimage* 13, no. 15 (December 1985): 19–20.

Desmond, Jane. "Yvonne Rainer and the Practice of Theory." Paper presented at the meeting of the Society for Cinema Studies, Montreal, May 10, 1987.

Devins, S. "*The Man Who Envied Women.*" *Variety* (October 2, 1985): 13.

Easterwood, Kurt; Susanne Fairfax; and Laura Poitras. "Yvonne Rainer: Declaring Stakes" (interview). San Francisco Cinematheque, 1990.

Fensham, Rachel and Jude Walton. "'Naming Myself,' an Interview with Yvonne Rainer." *Writings on Dance* (Melbourne), no. 7, (1991).

Field, Simon. "The State of Things." *Monthly Film Bulletin* 54, no. 636 (January 1987): 4–6.

Fischer, Lucy. "The Dialogic Text, an Epilogue." In *Shot/Countershot: Film Tradition and Women's Cinema.* Princeton: Princeton University Press, 1989.

Ford, Julie, "Yvonne Rainer . . . In Transition." *Siren* 1, no. 4 (October–November 1996): 14.

Foster, Susan Leigh. *Reading Dancing: Bodies and Subjects in Contemporary American Dance.* Berkeley: University of California Press, 1986.

Furlong, Lucinda, ed. *Set in Motion: The New York State Council on the Arts Celebrates 30 Years of Independent Film.* Catalogue, NYSCA, 1994.

Fusco, Coco. "Fantasies of Oppositionality." *Screen* 29, no. 4 (Autumn 1988) and *Afterimage* 16, no. 5 (December 1988).

Gentile, Mary C. "How to Have Your Narrative and Know It Too: Yvonne Rainer's *Film about a Woman Who . . .*" In *Film Feminisms, Theory and Practice.* London: Greenwood Press, 1985: 133–52.

Goldberg, Marianne. "The Body, Discourse and *The Man Who Envied Women.*" *Women and Performance* 3, no. 2, (1988): 97–102.

Goldberg, Rosalee. *Performance Art: From Futurism to the Present.* New York: Harry N. Abrams, 1996.

Goodeve, Thyrza. "Yvonne Rainer: Risks, between You and Me." *Declaring Stakes.* San Francisco Cinematheque.

———. "Rainer Talking Pictures" (interview). *Art in America* 85, no. 7 (July 1997): 56–63, 104.

Goodman, Saul. "Yvonne Rainer: Brief Biography." *Dance Magazine* 39 (December 1965): 110–11.

Green, J. Ronald. "The Illustrated Lecture." *Quarterly Review of Film and Video* 15, no. 2 (1994): 16–17.

Green, Shelley R. *Radical Juxtaposition: The Films of Yvonne Rainer.* Metuchen, N.J.: The Scarecrow Press, 1994.

Hecht, Robin Silver. "Reflections on the Career of Yvonne Rainer and the Value of Minimal Dance." *Dance Scope* 8 (Fall–Winter 1973–74): 12–25.

Hoberman, James. "All about Yvonne." *Village Voice* (Febrary 11, 1980): 47.

———. "Explorations: Our Movies, Ourselves." *American Film* 7, no. 1 (October 1981): 34.

———. "The Purple Rose of Soho" (review of *The Man Who Envied Women*). *Village Voice* (April 8, 1986): 64.

Holden, Stephen. "Time Bent, Love Tested and Illness Faced Down" (review of *MURDER and murder*). *New York Times* (June 20, 1997): C12.

Howell, John. "Ça Va? Pas Mal." *Art-Rite*, no. 8 (Winter 1975).

———. Review of *Work 1961–73. Art in America* 63 (May–June 1975): 18–21.

Hulton, Peter, ed. *Fiction, Character and Narrative: Yvonne Rainer.* Devon, England: Department of Theatre, Dartington College of the Arts, Theatre papers, 2d ser., no. 7, 1978.

James, David E. "Yvonne Rainer: *Film about a Woman Who . . .*" In *Allegories of Cinema: American Film in the Sixties.* Princeton: Princeton University Press, 1989: 326–35.

Jayamanne, Laleen, with Geeta Kapur and Yvonne Rainer. "Discussing Modernity, Third World and *The Man Who Envied Women*." *Art and Text* 23, no. 4 (March–May 1987): 41–51.

Johnston, Jill. "Judson 1964: End of an Era." *Ballet Review* 1, no. 6 (1967): 7–13.

———. "The New American Modern Dance." In *The New American Arts.* Edited by Richard Kostelanetz. New York: Collier Books, 1965: 162–93.

———. "Rainer's Muscle." In *Marmalade Me.* New York: E. P. Dutton, 1971: 36–40.

Jowitt, Deborah. "Two Choreographers." *Artscanada* 32 (March 1975): 46–47.

Kaplan, E. Ann. *Women and Film: Both Sides of the Camera.* New York: Methuen, 1983: 120–28.

———. *Looking for the Other: Feminism, Film, and the Imperial Gaze.* New York, Routledge, 1997.

Kaye, Nick. *Postmodernism and Performance.* New York. St. Martin's Press, 1994.

King, Kenneth. "Toward a Trans-Literal and Trans-Technical Dance-Theater." In *The New Art, a Critical Anthology.* Edited by Gregory Battcock, New York: E.P. Dutton, rev. ed., 1973: 119–26.

Klawans, Stuart. Review of *Privilege. The Nation* (January 28, 1991): 99.

Kleinhans, Chuck. "Lives of Performers." *Women and Film* 1, nos. 5–6 (Winter 1974–75): 51–54.

Koch, Stephen. "Performance: A Conversation." *Artforum* 11, no. 4 (December 1972): 53–58.

Kotz, Liz. "Loaded Questions." *San Francisco Weekly* (September 5, 1990).

———. "A Legend Comes Out." *The Advocate* (November 5, 1991): 82.

Kruger, Barbara. " 'Difference: On Representation and Sexuality' (review of film program), the New Museum/The Public Theater." *Artforum* (April 23, 1985): 94–95.

———. "Yvonne Rainer: *The Man Who Envied Women*." *Artforum* 24 (Summer 1986): 124.

Kuhn, Annette. *Women's Pictures: Feminism and Cinema*. London: Routledge and Kegan Paul, 1982.

———, ed. *Women in Film, An International Guide*. Fawcett Columbine, 1990, 333–34.

Laderman, David. "Interview with Yvonne Rainer." *Art Papers* 13, no. 3 (May–June 1989): 18–24.

Lant, Antonia. *Privilege* (review). *Women and Performance* 5, no. 2, issue 10: 213–18.

Lardeau, Yann. "Yvonne Rainer, *Journeys from Berlin/1971*." *Cahiers du Cinéma*, no. 316 (October 1980): x.

Larsen, Ernest. "For an Impure Cinevideo." *The Independent* (May 1990): 24–27.

Levin, David Michael. "The Embodiment of Performance." *Salmagundi*, nos. 31–32 (Fall–Winter 1975–76): 120–42.

Lippard, Lucy. "Talking Pictures, Silent Words: Yvonne Rainer's Recent Movies." *Art in America* 65, no. 3 (May–June 1977): 86–90.

———. "Yvonne Rainer on Feminism and Her Film." *The Feminist Art Journal* 4, no. 2 (Summer 1975): 5–11. Reprinted in *From the Center*. New York: E. P. Dutton, 1976: 265–79.

Livet, Anne. *Contemporary Dance*. New York: Abbeville Press, 1978.

Longfellow, Brenda. "*Privilege*: A New Politics of Difference." *Independent Eye*, (Canada) (Spring/Summer 1991): 40–47.

Lord, Catherine. "Journeys to the Other Side: Yvonne Rainer's *Privilege*." *Artpaper* 10, no. 6 (February 1991).

———. "Looking Like a Lesbian: Yvonne Rainer's Theory of Probability." *Documents* no. 10 (Fall 1997): 31–42.

MacDonald, Scott. "Text as Image in Some Recent North American Avant-Garde Films." *Afterimage* 13 (March 1986): 9–20.

———. "Demystifying the Female Body: Interviews with Anne Severson and Yvonne Rainer." *Film Quarterly* 45, no. 1 (Fall 1991): 18–32.

———. "Yvonne Rainer" (interview). *A Critical Cinema* 2. Berkeley: University of California Press, 1992, 344–54.

———. "Yvonne Rainer: *Journeys from Berlin/1971*." In *Avant-Garde Film/Motion Studies*. Cambridge: Cambridge University Press, 1993, 157–69.

————, ed. *Privilege* (script). In *Screen Writings: Scripts and Texts by Independent Filmmakers.* Berkeley: University of California Press, 1995, 270–331.

Mackay, Heather. "The Challenge of Rainer." *San Francisco Bay Guardian* 24, no. 48 (September 5, 1990).

Margulies, Ivone. "A Cautionary Tale: The Lure of Centre in Yvonne Rainer's Cinema." *Independent Eye* (Canada). (Spring/Summer 1991): 48–58.

————. "Expanding the 'I': Character in Experimental Feminist Narrative." In *Nothing Happens: Chantal Akerman's Hyperrealist Everyday.* Durham: Duke University Press, 1996, 100–109.

Mayne, Judith. "Screentests." In *The Woman at the Keyhole.* Bloomington: Indiana University Press, 1990: 75–85.

McDonagh, Don. "Yvonne Rainer: Why Does It Have To Be That Way." In *The Rise and Fall and Rise of Modern Dance.* New York: Outerbridge and Dienstfrey, 1970.

McGee, Mickee. "In Other Words: A Report on 'Sexism, Colonialism, and Misrepresentation.'" *Afterimage* (September 1988).

Mekas, Jonas. "Interview with Yvonne Rainer." *Village Voice* (April 25, 1974): 77.

————. "Yvonne Rainer's *Film about a Woman Who . . .*" *Village Voice* (December 23, 1974): 94–97.

Mellencamp, Patricia. "Images of Language and Indiscreet Dialogue: *The Man Who Envied Women.*" *Screen* 28, no. 2 (Spring 1987): 87–101. Reprinted in *Indiscretions: Avant-Garde Film, Video, and Feminism.* Bloomington: Indiana University Press, 1990: 173–87.

————. "Five Ages of Film Feminism." In *Kiss Me Deadly: Feminism & Cinema for the Moment.* Edited by Laleen Jayamanne. Sydney: Power Publications, 1995: 32–35.

Meyer, James. "Remembering the 60s." *Frieze,* no. 30 (September–October 1996): 41–43.

Michelson, Annette. "Yvonne Rainer, Part I: The Dancer and the Dance." *Artforum* 12, no. 5 (January 1974): 57–64.

————. "Yvonne Rainer, Part 2: *Lives of Performers.*" *Artforum* 12, no. 6 (February 1974): 30–35.

Mitchell, Robb. "Representing Women: An Interview with Yvonne Rainer." *Screenline* (Winter 1990/1991): 1–2, 10.

Mueller, John. "Yvonne Rainer's *Trio A.*" *Dance Magazine* 53, no. 3 (March 1979): 42–43.

Mulvey, Laura. "Feminism, Film and the Avant Garde." *Framework,* no. 10 (Spring 1979): 3–10.

Murray, Timothy. *Like a Film: Ideological Fantasy on Screen, Camera, and Canvas.* New York: Routledge, 1993, 25–64.

Nelson, Michael. *"The Man Who Envied Women." Experimental Film Coalition Newsletter* 2, no. 4 (October, November, December 1985): 6.

Nemser, Cindy. "Editorial: Rainer and Rothschild, An Overview." *Feminist Art Journal* 4, no. 2 (Summer 1975): 4.

Pahlow, Colin. *"Film about a Woman Who . . ."* *Monthly Film Bulletin* 44, no. 525 (October 1977): 211–12.

Phelan, Peggy. "Spatial Envy: Yvonne Rainer's *The Man Who Envied Women.*" *Motion Picture* 1, no. 3 (Winter–Spring 1987): 1, 16–19. Reprinted in *Unmarked: The Politics of Performance.* New York: Routledge, 1993: 71–92.

Pontbriand, Chantal. "Interview with Yvonne Rainer." *Parachute,* no. 10 (Spring 1978).

Pym, John. "Working Title: *Journeys from Berlin/1971.*" *Monthly Film Bulletin* 47, no. 558 (July 1980): 140–41.

Rabinovitz, Lauren. *Points of Resistance: Women, Power and Politics in the New York Avant-garde Cinema, 1943–71.* Urbana: University of Illinois Press, 1991: 192–94.

Rabinowitz, Paula. "National Bodies: Gender, Sexuality, and Terror in Feminist Counter-documentaries." In *They Must Be Represented: The Politics of Documentary.* London: Verso, 1994: 182–88.

Rainer, Yvonne. "Yvonne Rainer Interviews Ann Halprin." *Tulane Drama Review* 10, no. 2 (T-30) (Winter 1965) 142–67. Reprinted in *Happenings and Other Acts.* Edited by Mariellen R. Sandford. New York: Routledge, 1995, 137–59.

———. "Notes on Deborah Hay." *Ikon* (February 1967): 2–3.

———. "Some Retrospective Notes on a Dance for 10 People and 12 Mattresses Called *Parts of Some Sextets,* Performed at the Wadsworth Atheneum, Hartford, Conn., and Judson Memorial Church, NY, in March 1965." *Tulane Drama Review* 10, no. 2 (T-30) (Winter 1965): 168–78. Reprinted in *Work 1961–73.* Halifax: Press of the Nova Scotia College of Art and Design and New York: New York University Press, 1974, and in *Happenings and Other Acts.* Edited by Mariellen R. Sandford. New York: Routledge, 1995, 160–67.

———. "A Quasi Survey of Some 'Minimalist' Tendencies in the Quantitatively Minimal Dance Activity Midst the Plethora, or an Analysis of *Trio A.*" In *Minimal Art, A Critical Anthology.* Edited by Gregory Battcock. New York: E. P. Dutton, 1968, 263–73. Reprinted in *Work 1961–73.* Halifax: Press of the Nova Scotia College of Art and Design and New York: New York University Press, 1974, 63–69; in *Esthetics Contemporary.* Edited by Richard Kostelanetz. Buffalo: Prometheus Books, 1989, 315–19; and in *The Twentieth-Century Performance Reader.* Edited by Michael Huxley and Noel Witts. New York: Routledge, 1996, 290–99.

———. "From an Indian Journal." *The Drama Review* 15 (T-50) (Spring 1971): 132–38. Reprinted in *Work 1961–73.* Halifax: Press of the Nova Scotia College of Art and Design and New York: New York University Press, 1974, 173–88.

———. Letter to *Artforum* 12, no. 16 (September 1973): 10.

———. *Work 1961–73.* Halifax: Press of the Nova Scotia College of Art and Design; and New York: New York University Press, 1974.

———. "Kristina (For a . . . Opera)" (photo-romanzo), *Interfunkitionen* (Cologne), no. 12 (1975): 13–47.

———. *Film about a Woman Who . . .* (script). *October,* no. 2 (Summer 1976): 39–67. Reprinted in *The Films of Yvonne Rainer.* Bloomington: Indiana University Press, 1989, 77–97.

———. "Annotated Selections From the Filmscript of *Kristina Talking Pictures.*" *NoRose* 1, no. 3 (Spring 1977).

———. "A Likely Story." *Idiolects,* no. 6 (June 1978).

———. "Kristina Talking Pictures" (script). *Afterimage* (U.K.), no. 7 (Summer 1978): 37–73. Reprinted in *The Films of Yvonne Rainer.* Bloomington: Indiana University Press, 1989: 98–132.

———. "Paxton Untitled." *Soho Weekly News* 16 (November 1978): 31. Reprinted in *Dance Scope* 13 (Winter–Spring 1979): 8–10.

———. "Conversation Following Screening at Cinemateque of *Christina* [*sic*] *Talking Pictures,* April 6, 1978,*"* *Cinemanews* 78, nos. 3–4 (1978): 16–17.

———. "Backwater: Twosome/Paxton and Moss." *Dance Scope* 13, no. 2–3 (Winter–Spring 1979).

———. "Beginning with Some Advertisements for Criticisms of Myself, Or Drawing the Dog You May Want to Use to Bite Me With, and Then Going On to Other Matters." *Millennium Film Journal,* no. 6 (Spring 1980): 5–7.

———. "Incomplete Report of the First Week of the Edinburgh International Film Festival, August 17–30, 1980 and Musings on Several Other Films." *Idiolects,* nos. 9–10 (Winter 1980–81): 2–6.

———. "Looking Myself in the Mouth." *October,* no. 17 (Summer 1981): 65–76.

———. "More Kicking and Screaming from the Narrative Front/Backwater." *Wide Angle* 7, nos. 1–2 (Spring 1985): 8–12.

———. "Beyond Mythologies." *Experimental Film Coalition Newsletter* 2, no. 4 (October, November, December 1985): 3.

———. "Engineering Calamity with Trisha Brown: An Interview." *Update, Dance/USA* (October 1986): 20–22.

———. "Some Ruminations Around Cinematic Antidotes to the Oedipal Net(tles) while Playing with de Lauraedipus Mulvey, or, He May Be Off-Screen, but . . ." *The Independent* 9, no. 3 (April 1986): 22–25. Reprinted in *Psychoanalysis and Cinema.* Edited by E. Ann Kaplan. New York: Routledge, 1990, 188–97, and in French translation as "20 ans de théories féministes sur le cinéma," edited by Bérénice Reynaud and Ginette Vincendeau in *CinemAction,* no. 67 (1993): 177–82.

———. "Thoughts on Women's Cinema: Eating Words, Voicing Struggles." *The Independent* 10, no. 3 (April 1987): 14–16. Reprinted in *Blasted Allegories, An Anthology of Writings by Contemporary Artists.* Edited by Brian Wallis.

New York: The New Museum of Contemporary Art and Cambridge, Mass.: MIT Press, 1987, 380–85.

————. *The Man Who Envied Women* (script). *Women and Performance* 3, no. 2 (1988): 103–60. Reprinted in *The Films of Yvonne Rainer.* Bloomington: Indiana University Press, 1989, 173–218.

————. *The Films of Yvonne Rainer.* Bloomington: Indiana University Press, 1989.

———— with Ernest Larsen. "We Are Demolition Artists: An Interview with Alexander Kluge." *The Independent* (June 1989): 18–25.

————. "Response to Coco Fusco's 'Fantasies of Oppositionality,'" *Screen* 30, no. 3 (Summer 1989): 91–98.

———— with Simone Forti. "Tea for Two." *Contact Quarterly* 15, no. 2 (Spring/Summer 1990): 27–31.

————. "The Work of Art in the (Imagined) Age of Unalienated Exhibition." Preface to *Democracy: A Project by Group Material.* Dia Art Foundation, Discussions in Contemporary Culture Number 5. Seattle: Bay Press, 1990.

————. "Narrative in the (Dis)Service of Identity." *Agenda Contemporary Art Magazine* (Melbourne) (May 1991): 12–14.

————. Letter to Shu Lea Chang and Kathy High. *Felix* 1, no. 2 (Spring 1992): 27–29.

————. "Working Round the L-Word." In *Queer Looks: Perspectives on Lesbian and Gay Film and Video.* New York: Routledge, 1993, 12–20.

————. *Talking Pictures: Filme, Feminismus, Psychoanalyse, Avantgarde.* Vienna: Passagen Verlag, 1994.

————. Response to "Questions of Feminism." *October,* no. 71 (Winter 1995): 37.

————. *Privilege* (filmscript). In *Screen Writings: Scripts and Texts by Independent Filmmakers.* Edited by Scott MacDonald. Berkeley: University of California Press, 1995: 273–332.

————. "The Avant-Garde Humpty-Dumpty." WWW: http://thecity.sfsu.edu/users/XFactor/participants/participants.html (1996).

————. *MURDER and murder* (filmscript). *Performing Arts Journal,* no. 55 (1997): 76–117.

————. "Token Minimalist Dancing Girl: Yvonne Rainer talks with Linda Austin and Anya Pryor." *Movement Research Performance Journal,* no. 16 (Spring 1998): 15.

————. "Skirting." In *The Feminist Memoir Project: Voices from Women's Liberation.* New York: Crown Press, 1998, 443–49.

Ramsay, Margaret Hupp. *The Grand Union (1970–1976).* New York: Peter Lang, 1991.

Reynaud, Bérénice. "Petit dictionnaire du cinéma independent new-yorkais, II." *Cahiers du Cinéma,* no. 340 (October 1982): 35–47.

————. "Chorégraphie et cinéma: entretien avec Yvonne Rainer." *Cahiers du Cinéma,* no. 369 (March 1985): 43–45.

————. "Impossible Projections." *Screen* 28, no. 4 (Autumn 1987): 40–52. Reprinted in *The Films of Yvonne Rainer.* Bloomington: Indiana University Press, 1989: 24–35.

Rich, B. Ruby. "The Films of Yvonne Rainer." *Chrysalis,* no. 2 (1977): 115–27.

————. "Kristina: For an Introduction . . ." *Afterimage,* no. 7 (Summer 1978): 32–36.

————. "Yvonne Rainer" (monograph). Minneapolis: Walker Art Center, 1981.

Rosenbaum, Jonathan. "Regrouping: Reflections on the Edinburgh Festival 1976." *Sight and Sound* 46, no. 1 (Winter 1976–77): 2–8.

————. "Aspects of the Avant-Garde: Three Innovators." *American Film* 3, no. 10 (September 1978): 33–38.

————. "Explorations: The Ambiguities of Yvonne Rainer." *American Film* 5, no. 5 (March 1980): 68–69.

————. "Yvonne Rainer." In *Film: The Front Line—1983.* Denver: Arden Press, 1983, 132–40.

————. "Menopause and Racism" (review of *Privilege*). *Chicago Reader* 20, no. 22 (March 8, 1991): 27–29.

Rosenbaum, Mitchell. "Interview with Yvonne Rainer." *Persistence of Vision,* no. 6 (Summer 1988). Reprinted in *The Films of Yvonne Rainer.* Bloomington: Indiana University Press, 1989.

Rosovsky, P. *"Journeys from Berlin/1971." Variety* (February 6, 1980): 20.

Russell, Katie. "Yvonne Rainer Eats Her Cake." *Cinema Studies* (newsletter of the Department of Cinema Studies, New York University) 2, no. 3 (Fall 1986): 2.

Sagel, Hildegard. *"Film about a Woman Who . . .* von Yvonne Rainer: Bemerkungen zur Kamera, Aspekte einer Konstruktion." *Frauen und Film,* no. 10 (December 1976): 44–45.

Sharp, Willoughby, and Liza Bear. "The Performer as a Persona: An Interview with Yvonne Rainer." *Avalanche,* no. 5 (Summer 1972): 46–59.

Siegel, Marcia. *At the Vanishing Point: A Critic Looks at Dance.* New York: Saturday Review Press, 1972.

Silverman, Kaja. "Dis-Embodying the Female Voice." In *Re-Vision: Essays in Feminist Film Criticism.* Edited by Mary Ann Doane, Patricia Mellencamp, and Linda Williams. Frederick, Md.: University Publications of America and the American Film Institute, 1984, 131–49.

Smyth, Cherry. "No Place for Sissies" (interview). *Capital Gay* (London) (November 1991).

Soffer, Shirley. " 'You Gave Me So Much Room': A Reminiscence with Yvonne Rainer." *Helicon Nine,* no. 20 (Summer 1989): 92–107.

Stagow, Michael. "Rainer's Shooting Gallery" (review of *The Man Who Envied Women*). *San Francisco Examiner* (September 1985).

Steffenson, Jyanni. "Is This the Woman Who . . . ? A Review of Yvonne Rainer's *Privilege*." *Photofile* (Australia), no. 30 (Winter 1990): 34–37.

Stone, Judy. "Offbeat Film on Sex and Power" (review of *The Man Who Envied Women*). *San Francisco Chronicle* (September 1985).

———. "Documenting a Woman's Blues" (review of *Privilege*). *San Francisco Chronicle* (September 6, 1990).

Stone, Laurie. "Good Grief." *Village Voice* (June 24, 1997): 84.

Storr, Robert. "The Theoretical Come-on." *Art in America* 74, no. 4 (April 1986): 159–65.

Taubin, Amy. "Daughters of Chaos: Feminist and Avant-Garde Filmmakers." *Village Voice* (November 30, 1982): 80–81.

Tillman, Lynne. "A Woman Called Yvonne" (interview). *Village Voice* (January 15, 1991).

Trend, David. "True Stories." *Afterimage* 14, no. 6 (January 1987): 3–4.

Wallace, Michele. "Multiculturalism and Oppositionality" (review of *Privilege*). *Afterimage* 19, no. 3 (October 1991): 6–9.

Walworth, Dan. "A Conversation with Yvonne Rainer." *Psychcritique* 2, no. 1 (1987): 1–16.

Wikarska, Carol. *"A Film about a Woman Who . . ."* *Women and Film* 2, no. 7 (Summer 1975): 86.

Wollen, Peter. "Notes from the Underground: Andy Warhol." In *Raiding the Icebox.* Bloomington: Indiana University Press, 1993, 162–63.

Wooster, Ann Sargeant. "Yvonne Rainer's *Journeys from Berlin/1971.*" *The Drama Review* 24, no. 2 (T-86) (June 1980): 101–18.

Credits

Grateful acknowledgment is made for permission to reprint from the following writers and publishers: to Noel Carroll for "Interview with a Woman Who . . . ," from *Millennium Film Journal*, © 1980 Noel Carroll; to Camera Obscura Collective and *Camera Obscura* for "Interview by the Camera Obscura Collective," © 1976 *Camera Obscura*; to Thyrza Nichols Goodeve and *Art in America* for "Rainer Talking Pictures: Interview by Thyrza Nichols Goodeve," © 1997 *Art in America*; to Kate Horsfield for "Profile: Interview by Lyn Blumenthal," © 1984 Kate Horsfield; to Scott MacDonald and University of California Press for "Interview by Scott MacDonald," © 1992 The Regents of the University of California, and *Privilege*, © 1994 The Regents of the University of California; to The McGraw-Hill Companies for excerpts from Eldridge Cleaver, *Soul on Ice*, © 1968 The McGraw-Hill Companies; to Marian Reiner for "Grandmother, Rocking" from *Rainbow Writing* by Eve Merriam, © 1976 Eve Merriam; and to San Francisco Cinematheque for "Declaring Stakes: Interview by Kurt Easterwood, Susanne Fairfax, and Laura Poitras," © 1990 San Francisco Cinematheque.

The following have graciously given permission to reproduce their photographs: James Klosty, Esther Levine, Babette Mangolte, and the Peter Moore Archive.

Library of Congress Cataloging-in-Publication Data

Rainer, Yvonne, 1934–
    A woman who . . . : essays, interviews, scripts / Yvonne Rainer.
        p.   cm. — (PAJ books. Art + performance)
    Includes bibliographical references.
    ISBN 0-8018-6078-4 (alk. paper). — ISBN 0-8018-6079-2
(pbk. : alk. paper)
    1. Experimental films.   2. Rainer, Yvonne, 1934–   Interviews.
I. Title.   II. Series.
PN1995.9.E96R35   1999
791.43′3—dc21   99-20799 CIP